TO MARILYN,

MAY YOU FIND THE GREATEST SUCCESS IN ALL YOUR
EQUINE ADVENTURES. HOPEFULLY THIS BOOK WILL
INSPIRE YOU TO BRING OUT YOUR HORSE'S BEST
PERFORMANCE.

ENJOY!

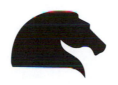

VETERINARY MANUAL

for the Performance Horse

ISBN 0-935842-06-3

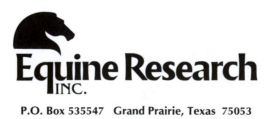

Equine Research
INC.

P.O. Box 535547   Grand Prairie, Texas 75053
Telephone (800) 848-0225

Author
Nancy S. Loving, DVM

Editing, Illustrations, Appendix
research staff of Equine Research, Inc.

Editor/Publisher
Don Wagoner

Disclaimer

Every effort has been made in the writing of this book to present scientifically accurate and up-to-date information based on the best available and reliable sources. However, the results of caring for horses depend upon a variety of factors not under the control of the author or publisher of this book. Therefore, neither Dr. Loving nor Equine Research Inc., assumes any responsibility for, nor makes any warranty with respect to, results that may be obtained from the procedures described or ingredients discussed herein. Neither Equine Research Inc., nor Dr. Loving shall be liable to anyone for damages resulting from reliance on any information contained in this book whether with respect to feeding, care, treatment procedures, drug usages and dosages, or by reason of any misstatement or inadvertent error contained herein.

Also, it must be remembered that neither Equine Research Inc., nor Dr. Loving manufactures any of the drugs, feeds, supplements, or products discussed in this book. Accordingly, neither Equine Research Inc., nor Dr. Loving offers any guarantees of any kind on such items—nor will they be held responsible for the results that may be obtained from the use of those items.

The reader is encouraged to read and follow the directions published by the manufacturer of each product, feed, supplement, or drug which may be mentioned herein. And, if there is a conflict with information in this book, the instructions of the manufacturer—or of the reader's veterinarian—should, of course, be followed.

To insure the reader's understanding of some technical descriptions offered in this book, brand names have been occasionally used as examples of particular substances or equipment. However, the use of a particular trademark or brand name is not intended to imply an endorsement of that particular product, or to suggest that similar products offered by others under different names may be inferior. Also, nothing contained in *Veterinary Manual for the Performance Horse* is to be construed as a suggestion to violate any trademark laws.

Table of Contents

7

SKIN AILMENTS: AVOIDING & CURING 333

15

22

23

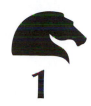

1

CONFORMATION
FOR PERFORMANCE

ANATOMY & FUNCTION

The *ideal* horse is an image to which we compare all others. There is no such thing as a perfect horse, but a horse with good conformation makes a durable athlete. Excellent conformation does not always guarantee excellence in performance; other talents such as temperament and trained abilities are usually needed to create a superior competitor. Each horse has strengths and weaknesses in different areas, both physical and mental.

A discussion of conformation is a study in anatomy and its relation to the function of each structure. Although various parts of a horse are isolated, scrutinized, and analyzed for their individual contributions to the abilities of that animal, each part influences the others as an interactive system. *(Anatomy, bone and muscle diagrams are located in the Appendix, starting on page 509.)*

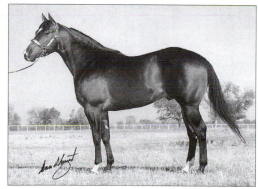

Fig. 1–1. Quarter Horse with good conformation.

1

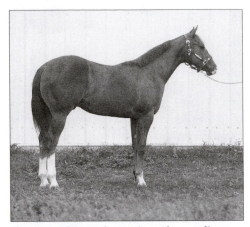

Fig. 1–2. The conformation of a yearling tells a lot about its potential for future athletic performance.

Muscles and tendons are responsible for motion. Think of the muscles as little levers and pulleys, moving different parts of the skeleton. The way the skeleton is put together, *conformation*, determines the strength and coordination of individual muscles. Muscle coordination is important for good performance. While different sports capitalize on strengthening some parts of a horse's body more than others, basic principles apply in creating any equine athlete.

To begin a conformation analysis, place the horse on a flat, level surface, and square it up. Stand back and survey the whole horse to gain an overall impression of its appearance and stance. Examine the horse's overall symmetry from front, back, and side. An asymmetric area like an atrophied leg muscle may hint at an old injury or limb disuse due to lameness.

Balance

A balanced horse makes a better athlete. Balance depends on the location of a horse's center of mass. As a rule-of-thumb, a horse with optimum balance is visually proportional into thirds:

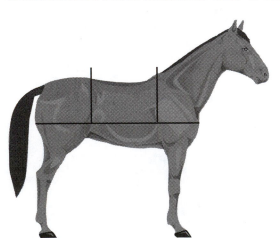

Fig. 1–3. The horse divided into thirds.

• the neck, from the poll to the withers
• the back, from the withers to the point of the hip
• the hindquarters

Of course, no horse can be divided exactly into thirds, but a horse that comes close to these guidelines will be well-balanced.

Another way to visualize the balance of a horse is with a box. The height at the withers, the height at the hip, and the length of the body should be *approximately* the same. There are variations among breeds, for example, some Arabians have one less thoracic vertebra than other breeds. Thoroughbreds come closest to meeting the "box" guidelines.

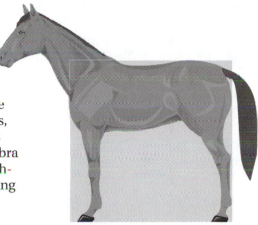

Fig. 1–4. An imaginary "box" for judging balance.

Whichever method is used, the imaginary dividing lines place the center of gravity of the well-balanced horse directly under a mounted rider, with 60% – 65% of the horse's weight falling on the forelegs. If a horse's head is too big or the neck is too long, it is difficult for the hindquarters to effectively counteract the extra weight up front. If the hindquarters are too small, there is no power to push the heavier front end.

Head

The head should be proportionate to the rest of the body, with ample length to provide room for strong teeth and the nasal passages. A head that is too large can create a heavy load on the front end, especially if attached to a relatively short neck.

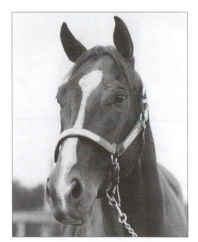

Nostrils

The nostrils should be generous in size so the horse can breathe plenty of oxygen to fuel performance. A deeply dished face pinches the nostrils and nasal passages, and limits the performance of a speed or endurance horse.

Fig. 1–5. Quarter Horse with a well-shaped head.

Nose and Jaws

A horse with narrow jaws may also have a narrow throatlatch, predisposing to nerve damage, which can lead to *roaring*. There should be enough space between the jaws to allow for an active and open airway. The nasal passages are filled with many blood vessels to cool or to warm incoming air to body temperature, preventing shock to the respiratory system.

Eyes

The eyes should be well placed for good vision. The ideal location is at the corners of the forehead. The eyes should have a nice soft expression, alert and interested. Poor eyesight may pose behavioral problems.

Neck

As a biomechanical structure, a horse's neck is the ultimate in design. The triangular shape enhances its function as a cantilever beam to evenly distribute the weight of the head. There is more variety in the necks of horses than in other species due to changes in breed and conformational characteristics developed through centuries of controlled breeding.

Neck Function

For the horse, a neck of proper length is necessary for survival. The neck lowers the head for grazing and drinking, and assists vision by swinging the head for accurate eye focus. The neck's large range of motion also enables a horse to shift and fine tune its center of gravity to maintain balance of its massive body. A horse with well-formed and coupled limbs and back can only achieve fine athletic potential if it can balance the body while in motion.

Neck as a Balance

What do all equine athletes have in common? Each uses its neck to shift the center of gravity in the necessary direction to maintain balance and maneuverability. Consider the following examples:

- A roping horse as it slides to an abrupt stop, the neck raised as it sinks onto the haunches.
- A dressage horse with an arched neck, as it executes precision movements of pirouette or piaffe which require collection and engagement of the hindquarters.
- A trail horse with head and neck extended, maneuvering up a steep embankment. As it descends a hillside, it raises the neck and head to lighten the front end, allowing the hindquarters to sink down for better stability on irregular footing.

- A cutting horse quickly shifting side-to-side to follow a cow's maneuvers, moving its head to facilitate shifts in direction.
- A racehorse at full gallop with neck and head extended to increase the length of stride and speed. This simple shift in the center of gravity enhances speed and also reduces fatigue.

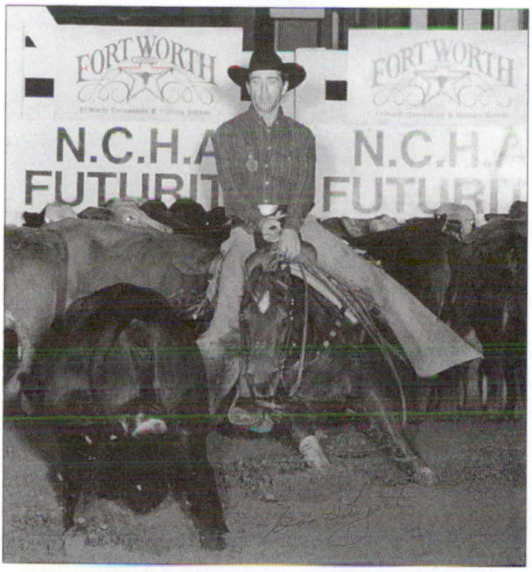

Fig. 1–6. A cutting horse moves its head to facilitate shifts in direction.

Bascule

A jumping horse must arch its neck into a *bascule*, which is an arc created by moving one end which is then counterbalanced by the other. This principle is the same as the seesaw. The bascule involves a series of steps: extending and lowering the head, arching the back, flexing the *lumbosacral joint* (L-S joint), and finally engaging the hindquarters. In this way, a horse translates horizontal forward movement into vertical motion up and over a jump.

Neck As A Counterbalance

Analysis of a horse's forward motion illustrates that the downswing of the head and neck is accompanied by a forward pull of the back muscles. As the body moves forward, propelled from the hind legs to the forelegs, the hindquarters lift from the ground to advance to the next forward stride. As the horse steps under itself, the neck and head continue to work as a counterbalance. With the hind legs supporting the horse, the head and neck rise, followed

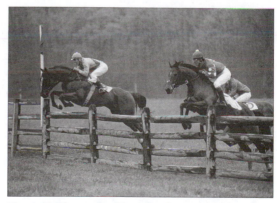

Fig. 1–7. The neck of jumping horses arching to function as a bascule.

by elevation of the forequarters and a forward swing of the forelegs to further advance the stride.

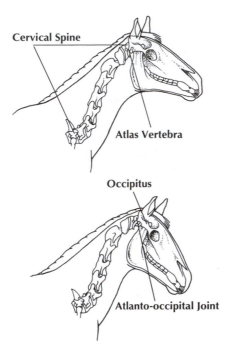

Fig. 1–8. The "Yes" joint showing flexion of the horse at the poll.

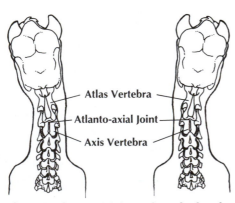

Fig. 1–9. The "No" joint swings the head from side-to-side.

Neck Structure

The bony spine is buried within the muscular structure of the neck. It provides a scaffold for attachment of all other ligamentous and muscular parts.

"Yes" Joint

The *cervical spine* is connected to the *occipitus*, or base of the skull, by the *atlas vertebra*, which is the first vertebra after the skull. The joint formed at their connection, the *atlanto-occipital joint*, moves up and down, like a hinge, earning it the name of the "yes" joint.

The head moves up and down without moving the rest of the neck or body, but the protrusions of the atlas vertebra restrict lateral, side-to-side movement of this joint. For riding purposes, the yes joint enables flexion at the poll to complete the stretch through the topline that aids self-carriage and can advance a horse to higher levels of performance.

"No" Joint

The *atlas vertebra* joins the *axis* (second) *vertebra* at the *atlanto-axial joint*, also called the "no" joint, because it rotates the head and neck side-to-side. The joint barely extends due to pressure against the atlas vertebra of another bony piece, the *dens*. *(The dens is the part of the axis vertebra which hooks under the atlas vertebra and cannot be seen in the illustrations.)*

Other Cervical Joints

The other cervical joints in the neck are similar to each other in shape and range of motion. They are capable of *flexion*, *extension*, and *lateral* movement. Throughout a horse's life, the flexion and extension capabilities of these joints remain relatively constant. However, there is an age-related reduction in axial rotation in the middle section of the neck, leading to reduced suppleness in later years.

Neck Length and Shape

Every horse has seven cervical vertebrae, and it is the length of each of these which determines if a neck is long or short. A horse's neck can be compared to a gymnast's balancing pole as it moves to accommodate shifts in equilibrium of the body.

Short Neck

A short neck limits the range of flexibility of the head and neck, and is less able to adjust rapidly, which is necessary to fine tune balance. Often, a short neck is also thick and muscular, which not only reduces the neck's suppleness, but adds substantial weight. A thick throatlatch, often associated with a thick neck, limits airflow through the windpipe. It can also limit flexion of the head when a rider asks the horse to go "on-the-bit."

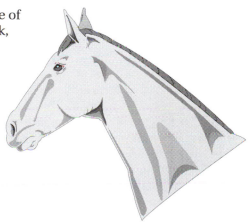

Fig. 1–10. A thick throatlatch limits air flow.

Neck Muscles and Stride Length

Neck muscles enable all body structures to work together to achieve balance. Interconnecting muscles between neck and shoulders swing a horse's forelegs through each stride. For the hindquarters to propel a horse forward, the shoulders and forelegs must swing freely.

The length of a horse's stride is closely correlated to neck length—in extended gaits the forelegs can never reach past the point of the nose.

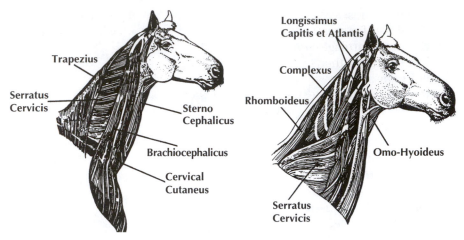

Fig. 1–11. On the left, superficial lateral cervical muscles. On the right, deep lateral cervical muscles.

Hence, a short neck limits the range of foreleg movement, and can increase wear and tear on the legs, because more steps are required to move a certain distance across the ground. Short, choppy strides result in wasted energy for movement and cause limb fatigue.

Long Neck

A horse performing at rapid speeds, such as a racehorse, eventer, or jumper, benefits from a moderately long and finely muscled neck. Too long a neck is a disadvantage as it adds extra weight to the front end, shifting the center of gravity forward. This shift forces a horse to travel on the forehand (front third in front of the shoulders), creating excess stress on the forelegs.

Neck muscles can contract and expand two-thirds of their natural length and in so doing advance the shoulder and forelegs through a stride. Muscles in a neck that is too long may have greater difficulty developing strength and are prone to fatigue. The neck and head might droop, forcing the horse onto the forehand and reducing efficiency of movement. If a horse does not have the strength to support its own head and neck, it tends to pull on a rider's hands, depending on them for support.

As an example of the relationship of form to function, horses with very long, slender necks may be predisposed to *roaring* syndrome, or *laryngeal hemiplegia*. To breathe efficiently, the larynx at the top of the trachea must be able to fully open with inspiration. The muscles which open the *arytenoid cartilages* are innervated by the two recurrent laryngeal branches of the *vagus nerve* on either side.

A longer neck is thought to increase tension on the vagus nerve, in most cases the left branch, leading to nerve damage and paralyzing the laryngeal muscle that opens the airway for breathing. The arytenoid cartilage controlled by this muscle then collapses into the airway on the left side. As air passes through the restricted opening it produces turbulence and creates a "roaring" sound. Exercise tolerance and stamina are compromised. *(See more information in Chapters 5 and 6.)*

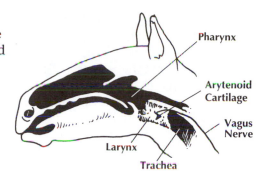

Fig. 1–12. Side view of the throat.

Low-Set Neck

Ideally, the neck should join the chest just above the point of the shoulder. A low-set neck throws a horse onto the forehand by shifting the center of gravity forward and down, restricting shoulder movement and mobility as well as stride length. For a show hunter or western pleasure horse, traveling "long and level" is ideal for competition, but it can seriously compromise the performance and coordination of a jumper, eventer, or dressage candidate.

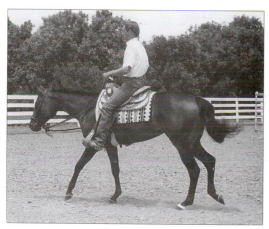

Even in sports where a level neck is desirable, training a horse to carry its neck too low is dangerous to both horse and rider. The horse falls heavily on the forehand, increasing concussion to the forelegs. A low

Fig. 1–13. A Western Pleasure horse with a low and level neck.

neck set reduces the shoulder's freedom of movement, so the horse tends to shuffle and frequently stumbles.

The external shape of the neck depicts the internal configuration of the cervical spine. Over time, training methods build individual muscle groups, but the bony vertebral scaffold is unchangeable. The neck's actual *shape* has more influence on the way a horse travels than does its length.

Neck Influence on Head Carriage

The shape of the neck and its connection to the head and withers determine normal head carriage in a horse. Normal head carriage at a 45° angle to the ground optimizes a horse's field of vision while allowing the head and neck the mobility necessary to retain body balance. In this position, the larynx is open to promote efficient breathing. The bit falls on the bars of the mouth rather than sliding into the cheeks so the rider has more control.

Carrying the head at this natural angle enables the neck muscles connected to the shoulder to lift the shoulder so the forearm can freely swing, increasing limb advancement across the ground.

Ewe-Neck

A horse with a *ewe-neck* is predisposed to high head carriage, resulting in a hollow back and an inability to engage the hindquarters or move forward onto the bit. A horse with its head in the air is unable to move effectively because its rear end is poorly connected to its front end. Therefore, it is unbalanced. Such a ride is uncomfortable to both horse and rider. With the head in a "star gazing" position, the bit does not properly contact the bars of the mouth. The situation is further aggravated as the horse throws its head higher to escape the irritating bit pressure.

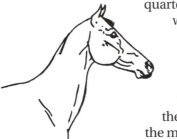

Fig. 1–14. Ewe neck.

Arched Neck

If the neck is arched, the head is in a vertical position which limits the horse's range of vision. The cervical vertebrae in the neck assume an "S" curve that functionally shortens neck length. These factors are important to advanced levels of dressage. A collected head carriage benefits performance of lateral precision movements. Shortening the neck length moves the center of gravity towards the hind end. Shifting the center of gravity backwards frees the head and neck to move up and down. Therefore, suppleness increases from side-to-side. The shoulders and forelegs also move with greater freedom.

Withers

Stretch Through the Topline

For many equine athletic endeavors, the aim is to achieve longitudinal flexion (arching of the spine) through the entire back and topline.

Stretched muscles are relaxed muscles. Consequently, they are less prone to fatigue and injury. Interactive use of muscle groups adds strength to a horse's movements. Stretch through the entire topline and neck starts at the withers. (The withers are formed by the top portions of the 3rd through 8th thoracic vertebrae of the spine.)

The Role of the Withers

The *scalenus muscles* of the neck connect to the first rib. As these muscles raise the base of the neck, an increase in the lever arm at the withers improves stretch through the topline. As the first rib is pulled forward, the rib cage expands and increases respiratory capacity for speed and stamina.

The fibroelastic *nuchal ligament,* an extensive fan-like structure forming the crest of the neck, extends from the base of the skull and anchors onto the withers. The nuchal ligament passively supports the head and neck to distribute the mechanical load, and assists extensor muscles of the head and neck. Additional neck muscles that raise the head and neck, or move them from side-to-side, anchor to the withers. Muscle groups that elevate the shoulder and extend the spine also anchor here.

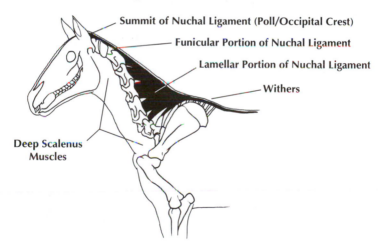

Summit of Nuchal Ligament (Poll/Occipital Crest)

Funicular Portion of Nuchal Ligament

Lamellar Portion of Nuchal Ligament

Withers

Deep Scalenus Muscles

Fig. 1–15. The nuchal ligament supports the head and neck.

A proper crest of the neck that carries well back over the withers enhances the fulcrum effect of the withers. As the withers rise when a horse stretches through its neck, the back and spine arch, engaging the hindquarters with hocks and stifles moving well underneath the body.

This specific arching movement is important not only to dressage horses, but to cutting, reining, jumping, and trail horses as well. Such flexibility and suppleness are not only dependent upon conformational structure, but require conditioning.

High Withers

The withers should sit about 1 inch higher than the horse's croup. A high withers allows a greater range of movement for the neck and back muscles that attach to it. Like a seesaw, the higher the fulcrum point (withers), the more freedom both sides of the seesaw (neck and back) have to move up and down. A high, broad withers provides greater flexibility through the back and spine. As a horse lowers and extends the neck, the back rises.

Low Withers

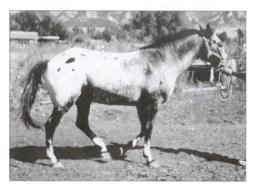

Fig. 1–16. An example of low withers.

If the withers are too low, the saddle and rider slide forward, shifting the center of gravity forward and increasing impact to the forelegs. The saddle and rider may also injure poorly muscled withers.

Chest

A good chest is deep and well-defined to allow for a large respiratory capacity and a well-developed heart. The depth of a horse's chest is more important than width. The ribs should have ample space between them and project backwards. Such ribs improve chest depth and allow for excellent lung expansion during athletic pursuits.

Proper Width and Depth of Chest

A chest that is too wide does not allow good clearance for the elbows, and the horse is prone to girth gall. The greatest width of the barrel should lie behind the

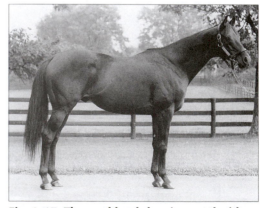

Fig. 1–17. Thoroughbred showing good withers and chest depth.

girth so shoulder movement is not restricted. A narrow chest can result in limb interference like *plaiting*, which is crossing one foot over the other while in motion, or striking the inside of a leg with the opposite foot.

For example, a horse with *base-narrow*, toed-out conformation where the hooves are closer together than the shoulders, will wing with its feet as it moves. (If it was pigeon-toed, it would paddle instead.) Winging results in limb interference, potentially injuring the splint bones. The base-narrow stance also creates pressure on the inside of the knee joints and inside splint bones, increasing the chance of developing *splints*.

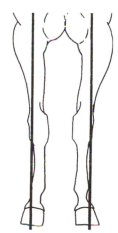

Fig. 1–18. Base-narrow and toed-out.

Shoulder

Bones that are located higher in the leg have greater influence on the freedom of limb swing. It is actually the relationship of the shoulder bone *(scapula)* to the arm bone *(humerus)* that has the most influence on arm swing and stride length. Ideally, the angle between the scapula and humerus should be greater than 90°, preferably nearing a more open angle of 105°.

Stride Length

A horse's stride length depends on the conformational angles of its shoulder and foreleg. The longer a horse's stride, the faster it can cover ground, and the fewer steps the horse takes to get from point to point. If the number of steps is greater, the horse fatigues faster, and experiences more stress and strain on the limbs. Therefore, a shorter stride length increases the possibility of lameness since the forelegs absorb up to 65% of the weight-bearing impact.

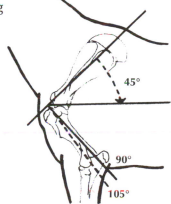

Fig. 1–19. The scapulo-humeral angle should be greater than 90°.

Sloping Shoulder

A sloping shoulder at an angle of 45° to the ground anatomically moves the withers further back to relieve the shock of impact for the rider. A sloping

13

shoulder distributes the attachment of muscles and ligaments over a greater area, diffusing the impact on the horse's musculoskeletal system.

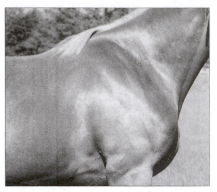

Fig. 1–20. A sloping shoulder.

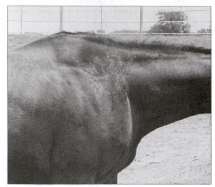

Fig. 1–21. A vertical shoulder.

Vertical Shoulder

If the shoulder is vertical and upright, a horse will have greater knee action. The knees will be lifted high with each step, creating a rough, inelastic ride that transfers concussion to the rider while the horse covers less ground with each stride. Again, the greater the number of steps taken, the faster the onset of fatigue.

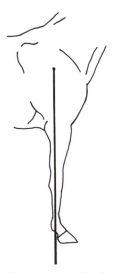

Fig. 1–22. A plumb line intersecting all parts of the foreleg.

Forelegs

Viewed from the side, the foreleg should be a straight column from the elbow to the fetlock. Straightness of this column promotes equal loading, or axial compression forces moving down the leg with weight-bearing, across the joints and bones.

Looking at the side of a horse, a plumb line dropped from the middle of the shoulder blade and bisecting the fetlock should fall directly behind the heel. Any deviation from the straightness of the column predisposes to degenerative joint disease (DJD), known as arthritis. Abnormalities in bone growth plates lead to *angular limb deformities*. These deformities predispose to DJD because of abnormal loading forces on the joint. Examples of these syndromes are: knock-knee *(carpus valgus)*, bowlegged *(carpus varus)*, splay-footed *(fetlock valgus)*, and pigeon-toed *(fetlock varus)*. The pigeon-toed horse is often afflicted with ringbone, a DJD of the pastern or coffin joint.

Upper Arm

The humerus should be at least half as long as the scapula. If the point of the shoulder is high, the humerus is long and steep, creating a more open shoulder angle. The longer the humerus, the

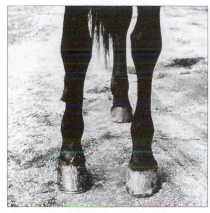

Fig. 1–23. A pigeon-toed horse.

greater a horse's ability to move the elbow away from the body. If a horse can move the elbow forward with greater freedom, it improves things such as better racing stride, jumping, and crouching low to head a calf.

If a horse can move the elbow sideways, it executes lateral movements important to dressage, polo, and cutting.

A horse with a short humerus has short, choppy strides, and does not easily perform speed or lateral work. If the humerus lies in a horizontal plane, the *scapulo-humeral* angle closes. The limbs cannot fold tightly, and the horse has difficulty with sports like cutting, barrel racing, jumping, or polo.

The elbow should be in front of the peak of the withers so the humerus does not fall horizontally. A horizontal humerus produces a pigeon-breasted horse that stands with the forelegs too far under the body. It is hard for a pigeon-breasted horse to move in balance.

Forearm

The muscles in the forearm extend the limb forward and absorb the shock of impact. It is preferable to have strong, well-developed muscles. A long forearm increases the length of a horse's stride. A long forearm coupled with a short cannon bone and a medium length pastern creates structural stability in the limb, while achieving optimal leverage and strength of the *musculotendinous* attachments.

Knees

Normally a horse's knee *(carpus)* is slightly sprung and not entirely straight due to the normal curvature of the forearm bone *(radius)*. The front contours of the knees should be flat and shield-shaped, with well-defined corners.

Problem Knees

Bucked Knees

Excessive curvature of the radius leads to bucked knees or *over at the knee*, and places strain on the flexor tendons. An enlarged and thickened tendon, or *bowed tendon* can result as it prematurely flexes with each weight-bearing stride.

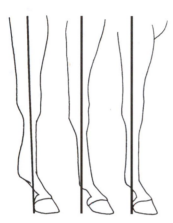

Fig. 1–24. From left to right: tied in behind the knee, calf knee, normal limb.

Calf Knee

A knee that is set too far back is called a *calf knee*, a major flaw that often leads to fractured knee bones in the racehorse, and degenerative joint disease in other athletes. An upright pastern and a long-toe – low-heel foot configuration create a functional calf knee, stressing the knee joints and flexor tendons, and delaying *breakover* of the foot.

Other Knee Problems

Knock-knee *(carpus valgus)*, occurs when the knees deviate toward each other. Bowlegged *(carpus varus)* horses have knees which deviate away from each other. Both of these abnormalities predispose to DJD.

Cannon Bone

If the measurement at the top of the cannon bone is less than at the bottom of the cannon bone, the horse is *tied in* behind the knees. The width of the flexor tendons and suspensory ligaments is smaller at the top of the cannon area, predisposing them to strain and injury.

When the cannon bone is offset to the outside of the forelegs, known as a *bench knee*, greater stress is placed on the inside of the knee joint.

Pasterns

The angle of the pastern's slope to the ground is important to the stability of the joints in the lower legs and smoothness of stride. In general, the angles of the hoof, pastern, and shoulder to the ground should be the same. The pasterns should be of medium length. A short pastern is upright, while a long pastern tends to slope toward the ground.

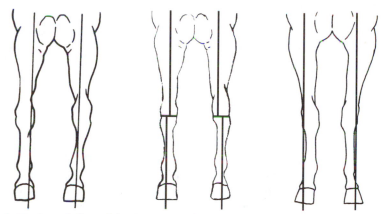

Fig. 1–25. From left to right: bow-legged, bench knees, knock-knee.

Short Pastern

A short pastern acts as a poor shock absorber. Not only does this configuration result in an uncomfortable ride, but the horse receives added concussion to the middle third of its feet, predisposing it to navicular disease.

Long Pastern

A long pastern provides a comfortable ride, but it predisposes to tendon injury because the fetlock drops further with each weight-bearing stride. Excessive fetlock drop increases the pull on the flexor tendons. A horse with a long pastern often develops *windpuffs* (inflammation) of the fetlock joint and flexor tendon sheath. It is also at risk for a bowed tendon, *sesamoiditis* (inflammation of the fetlock sesamoid bones), or *suspensory desmitis* (inflammation of the suspensory ligament).

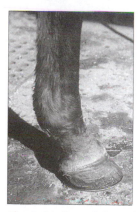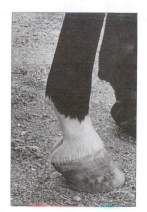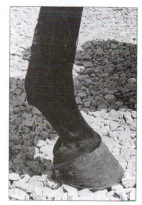

Fig. 1–26. From left to right: short pastern, medium pastern, long pastern.

Back

How the muscles of the hindquarters connect to the back at the lumbosacral joint is called *coupling*. To achieve the greatest strength and flexibility, hindquarter muscles should be carried well forward into the back. The loin is unable to flex from side-to-side, therefore a long lumbar span creates a weak back. A short back limits the range that a horse can move the legs and elbows vertically, or *scope*. Scope is important in events such as racing, jumping, hunting, and cutting.

A back that is too long may eventually develop a *sway back* as muscular attachments weaken with age and use. A swaybacked horse is often plagued with chronic back pain. A long back also prevents a horse from executing lateral movements with ease. Ribs and interlocking facets of lumbar vertebrae prevent a horse from rotating sideways in the area in front of the ninth thoracic vertebra. Maximum bending and rotation lie behind the area under the saddle and behind the rider's leg.

Loins

Ideal loins are short and only encompass a handspan, or about 8 inches, between the last rib and the point of the hip. The horse that uses its loins well also has rounded *gluteal* muscles for upward thrust of the leg off the ground, and developed *quadriceps* muscles on the thigh that pull the hind leg forward. A weak loin that is too long results in a lack of drive in the hindquarters, with underdeveloped gluteals and quadriceps.

Loins and Body Carriage

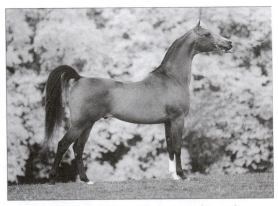

Fig. 1–27. An Arabian with nice conformation showing a good back with short loins and rounded gluteal muscles.

As the horse carries its head and neck in the correct position for bit contact, it engages the hindquarters to relax and round the back, allowing the forelegs to be used most efficiently. Weight is distributed evenly fore and aft, and a horse in this frame is balanced and agile. A balanced frame permits shoulders to extend and flex to their full potential, not only lengthening the stride but adding to suspension and smoothness of the stride.

Hindquarters

Many equine sports require quick turns, sudden stops, and perfect balance. A horse normally carries as much as 65% of its weight on the front end. Events like reining, roping, cutting, trail riding, polo, jumping, and dressage have at least one similar characteristic. These sports transfer a horse's center of gravity toward the rear end. Without strong hindquarters, it cannot perform well. The propulsive muscles of the body originate on the pelvis, so a strong hind end means greater power and drive.

Effects of Exercise on Hindquarters

Just as calisthenic exercises for people strengthen the attendant muscle groups, a horse in training improves muscle condition to retain balance through gait transitions and various movements.

Collection of a horse starts in the hindquarters, specifically at the lumbosacral joint (L-S joint) at the top of the croup, and is carried on through the back, withers, and neck, to the poll. If a horse's hindquarters are likened to an engine because they propel the horse into motion, then the L-S joint at the top of the croup is the transmission. The L-S joint pivots and rotates the hindquarters and pelvis forward under the body. The abdominal muscles help pull the pelvis forward to engage the hindquarters.

Angle of Croup and Pelvis

The slope of the pelvis bone from the point of the hip to the point of the buttocks determines the slope of a horse's croup. The more slope and length to the pelvis, the greater the horse's *power*. A horse with a very steep pelvis generates a greater upward thrust, although its steps are small. Consider the slope and width of a working draft horse that is the essence of power and push from the hindquarters.

On the other hand, a pelvis that inclines towards the horizontal enhances *speed*, especially at the trot. A more horizontal pelvis allows the hip joint to

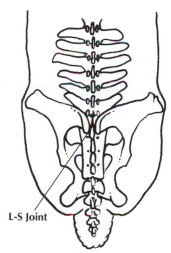

L-S Joint

Fig. 1–28. The L-S joint pivots and rotates the hindquarters.

19

lengthen when the hind leg is extended. Therefore, a horizontal pelvis results in a greater push forward. This configuration gives a fluid, ground covering stride.

The ideal croup inclines about 25° and is relatively long in proportion to the body. Long muscles over the croup have a greater range of muscle contraction across the skeleton, improving speed, which is important to the racehorse. A shorter croup decreases leverage and muscle power.

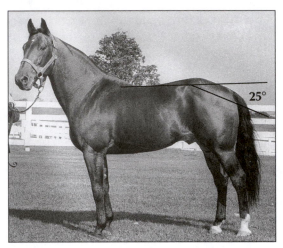

Fig. 1–29. Standardbred with nice conformation showing a good croup angle.

The hindquarters should have ample vertical depth as defined by a triangle formed by the point of the hip, the point of the buttock, and the stifle joint. For the athletic horse, the best results are obtained by a long, perpendicular thigh and a gaskin that is a bit shorter than the length of the thigh.

The Stifle

The stifle should sit at the same height as the elbow. The stifle is turned slightly out so a horse can move forward freely without physical interference from the flank. This preferred position of the stifle causes many horses to slightly toe out on the hind legs.

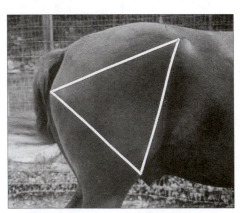

Fig. 1–30. Triangular shape of the hindquarters.

A long thigh and short gaskin with good muscling are advantageous in any athletic endeavor except for the racehorse. For racehorses, especially sprinters, a long hip, gaskin, and thigh increase the muscle leverage for optimal stride length, power, and speed during a sprint effort.

A relatively straight hind leg is more efficient at thrusting at the ground for pushoff. This characteristic can be helpful for events such as jumping, Quarter Horse racing, roping, etc. However, if the limb is too straight, excess stress on both stifle and hock joints can lead to arthritis. These horses are also prone to *upward fixation of the patella* where a ligament of the stifle locks over the kneecap, and *thoroughpin,* which is a windpuff of the Achilles tendon behind the hock.

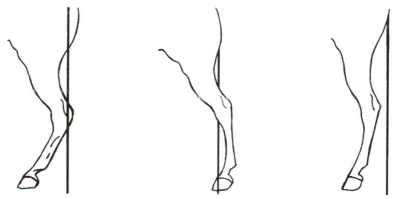

Fig. 1–31. Poor hind leg conformations, from left to right: sickle hocked, camped out, and camped under.

In contrast, a longer, angled hind leg helps the horse bring the hocks under the body which is important for dressage, cutting, and reining sports. Stride length increases with a more angled hind leg. When this characteristic is extreme, the horse may be *camped out* where the hind legs stick out behind, or *sickle hocked* where the hind legs angle beneath the horse.

Horses with these conformation problems are prone to:

- *bog spavin*—excess joint fluid in the hock from inflammation
- *bone spavin*—DJD of the hock
- *curb*—strain of the plantar ligament on the back of the hock

If the limb is too long and angled, the croup may rise higher than the withers with each stride, resulting in a rough, uncomfortable ride.

More than 80% of hind leg lameness develops in the hock or stifle joints, therefore conformation of

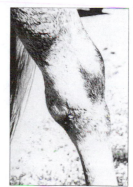

Fig. 1–32. Bog spavin.

these structures is very important to continuing soundness in the performance horse. Any athletic pursuit that moves the horse's weight towards the hindquarters, for example, dressage, cutting, roping, and reining, amplifies the stress on these joints.

Hind Legs

From the side, a plumb line dropped from the point of the buttocks to the point of the hock should fall along the back of the tendons to the fetlock.

Post-Legged

A horse with hind legs that are too straight is *post-legged*. This conformational flaw increases concussion and loading of the joints. The tendon sheaths therefore have a tendency to puff from poor circulation. A post-legged horse is predisposed to upward fixation of the patella, DJD, thoroughpin, and bone spavin in the hocks.

The Hocks

The hocks alternately flex and swing and then support and push the limbs to produce drive. A "low-set hocked" horse (which results from a relatively short cannon bone) has more power for pushing and quick turns. This power is important in all sprint efforts. It is also desirable to have open angles on the front face of the hind legs approximating 160°.

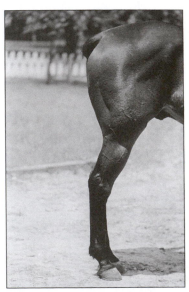 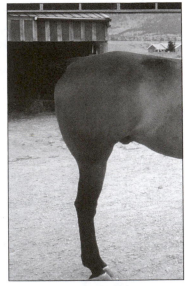

Fig. 1–33. On the left, a normal hind leg. On the right, a post-legged horse.

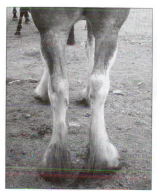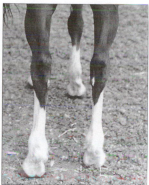

Fig. 1–34. On the left, true cowhocks of a draft horse. On the right, the hind leg stance of an Arabian.

Cowhocks

A horse with **true** *cowhocks* has limbs very different from the normal toed-out conformation seen with Arabians and Trakehners. As seen from behind, the cowhocked horse has fetlocks that reach much farther apart than do the point of the hocks. A toed-out horse has fetlocks placed underneath the hocks, yet the toes turn out from below the fetlocks. Cowhocks place excessive strain on the insides of the hocks and stifles, predisposing to DJD.

Similar characteristics for the lower part of the forelegs apply to the hind legs for mechanical efficiency. As in the foreleg, it is preferable to have short cannon bones in the hind leg so that tendons can effectively pull on the point of the hock to create drive. The fetlocks should be clean and tight, without bumps or nicks, and the pasterns should be strong, well-defined, and of medium length.

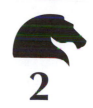

2

DEVELOPING STRONG BONES

Bones provide a mechanical scaffold from which muscles, ligaments, and tendons are supported. Efficiency of movement depends on how the skeleton is conformed. The muscles work like levers and pulleys as they are superimposed on the skeleton. The visible size, shape, and structure of bone in each horse is the subject of much debate regarding conformation and its relation to performance. Yet, there is no question that the internal architecture of bone is important to a horse's ability to absorb impact without developing lameness. *(See anatomy, bone and muscle diagrams in the Appendix, starting on page 511.)*

BONE STRENGTH
Internal Remodeling

Lameness is the primary cause of poor performance in the equine athlete. Prematurely subjecting a horse's bones to stressful exertions can permanently affect its potential.

Bone, as a dynamic organ, continually alters its shape and mass according to the stresses placed upon it. By understanding a little about the microscopic changes that occur, an owner or trainer can modify bone strength with conditioning.

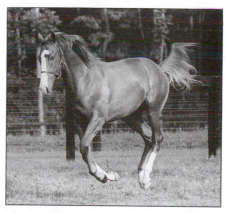

Fig. 2–1. Bone continually alters shape and mass according to the stresses placed upon it.

Bone changes itself, conforming to stress by increasing or decreasing its mass accordingly. Cells that form new bone are called *osteoblasts*. New bone is produced in weaker areas. Bone is one of the few tissues in the body capable of *regeneration* rather than repairing with a scar. *Resorption*, or removal of bone by cells called *osteoclasts,* occurs in areas that no longer need to respond to stress.

These active processes are called *remodeling*. Bone has abundant blood vessels that supply nutrients and oxygen to support remodeling and mineralization in adapting to physical stress.

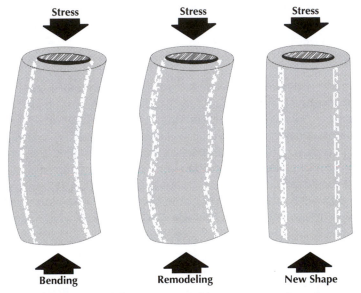

Fig. 2–2. The remodeling response of bone to stress. Bone becomes stronger and no longer bends when stressed.

Bone is also a storage reservoir for calcium and phosphorus. The deposit or removal of these minerals is controlled by:

- physical stress on the bone
- hormonal influences from the endocrine glands
- nutrition

Bone responds to stress by changing the arrangement, type, and amount of bone. Age determines which hormones are more active; for example, a growing skeleton is affected by hormones that encourage the deposit of minerals into bone.

As bone matures, minerals (calcium and phosphorus) are deposited into the bone at the expense of *cellular fluid* to occupy up to 65% of the space. By the time a horse is fully mature, the minerals make up 95% of the bone. The amount of these minerals in a bone determines its *bone mineral content* (BMC).

Internal remodeling proceeds without changing the observable shape of the skeleton. However, these invisible changes in the bones greatly affect intrinsic strength and skeletal maturity of a horse.

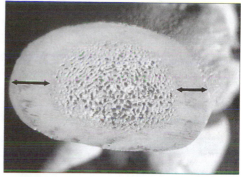

Fig. 2–3. Cross section of a cannon bone. Greater bone deposition on the left shows effects of internal remodeling.

Bone Strength Indicators

At one time, the skeletal maturity of a horse was estimated by radiographic assessment of closure of the growth plates, and by subjective evaluation of body growth and development. Recent research on athletic stress of young racehorses indicates that bone strength depends on more than growth plate closure. Bone strength depends on its cross-sectional area and bone mineral content.

Cross-sectional area increases with skeletal maturity, especially if coupled with intelligent conditioning methods for a young horse. An increase in cross-sectional area logarithmically increases bone strength so it can ultimately sustain more stress.

Measuring the cannon bone just below the knee helps determine the horse's current structural strength. For optimal strength, the measurement of the cannon bone should yield *at least* 7 inches circumference for every 1,000 pounds of body weight. Using these figures as guidelines, the ideal circumference of an individual horse's cannon bone can be determined. The formula looks like this:

$$\frac{\text{7 inches}}{\text{1,000 lbs}} \times \text{body weight of horse} = \text{ideal circumference}$$

For example, if a horse weighs 750 pounds the formula would be:

$$\frac{\text{7 inches}}{\text{1,000 lbs}} \times 750\ \text{lbs} = \text{ideal circumference}$$

Then, $0.007 \times 750 = 5.25$ inches

Therefore, the ideal circumference of the cannon bone of a 750-pound horse is 5¼ inches. This formula helps an owner or trainer set conditioning goals for an individual athlete. If the result is more than the actual circumference, the horse should undergo bone strengthening exercises. Both cross-sectional area and bone mineral content are also influenced by the horse's age and physical maturity. These factors determine the ability of the bones to withstand stress.

How can the body and mind of a young horse be strengthened without overtaxing the musculoskeletal system? Nutritional manipulation or exercise regimens cannot hasten growth and maturation. Genetics and breed determine skeletal maturity, and these factors are dictated by time. Yet, conditioning programs can improve ultimate bone strength and build a durable athlete. **Taking time to properly condition** the young athlete will pay high dividends in future soundness.

Exercise and Bone Strength

The mechanical forces of exercise stimulate change in weight-bearing bones. Exercise increases bone strength by increasing mineral deposition and bone mass. The *quantity* of bone, but not necessarily the *quality,* increases with exercise. Human sports medicine studies show increases of up to 20% in bone mass of active athletes as compared to non-athletes.

The Importance of Consistent Exercise

Sports medicine research reveals another significant factor that is most applicable to the equine athlete. Not only does exercise enhance bone mineralization, but, more important, the *rate* at which a mechanical force is applied to the bones greatly influences the degree of bone development. For instance, consistent running with gradual increases in distance effectively increases bone min-

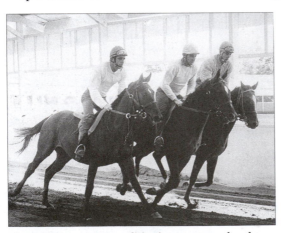

Fig. 2–4. A proper conditioning program for the young horse builds a durable athlete.

eral content, whereas occasional and sporadic exercise has little effect on bone mineral content. A *routine* of conditioning is essential to increase bone strength.

Daily exercise does not need to be excessive or prolonged. There is a threshold that stimulates deposit of minerals into the bone. Once the threshold is met, more exercise does not further increase bone mineral content. Loading bone with exercise for a short time each day (i.e., 20 – 30 minutes), stimulates as much new bone development as a lengthy workout. The actual time required to strengthen bone may be more or less, depending on the individual's maturity and fitness level.

Training Techniques

To most effectively increase the cross-sectional area and bone mineral content of equine bone, a vigorous, intermittent exercise of short duration is best. After a warm-up of 10 – 15 minutes, a short sprint or 20 minutes of hill work is more effective than a 3-mile slow gallop. Gradual increase in incremental exercise also strengthens the ligaments, tendons, and muscles of a horse. Such a program resembles *interval training* techniques that build, but do not overtax, the musculoskeletal system of a young horse. *(See Chapter 6 for more information on interval training.)*

Inactivity

The opposite effect, demineralization, occurs when the skeleton is subjected to weightlessness or reduced gravitational loading. The extreme case occurs in the human example of space flight and to a lesser degree with bed rest. Of course, these specific phenomena are of no concern in caring for the equine athlete. However, applying a cast or disuse of an injured limb for an extended period similarly decreases bone strength. Bone mineral content diminishes: cells dissolve existing bone while bone-forming cells remain quiescent. With this caution in mind, rehabilitation of an injured horse must proceed slowly.

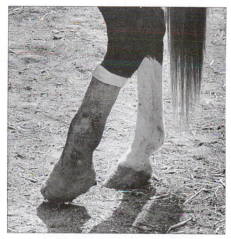

Fig. 2–5. Immobilization caused by an injury can decrease bone strength.

A loss of bone, or lack of development, can also result from administering excessive amounts of corticosteroids. Such problems can also result from the body's manufacture of corticosteroids when a horse is subjected to mental stress. Mental stress develops from chronic pain, overtraining, and competition.

BONE RESPONSE TO BIOMECHANICAL STRESS

The term biomechanical stress refers to all the forces applied to a bone during weight-bearing. The laws of physics define the way different forces affect the bone. *Stress* measures force per unit area; the degree to which a bone deforms to the stress is termed *strain*. Removing a stress allows a bone to return to its original shape—this is its *elasticity*. The ability of a bone to resist being deformed is defined as *stiffness*.

For example, since a horse bears more than 60% of the weight-bearing force on the forelegs, the cannon bone reflects changes in bone from consistent biomechanical stress. The cannon bone resembles a cylinder. According to the laws of physics, the total strength of a cylinder is a function of its cross-sectional area and the elastic strength of its component materials. In a growing horse, the cross-sectional area enlarges while the elastic component essentially remains the same. As a horse increases in body weight and mass, the total weight-bearing capabilities of the bones adapt correspondingly.

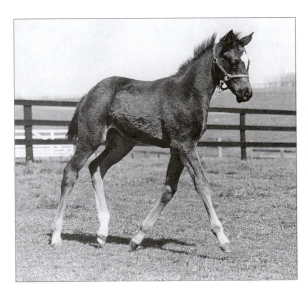

Fig. 2–6. As young horses mature, their bones become stronger by increasing in cross-sectional area.

Mineral Reinforcement

Mineral reinforces the connective tissue of fibrous collagen in the bone. Not only does bone *density* increase with bone mineral content, but stiffness also increases, improving a bone's resistance to deforming forces.

As a young horse matures, its bones become increasingly strong and able to withstand more axial loading down the limbs. Again, this strength is accomplished by increases in cross-sectional area and bone mineral content, and by conversion of randomly arrayed immature bone cells into highly structured mature bone cells.

Forces That Stress Bone

The impact of exercise exerts varied biomechanical stresses on bone:

- axial compression (squeezing together directly down the bone)
- axial tension (pulling apart)
- torsion (twisting)

The structural complexity and internal organization of a bone determine its ability to resist injury and microscopic damage from biomechanical stresses.

Compression and Tension

Collagen, the connective tissue of bone, accounts for tensile (stretch) strength while the mineral content determines compressive strength and stiffness. Bone mineral content provides maximal strength to a bone since it is most adept at resisting compressive forces.

Excessive and repeated concussion to a limb results in a progressive loss of stiffness and decrease in strength, inviting bone fatigue and failure. With fatigue, a horse's performance suffers, and it is prone to injury and lameness.

Torsion (twisting)

An equine limb can withstand large amounts of compressive force, but the torsional strength is only one-third as strong as the compressive strength. Torsion results from:

- abnormal conformation
- angular limb deformities
- rutted ground
- inconsistent composition of the ground surface

31

- lack of uniformity in the moisture content and cushioning features of the ground
- caulks or toe-grabs on horseshoes

A horse in any of these situations is particularly prone to bone injury.

Propulsive Forces

At a walk, most limb strain occurs in the swing phase when the foot is off the ground. The predominant force on the limb is the tension of tendon pull. At a gallop, reaction forces from the ground contribute to bone strain. These strains occur as the limb is loaded when the foot hits the ground.

Multiple Forces

A bone is not uniform in cross-sectional area. Its shape varies along the shaft, and *cortical walls* vary in thickness. Because of these variations, different forces are applied simultaneously within a single bone.

Stresses and strains on bone result from multiple forces at one time:

- the pull of tendons, ligaments, and muscles
- the effect of weight-bearing and the support of body mass
- the forces created from impact with the ground

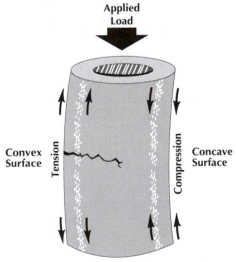

Fig. 2–7. If the tension side fails, the bone will fracture.

Bone Fracture

When simultaneous forces on a bone overcome its inherent strength, the bone fails, or fractures. A bone's ability to withstand tension (stretching) forces is only two-thirds of its ability to withstand compression. As bone is compressed, it expands, causing the compression side (concave surface) to push or bend the tension side (convex surface). As the tension side fails, it moves outward, creating a break.

MANAGING YOUNG BONE
Dangers of Excessive Biomechanical Stress

From 3 months of age up to 1 year, equine bone increases in compressive strength due to increased bone mineral content. Compressive strength stabilizes at this level until 3 years of age. Between 4 and 5 years of age, compressive strength again improves as bone mineral content continues to increase until a horse is about 7 years old.

Bone Failure in Young Athletes

Excessive and repetitive stresses to *young* limbs cause failure. Of 3-year-old racing Thoroughbreds, 70% suffer from *bucked shins* (microfractures in the cannon bone along the front and inside surfaces). In humans, a similar phenomenon called *shin splints* occurs along the lower tibia. Initially, microscopic fractures appear in the bone cortex, but with an eventual overload, a total stress fracture results.

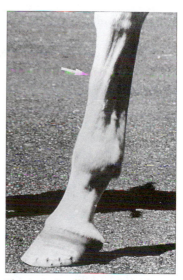

Fig. 2–8. Swelling typical of bucked shins.

Activities Which Increase Risk

Certain types of activities should be avoided or carefully controlled to protect young horses from significantly increased biomechanical stress:

- weight-bearing stress of carrying a rider
- longeing, even in large circles, which exerts twisting forces on bones and particularly on immature joints
- jumping a young horse, which radically overloads the limbs
- long distance work, particularly at speed, which is especially detrimental to a growing skeleton

Bone Fatigue

When bone begins to lose elasticity after being deformed by loading and unloading cycles, it has reached its *fatigue state*.

To illustrate how differently applied loads on a limb affect strength, consider the following example. If a Thoroughbred runs at top speed on a straight line, assuming all else is normal, it can run for 19 miles before fatigue failure of the cannon bone. Yet, running through a turn dramatically increases the load per unit area. Instead of 19 miles, bones subjected to uneven loading in the turn can travel only 0.2 miles before fatigue develops. There is a level of exercise that brings bones past a fatigue state, into an overload range, with subsequent disaster.

Skeletal Maturity

Different breeds mature at different rates. Closure of the growth plates of the long bones is not the only criterion used to determine the age at which a horse can begin competitive athletics. One long bone, the *distal radius* above the knee, has previously served as a monitor for the entire body. In most horses, the growth plates of the long bones close by 3 years of age. For example, in a Thoroughbred or Quarter Horse the radial growth plate closes by 2 – 3 years. Once the growth plate closes, a bone stops growing longer. It instead concentrates on converting to mature and more mineralized bone, and remodeling to conform to biomechanical stresses.

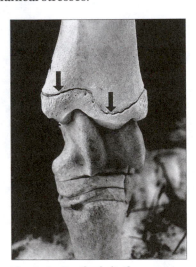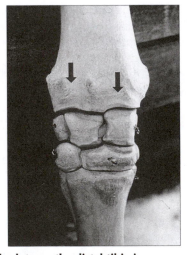

Fig. 2–9. On the left, the open growth plate on the distal tibia in a young horse. On the right, the closed growth plate of the distal radius in a mature horse.

The AERC *(American Endurance Ride Conference)* and the NATRC *(North American Trail Ride Conference)* recognize the need for a horse to reach skeletal maturity before exposing it to the rigorous exertion of long distance riding. The AERC regulations require that a horse must be 5 years old before competing in a 50-mile endurance race, and 4 years old before attempting a 25-mile ride. Allowing a horse to mature skeletally to at least 5 years of age before demanding severe exertion tremendously prolongs its durable athletic life.

Dietary Requirements for Young Horses

While a young horse is growing, careful dietary management encourages young bones and joints to develop normally. Feed a proper calcium to phosphorus ratio of 1.5 : 1, and safe levels of protein and minerals. Excesses of certain minerals, energy, and protein, or a calcium to phosphorus ratio that exceeds 2 : 1, can create serious orthopedic problems. Examples of these developmental abnormalities include:

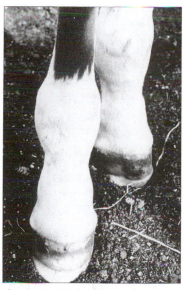

Fig. 2–10. Epiphysitis in the fetlock of a foal.

- *epiphysitis* (inflammation of the growth plate)
- *osteochondrosis* (failure of complete ossification, or bone formation, beneath the joint cartilage, leading to cystic defects or incomplete cartilage flaps)
- *contracted tendons*
- acquired *angular limb deformities*

To guarantee feeding a balanced diet, consult with a veterinarian or an equine nutritional specialist. Good nutrition promotes stronger and healthier bone development, allowing genetic potential to be achieved. More important, an erratic and unbalanced nutritional source adversely affects the alignment and strength of the maturing skeleton. *(For more dietary information see Chapter 7.)*

Early Training

A youngster can be trained without subjecting it to extreme physical stress. Penning one up and allowing it to lie fallow wastes an opportunity to build a foundation for athletic development. A young foal should be turned out to pasture and allowed to play. This activity strengthens bones and muscles, and builds reflexes. The foal learns to use its body athletically. Ponying a foal behind the mare on short rides is another way to build stronger bones.

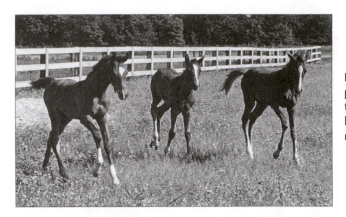

Fig. 2-11. Foals playing in a pasture build strong bones and muscles.

One to Three Years

To properly prepare, and also to protect yearlings to 3-year-olds for many future events, long lining and driving a light cart in harness are excellent ways to supple and strengthen a growing horse. The young horse learns discipline and obedience, and the feel of tack and equipment. From this type of work it learns voice commands, and the subtle feel of a bit and reins. As a teaching method, driving allows an equine body to grow, while exercising mental concentration and acceptance of authority.

Three to Four Years

For many breeds, weight carrying should be delayed until between 3 and 4 years of age. Leave any tight circle work for even later years. Show the young horse big, open spaces, and slowly increase the duration and distance of a ride. This method will optimize the principles of consistent exercise that build bone mass. Gradually introduce speed training over the year after a foundation has been built with long, slow distance conditioning. As the musculoskeletal system matures and adapts to increased physical demands, the cardiovascular system also matures and adapts to conditioning by increasing capillary beds and enzymatic biochemical functions. Stamina slowly develops in the whole body and mind.

Raising a young horse is a slow process, but a horse is a misleading animal to train. Because of a horse's size and brute strength it is easy to ask for more than it has to offer—long before its body and mind are capable. Prevent problems by applying an intelligent conditioning program and quality nutrition during a horse's growing years so it can realize its full athletic potential.

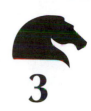

3

IMPROVING MUSCLE PERFORMANCE

An athletic equine body displays firm, well-defined skeletal muscle. The horse depends on skeletal muscle to hold the body together, to maneuver, to support joints, and to convert stored food energy into mechanical motion. More than one-third of a horse's weight consists of skeletal muscle. It is a tissue capable of varied adaptation in response to training and conditioning. *(See anatomy, bone and muscle diagrams in the Appendix, starting on page 511.)*

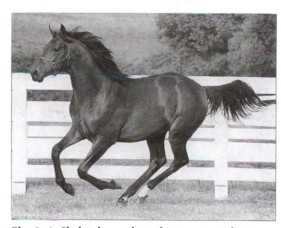

Fig. 3–1. Skeletal muscle makes up more than one-third of total body weight.

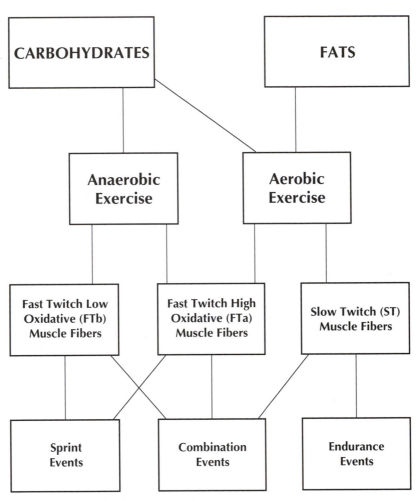

Fig. 3–2. Primary Muscle Fuels.

FOOD FOR ENERGY

To achieve its athletic potential, a horse involved in a rigorous conditioning and training program must be fueled with high-energy food. Food becomes fuel for everyday living and normal biological functions, as well as for hard-working muscle. The main types of fuel derived from food are carbohydrates, fats, and proteins. Protein is a metabolically expensive food source to generate energy. It costs more energy to metabolize than other food fuels, while at the same time it creates very little energy for working muscles as compared to carbohydrates and fats. Its use as a muscle fuel therefore has limited application to the adequately fed performance athlete. Therefore, the most important fuels for working muscles are carbohydrates and fats.

Muscle Fuels

Carbohydrates are organic compounds that are composed of carbon, hydrogen, and oxygen. Fats are made up of *glycerol* and *fatty acids.* Grain, hay, and forage provide carbohydrates and fats which are digested by bacterial residents of the bowel. Vegetable oil is also an important fat supplement for the performance horse. Carbohydrates and fats supply fuel for the muscle cells to produce energy for exercise. As the food travels through the intestines, *glucose* and fatty acids are absorbed into the bloodstream.

Glucose/Glycogen

Glucose is a carbohydrate obtained from digestion of grain, hay, and forage. Glucose in the bloodstream is either used immediately by muscle tissue to produce energy, or it can be stored as *glycogen* in skeletal muscle and in the liver. Glucose can also be stored in fat reserves *(adipose tissue)* as *triglycerides* or fat for later use. (A triglyceride is composed of one molecule of glycerol joined to three molecules of fatty acid.) Glycogen is a connected chain of glucose sugar molecules. To be used by muscle cells, stored glycogen must broken back down into sugar molecules.

Fatty Acids

Another source of fuel, volatile fatty acids (VFAs), are produced from carbohydrates as they are fermented in the large intestine. VFAs can be used immediately to fuel muscle contraction. If they are not needed immediately, they are stored in adipose tissue as triglycerides.

Likewise, the fats in the horse's feed (or vegetable oil) are digested, and formed into triglycerides. Their fatty acid components can be used immediately as muscle fuel or stored in adipose tissue. Later, when the horse needs more fuel, the triglycerides are released from the adipose tissue into the bloodstream, and then they are called *free fatty acids. (See more about supplementing dietary fats in Chapter 12.)*

Muscles Produce Energy

For a muscle to provide locomotion, it must contract, which requires energy. Muscles cannot store enough energy for more than a few seconds of forceful contractions. With glucose and fatty acids, the muscle cells produce and consume millions of energy molecules called ATP *(adenosine triphosphate).* An ATP energy molecule consists of an amino acid attached to three phosphate molecules.

To create energy, muscle enzymes break apart the bond between two of these phosphate molecules. This action creates energy for muscle contraction. Left over is ADP (adenosine diphosphate), which is an amino acid attached to two phosphate molecules, and the unattached, free phosphate molecule.

To produce more ATP energy molecules, the above process is reversed. The muscle cells use glycogen and fatty acids as fuels to reattach a free phosphate molecule back onto an ADP, creating ATP.

These processes occur within the muscle cells thousands of times each microsecond. Without fuel, the phosphate molecule cannot be reattached. ATP would not be formed, so there would be no phosphate bond to break, and no energy for muscle contraction.

Fatty Acid Versus Glycogen

Fatty acids, both VFAs and free fatty acids, are more efficient at generating ATP energy molecules than glycogen, which is why fatty acids are the preferred fuel for muscle contraction. A diet that is supplemented with fats allows the muscles to create more energy during hard work.

ENERGY PRODUCTION

Muscle fibers contracting and relaxing consume large amounts of energy. The processes of energy production and consumption are called *metabolism.* How the muscles produce and consume energy distinguishes certain muscle fiber types from each other. There are two basic types of muscle metabolism. *Aerobic metabolism* uses oxygen to produce energy, while *anaerobic metabolism* does not.

Aerobic Metabolism

Aerobic metabolism means the muscle cell burns fuels using oxygen and enzymes to produce energy. Both of the muscle fuels, glycogen and fatty acids, can be burned aerobically. This method is the most efficient way of producing energy, because it completely burns these fuels without creating toxic by-products. The by-products of aerobic metabolism are carbon dioxide and water, which are non-toxic, and are easily carried from the muscle by the circulatory system. For this reason, all performance horses, regardless of their specific event, should be involved in aerobic training.

Muscle cells that function aerobically produce energy in specialized cellular "factories" called *mitochondria*. Mitochondria break down fuels fatty acids and glycogen, forming energy, carbon dioxide, and water. Because these processes are so complicated, aerobic metabolism produces energy relatively slowly. With greater exertional demands on the muscles, energy must be generated more quickly. This is done by anaerobic metabolism.

Anaerobic Metabolism

Anaerobic metabolism means the muscle cell burns fuel using enzymes, but without using oxygen, to produce energy. Anaerobic metabolism produces energy faster but less efficiently than aerobic metabolism. Fatty acids cannot be burned anaerobically, but glycogen can be used either aerobically or anaerobically. There are two types of anaerobic metabolism, each using a different fuel, phosphocreatine or glycogen.

Sudden, High Intensity Work

The first type of anaerobic metabolism occurs as a horse accelerates with a burst of speed from the starting gate or roping box. At this point in the event, the muscles are fueled by *phosphocreatine*. High energy phosphocreatine can support the high intensity work required of a sprint acceleration or jumping effort for only a few seconds. The energy is provided by breaking apart the phosphocreatine molecule's bonds and does not require oxygen. It also does not produce toxic by-products. Although great thrust and rapid speed are possible when muscles are fueled by phosphocreatine, its supply is extremely limited.

After several seconds the phosphocreatine supply is depleted in the muscles; the muscles then depend on aerobic metabolism or the second type of anaerobic metabolism for continued sprint performance. Phosphocreatine is replenished in about 3 minutes, but by then the sprint activity (such as Quarter Horse racing, roping, or barrel racing) is finished. Neither conditioning nor dietary strategies can increase phosphocreatine stores in the muscles.

Lack of Oxygen During Strenuous Work

The second type of anaerobic metabolism occurs when the horse cannot breathe in enough oxygen to support strenuous work. Muscle enzymes break down glycogen into energy without using oxygen. The toxic by-product of this type of anaerobic metabolism is *lactic acid*, which if produced in excessive amounts, will depress enzyme systems and limit the amount of ATP that is produced. With a limited energy supply available for contraction, muscles rapidly fatigue and performance suffers.

USE OF ENERGY

Remember that one energy form is not used exclusively by working muscle; however, the longer the muscles can use fatty acids to fuel exercise, the more glycogen is spared for later use, and the longer fatigue is delayed. Depending on blood circulation and oxygen supply in the muscles at any given moment, fats or carbohydrates (fatty acids, glucose, and glycogen) will be used as needed. Oxygen supply depends on the horse's level of fitness and the type of activity. Some sports are primarily aerobic, others are primarily anaerobic, and some depend on a balance between the two types of metabolism.

Endurance Type Activities—Aerobic

Endurance type sports consist of prolonged activity at steady paces of walk, trot, and slow canter averaging 8–12 m.p.h. Horses involved in these activities primarily use aerobic metabolism, relying on fatty acids and glycogen as energy sources. They include:

- trail riding
- combined driving
- dressage
- competitive trail events
- pleasure riding
- the roads and tracks phase of eventing

Sprint Type Activities—Anaerobic

Sprint type activities demand intense efforts of short duration (up to 1 minute) at or near maximum speed. A horse depends heavily on anaerobic metabolism during a short sprint. The muscles are fueled from

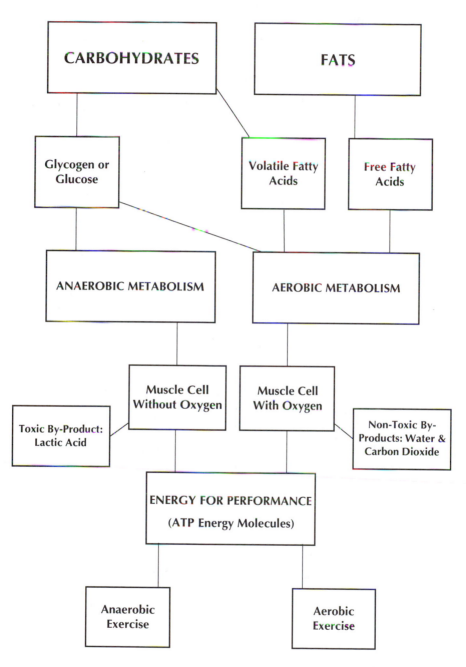

Fig. 3–3. Muscle Metabolism.

sources that do not require oxygen, such as glycogen and phosphocreatine. Examples of sprint activities include:

- roping
- barrel racing
- Quarter Horse racing

Combination Activities

Other activities balance both aerobic and anaerobic metabolism. These activities include:

- steeplechasing
- Standardbred racing
- reining
- polo
- three-day eventing
- Thoroughbred racing
- jumping
- cutting

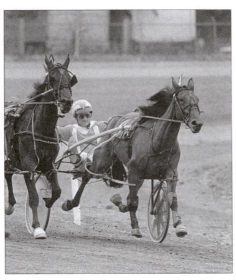

Fig. 3–4. Standardbred racing is a combination activity.

In Thoroughbred and Standardbred racing, the initial sprint is anaerobic, using the phosphocreatine method of energy production. Then the horse begins using aerobic metabolism of fatty acids and glycogen. When aerobic metabolism is no longer sufficient for the racehorse's energy needs, it again depends on anaerobic metabolism, using glycogen for fuel. Of course, these processes happen simultaneously in the muscles. At any one point in the event the horse may depend *more* on one type of muscle metabolism than another type.

Muscle Fiber Types and Metabolism

The contraction and relaxation of a muscle fiber is called a *twitch*. How fast a certain fiber twitches defines its type. There are three possible muscle fiber types:

- *slow twitch* (ST)
- *fast twitch high oxidative* (FTa)
- *fast twitch low oxidative* (FTb)

Each of these three fiber types contracts at different rates and in environments varying in oxygen content. Most muscles contain a mixture of all three fiber types. Studies in equine sports physiology show how different types of muscle fibers, and their production and consumption of energy, influence athletic potential. One athlete may have a higher proportion of a certain type of muscle fibers than another athlete, which is suited for a different performance effort.

For example, slow twitch muscle fibers contract at one-third the rate of fast twitch muscle fibers, and are particularly suited to endurance work. The faster contraction rates of fast twitch fibers produce the speed and power required by sprint work.

Slow Twitch Muscle Fibers

Slow twitch muscle fibers use oxygen to produce energy. Each ST fiber has a considerable blood supply and special cellular factories (mitochondria) to take in and use oxygen to burn fatty acids and glycogen. These fibers are small in cross-sectional diameter and surrounded by capillaries (tiny blood vessels) so oxygen can quickly reach them. ST fibers are the muscle type best suited for endurance sports. Up to 50% of an elite endurance athlete's muscle may be ST fibers.

Slow twitch fibers, however, produce energy so slowly that they cannot meet the intense energy demands of short, rapid bursts of speed or quick thrusts required by racing, cutting, or polo.

Fast Twitch Muscle Fibers

Fast twitch muscle fibers have high concentrations of enzymes that rapidly produce energy from glycogen in the muscle cells during exercise. The faster the twitch, the greater the muscle cell's ability to contract rapidly and forcefully to create the speed and power so important for sprint type sports. Horses with up to 80% FT muscle fibers, like Quarter Horses, Standardbreds, and Thoroughbreds, have excellent speed potential.

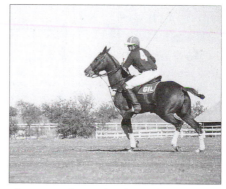

Fig. 3–5. Polo ponies depend on fast twitch muscle fibers for quick accelerations.

Fast Twitch High Oxidative

Fast twitch fibers are further divided into two subtypes: fast twitch high oxidative (FTa) and fast twitch low oxidative (FTb). FTa fibers can use oxygen to some degree to produce energy. When at least 50% of the FT muscle fibers are FTa, the horse performs well at high speed over limited mileage (less than 5 miles), as in Thoroughbred and Standardbred racing.

Fast Twitch Low Oxidative

Fast twitch low oxidative muscle fibers work in an anaerobic muscle cell environment. FTb fibers are unable to use oxygen even if it is available because they lack certain enzymes. An example of horses with high proportions of FTb fibers are Quarter Horse racing competitors that sprint for less than 30 seconds.

OVERVIEW OF MUSCLE FIBER TYPES		
Fiber Type	**Metabolism**	**Activity Examples**
ST— Slow Twitch	Aerobic—Breaks down glycogen or fatty acids to produce energy using oxygen	Competitive Trail Combined Driving Dressage Pleasure Riding
FTa— Fast Twitch high oxidative	Both Aerobic and Anaerobic	Three-Day Eventing Polo Jumping Reining Cutting Thoroughbred Racing Standardbred Racing
FTb— Fast Twitch low oxidative (Can convert 7% to FTa.)	Anaerobic—Breaks down glycogen to produce energy without using oxygen	Roping Barrel Racing Quarter Horse Racing

Fig. 3–6.

Fiber Types, Genetics, and Conditioning

All three muscle fiber types exist in all horses. The ratio of ST to FT fibers is genetically determined. The horse's genetic predisposition for certain muscle fiber types is based on breed and heritable tendencies. Aerobic conditioning can slightly alter ratios among FT fiber types, with potential conversion of some FTb to FTa. The slower contracting ST fibers cannot be trained to contract faster.

The Process of Exercise

When a horse first begins exercising, capillaries have not yet opened to feed oxygen to the muscles. Initial muscle metabolism relies on an anaerobic fuel source, phosphocreatine, in the fast twitch muscle fibers. Within a few minutes of warm-up, circulation is active in the muscles and aerobic sources of energy are tapped. If the horse continues at slow speeds at a heart rate less than 150 – 160 beats per minute (using aerobic metabolism), fatty acids initially provide the primary fuel source for the muscle.

As a horse continues to exercise, different muscle fibers are selectively recruited according to need. A certain muscle may rely on aerobic fuel supplies (fatty acids or glycogen) or anaerobic fuel supplies (glycogen) at various times in the activity, depending on the work intensity each individual muscle tissue is asked to do.

For example, endurance performance calls on slow twitch and fast twitch high oxidative fibers. With a longer or faster effort, an increasing dependency on anaerobic fuel supplies calls more FTa and FTb fibers to work. Once glycogen is depleted, the muscles run out of fuel, and fatigue sets in. As an endurance horse nears exhaustion, all three muscle fiber types have been used, with depletion of all forms of fuel.

Sprint events, such as Quarter Horse racing, barrel racing, or roping, recruit all three muscle fiber types at the same time throughout the effort, although these horses have a greater proportion of FT than ST fibers. Because they use more anaerobic than aerobic metabolism, lactic acid may accumulate in the working muscles of these horses, which causes fatigue.

Fiber Type Correlated With Activity

Many studies of muscle composition have tried to correlate an individual horse's abundance of one muscle fiber type with excellence in a specific event. The studies have not yielded reliable results on the individual level. However, if a breed *in general* has more ST fibers, those horses are more suitable for performance in endurance type events. Breeds with greater numbers of FT fibers are more suitable for performance in sprint type events.

Muscle Contraction

An equine muscle is composed of thousands of individual fibers. Organized contraction of stimulated muscle fibers creates movement of a muscle. A tendon connects a muscle to a bone. Movement of a muscle moves the complementary bone and joint. Large muscle groups working together propel a horse into motion or slow it down. Muscle control and coordination improve with practice and training to produce greater precision, power, and speed.

Concentric Contraction

Concentric contractions shorten the muscles. As a simple analogy of muscle contraction, think of a fully elongated extension ladder—a relaxed muscle fiber. A muscle contraction shortens the ladder as the rungs slide over one another. As parts of the ladder overlap, it thickens as it shortens; so does a muscle fiber in concentric contraction. Pulling apart the extension pieces once again lengthens (or relaxes) the ladder (or muscle fiber). Pulling a ladder apart or pushing it together requires work, as does moving a muscle to flex a joint.

Eccentric Contraction

Another common type of muscle contraction is an *eccentric* contraction that lengthens the muscle. It is used to overcome the pull of gravity as a horse's full weight is supported by a limb. If extensor muscles did not perform this protective kind of work, then joints could overflex and be damaged. A horse that travels down a steep hill uses eccentric muscle efforts to slow the descent.

Isometric Contraction

Some muscle fibers do not change length with contraction. If the length remains the same because of an opposing pull from another muscle, it is called an *isometric* contraction. Isometric contractions occur in a horse that is on the verge of moving. For example, a roping or event horse that is tensely poised in the start box, or a racehorse poised at the gate, is using isometric contraction. A cutting horse, when hunkered down, anticipating the calf to move, is also using a form of isometric contraction.

MUSCLE FATIGUE

In any equine sport, muscle fatigue develops due to several factors:
  • lack of fuel, especially glycogen

- lactic acid accumulation in working muscle
- imbalances in body fluids and electrolytes
- heat build-up in working muscle

Intense speed workouts accumulate lactic acid in the muscle faster than endurance events because at speed the muscles must produce energy without oxygen. Excessive lactic acid in the muscles can lead to soreness, fatigue, exhaustion, or tying-up *(myositis)* in any type of sport.

Aerobic Conditioning of Muscles

Aerobic metabolism produces energy using oxygen. Oxygen is an essential ingredient for sustained exercise of muscles. After 3 or 4 months of steady aerobic conditioning, capillary beds expand in size and quantity to supply greater blood and oxygen circulation to the muscles. Then removal of toxic by-products, like lactic acid, also improves.

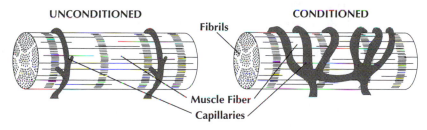

Fig. 3–7. After 3 or 4 months of steady aerobic conditioning, capillary beds expand in size and quantity.

The aerobic conditioning process also doubles the activity of aerobic enzyme systems for more efficient energy production in the muscles. Muscles are therefore able to function for longer periods before energy reserves are depleted. This efficiency delays the need for anaerobic metabolism and therefore delays lactic acid accumulation in the muscles.

Conserving Glycogen
Using Fatty Acids as Fuel

According to Dr. Philip Swann in his book, *Racehorse Training and Sports Medicine*, more than 30 times the energy is stored in a horse's fat depots than in all the glycogen reserves in the skeletal muscles and liver. The primary benefit of aerobic conditioning is that it promotes the use of fatty acids as an energy source. Fatty acids are released into the bloodstream from adipose tissue storage, and carried to the muscles for fuel. Using fatty acids conserves glycogen stores and delays muscle fatigue so a horse can perform for a longer time without accumulating lactic acid. An aerobically-trained horse can better convert fatty acids into energy instead of using glycogen as fuel.

However, fatty acids cannot provide an exclusive energy source because their rate of uptake by muscle tissue is limited. If exercise intensity increases and oxygen supplies decrease, then the muscles must rely on glycogen as a fuel source. The depletion of glycogen reserves leads to exhaustion. This lack is what ultimately limits the endurance athlete's performance.

Increasing the fat stores in the horse by allowing it to gain weight will not improve the body's ability to use fatty acids for energy production. Only aerobic conditioning can accomplish this goal. In fact, extra body weight is detrimental because the horse uses more energy to carry the extra weight around, and a layer of stored fat prevents heat dissipation from working muscles. Both of these factors lead to fatigue.

Increased Glycogen Storage

Not only do a horse's muscles learn to more efficiently metabolize fatty acids as an energy source, but conditioning also creates more glycogen stores in the muscles. Over a 10-week conditioning period, glycogen reserves may increase by as much as 33%.

Anaerobic Conditioning of Muscles
Increased Muscle Mass

Anaerobic conditioning builds muscle mass because the cross-sectional areas of the fast twitch muscle fibers increase to improve muscle strength and power. For example, compare the heavy muscling of a Quarter Horse to the lean, flat muscling of an Arabian. The large hindquarter muscles of the Quarter Horse athlete is partially a result of anaerobic muscle conditioning, and partially a result of genetics.

Lactic Acid Tolerance

During intense bursts of exercise, anaerobic metabolism of muscle glycogen is the main source of energy. Because energy demands increase 200-fold during these intensive exertions, the high rate of energy production provided by anaerobic metabolism is essential to a sprinting horse. During most anaerobic metabolism, glycogen is broken down into energy and lactic acid.

At first, this toxic by-product is carried away from the muscle by the bloodstream. As energy demands increase, however, more lactic acid is produced than the circulation can remove. Lactic acid accumulation in the muscles slows energy production and weakens the contractions of muscle fibers. Therefore, accumulating lactic acid causes fatigue and muscle soreness.

Anaerobic Threshold

The *anaerobic threshold* is the point at which lactic acid begins to accumulate in the muscles and bloodstream. Sprint conditioning can raise the anaerobic threshold by making anaerobic energy production more efficient. It also trains specific enzyme systems to buffer, or neutralize lactic acid. Raising the anaerobic threshold delays the onset of fatigue. With a higher anaerobic threshold, a racehorse can travel at faster speeds or an endurance horse can go longer distances before excessive lactic acid accumulates in the muscles.

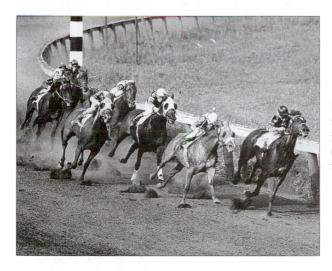

Fig. 3–8. Increasing the anaerobic threshold delays muscle fatigue in the racehorse.

Sodium Bicarbonate

Before a race, racehorses are commonly treated with a sodium bicarbonate (baking soda) drench, called a "milkshake," in an attempt to counteract the lactic acid and enhance race performance.

Although sodium bicarbonate does seem to improve the buffering capacity of the blood, recent studies report no statistical differences in racing times of horses receiving milkshakes before racing, particularly in studies with Quarter Horse or Thoroughbred racehorses.

The use of sodium bicarbonate is still controversial. It is thought that high intensity exercise of 2 – 9 minutes, such as Standardbred racing, may be enhanced with sodium bicarbonate. Quarter Horse and Thoroughbred races are finished in less than 2 minutes, and the value of milkshakes for these horses is as yet inconclusive. Many other variables such as environmental conditions, track surface, and jockey experience also influence racing results. Some milkshakes also contain electrolytes, and can actually be detrimental if the horse has no access to water before the race.

Studies with human athletes indicate that for events involving multiple bouts, performance is enhanced with sodium bicarbonate. The use of multiple bouts is an important element in Standardbred racing and training. The longer duration of exercise coupled with multiple workouts may make milkshakes beneficial to the Standardbred racehorse.

To be effective, (if it is indeed effective) the horse must be drenched at a dose of 0.4 grams of sodium bicarbonate per kilogram of body weight. The maximal buffering effects are attained approximately 3 hours after drenching, so plan to drench the horse about 3 hours before race time.

Sodium bicarbonate should *never* be administered to the long distance horse, as losses of electrolytes in the sweat for several hours tend to excessively alkalinize the bloodstream.

Other Benefits

The horse evolved as a flight and flee animal able to escape from predators by fast bursts of speed. Studies confirm that training specifically for intense bursts of speed does not change the metabolism of glycogen. However, conditioning does improve nerve signals, coordinating muscle movement. The rate of muscle contraction and the removal of lactic acid are also improved by anaerobic conditioning of muscles.

MUSCLE STRENGTHENING

All forms of conditioning strengthen a horse's muscles. Along with improved oxygen use and lactic acid tolerance, the muscles learn to contract faster and with more force to enhance speed. In addition, nerve control to the muscles is fine tuned, improving muscular coordination.

General muscle strengthening is as important to a horse's performance as learning the skills of the athletic endeavor. Strength in the muscles makes the task easier. Muscle strength delays the onset of fatigue, particularly during the demands of a competition. Strong muscles reduce the risk of a misstep that could strain tendons, ligaments, or joints.

It is equally important to train for the specific athletics a horse will perform. An endurance horse must train over irregular terrain and at competition speeds. On the other hand, endurance training cannot sufficiently educate muscles to respond to the quick energy bursts required by such events as racing, cutting, or jumping. If a horse is to accomplish these tasks, it must practice them.

Muscle strengthening is a process requiring many months. It is also cumulative over years. Living tissues return to fitness faster after short periods (weeks) of layoff than they did at the beginning of training. Along with the horse's genetic and psychological predisposition, the amount of effort put into the horse's training determines its durability and ability to perform.

Muscle Exercises

Aerobic Exercise

Muscles adapt to the type of stress applied to them. A horse that exclusively performs aerobic exercises does not build power or bulk in muscle. An example of the effect of aerobic exercises is the flat muscling typical of Arabian endurance horses. Aerobic exercises are low resistance but highly repetitive, like trotting down a level trail at the same rhythm and speed for miles. This exercise improves stamina, neuromuscular precision, and economy of movement. The range of movement and the elasticity of muscles also improve. The slow twitch fibers benefit from aerobic conditioning by improving their use of oxygen.

Anaerobic Exercise

In contrast, anaerobic exercises are high resistance efforts with fewer repetitions, and lasting up to 30 seconds. Short brisk gallops or rapid hill climbs are examples of anaerobic drills. During each intense exercise, muscles are quickly depleted of stored energy, and then rested between bouts. These exercises increase the bulk and substance of fast twitch muscle fibers.

Resistance

As an example of the effect of resistance on muscles, consider the development of a horse's neck muscles as it is trained to accept bit contact. With the neck in a normal, relaxed position, the nuchal ligament stretching from the poll to the withers passively assumes the load of the head. The muscles along the top of the neck are not stressed when the neck is in a relaxed position. When the horse is asked to go on bit contact, its neck and head arch and activate those muscles on the top of the neck. The head acts as a "weight" to provide some resistance to the exercise. The horse then actively holds the head and neck with muscular effort rather than by passive support from the ligaments. Continual exercise of the neck muscles develops them over time and bulks up the neck.

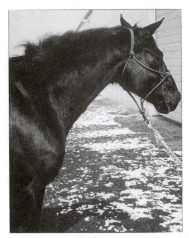 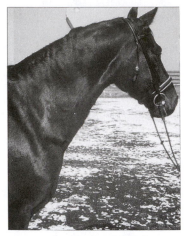

Fig. 3–9. On the left, an untrained horse's neck. On the right, the muscular neck of a trained dressage horse.

Faster Gait

To increase the resistance of an anaerobic exercise, add a faster gait to the muscle training period. For example, trotting up a hill places more demand on muscle tissues than walking up a hill.

Hill Work

An inclined grade or a hill challenges and strengthens body muscle. The resistance of a horse's body weight as it climbs a hill develops hind leg, forearm, and shoulder muscles. Walking or trotting a hill develops independent muscles in each hind leg.

As the horse accelerates into a canter or gallop, it propels itself forward by pushing off the ground with both hind legs at about the same time. A hill climb in a canter or gallop exercises the hind legs as a unit, with considerable strain on the rump and back muscles. These muscles strengthen accordingly.

Downhill work strengthens pectoral, shoulder, and forearm muscles, while the quadriceps muscles in the hind legs are strengthened by a braking motion.

Hill work has more advantages besides muscle strengthening. A horse gains as much training effect on the muscles and cardiovascular system doing a hill climb as it would covering three times the distance on flat ground. Also, bones and joints do not receive as great an impact stress with hill work as with flat work, which attempts to reach the same heart rate by increasing speed.

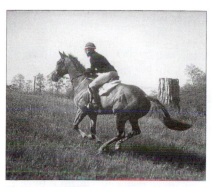

Fig. 3–10. Hill work at the canter strengthens the hind legs, rump, and back muscles.

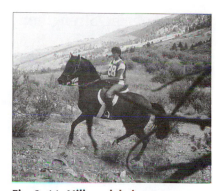

Fig. 3–11. Hill work helps prepare a horse for rocky, mountainous terrain during a competitive trail event.

Deep Footing

Work in deep footing, like sand, snow, or a spongy meadow, creates resistance in thigh and pectoral muscles. Mud is not a good medium for this type of training as it can cause tendon injuries and even bone fractures. If mud is incorporated into a training routine, work at the walk, never at the trot or canter. Slow and careful conditioning accustoms a horse to deep footing, preventing tendon strain.

Benefits of Cross Training

Sprint work benefits endurance performance by improving the efficiency of the fast twitch fibers. These fibers contribute to the staying power of a long distance horse as it eventually depletes aerobic fuel supplies and resorts to the recruitment of FT fibers.

Endurance conditioning benefits a sprint horse by improving aerobic metabolism, which reduces the horse's dependency on anaerobic energy production. Then less lactic acid is produced. In addition, aerobic conditioning develops the capillary beds, which makes removal of lactic acid more efficient. Also, aerobic conditioning increases muscle glycogen stores. A sprint horse relies almost exclusively on glycogen metabolism for energy.

The abundance of equestrian sports provides a variety of exercises to develop and strengthen muscles. Long rides stretch and supple muscles, teach balance and rhythm, and strengthen all body systems. Obstacles such as cavaletti poles teach precision through a gymnastic routine. The even footing of a track is excellent for speed workouts. Cross training builds a versatile and durable athlete.

Sports-Specific Strengthening Exercises

Dressage

Combining calisthenics (developing muscular tone) with strength training improves the back, belly, and hind leg muscles in the dressage

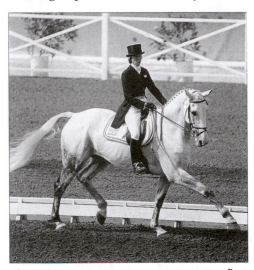

Fig. 3–12. Dressage movements create a fit and responsive horse.

horse, making it capable of performing precision movements with ease. Work the horse on bit contact and in a dressage frame, and then allow it to relax and stretch between difficult exercises. Repetitive practice and correct execution of advanced movements of half-pass, piaffe, passage, and pirouettes strengthen the associated muscles. Trotting cavalettis teaches rhythm and balance, and also teaches the horse to work with the hocks up and under the body. Cantering 2-foot fences spaced one stride apart encourages simultaneous hind leg use, developing croup and back muscles. Downhill walking also teaches a horse to balance with its hindquarters, an important element of collected work.

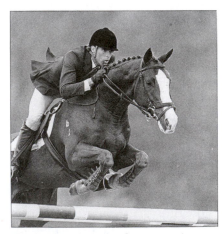

Fig. 3–13. A jumping horse requires strength in the hindquarters.

Jumping

A jumping horse not only propels off the ground with strong hindquarter muscles, but landing exerts considerable force on shoulder and neck muscles. These horses particularly benefit from hill climbs at a canter, with slower downhills to rest the muscles between strengthening exercises. Cavaletti work and dressage exercises also strengthen hindquarter muscles.

Racing

Two of the most beneficial exercises for the racehorse are hill climbs and interval training. Hill work strengthens the hindquarter muscles for acceleration and drive. It also provides aerobic conditioning, which is an important factor in racing.

Interval training consists of repeated sets of speed work and partial heart rate recovery periods. Interval training increases speed and promotes lactic acid tolerance. *(See Chapter 5 for more information on interval training.)*

Reining

A reining horse executes sudden stops and roll backs, and should strengthen the muscles over the croup and back. These muscles tuck the hindquarters beneath the body for such abrupt efforts. Besides practicing sliding stops and spins, a reining horse may benefit from hill work at a canter or slow gallop to build buttock muscles. Downhill walking improves balance and coordination. Exercise in deep footing strengthens thigh muscles.

Cutting

A cutting horse relies on strength in the shoulder and chest muscles, as well as buttock and thigh muscles that enable it to move quickly in front of the calf. Hill work, both ascents and descents, exercises all these muscles, and provides a break from the mental pressure that comes from persistent cutting practice.

MYOSITIS

The hard-working performance horse is subject to a skeletal muscle disease syndrome, generally called *myositis*. This syndrome also goes by other names: "tying-up," "Monday morning disease," exertional rhabdomyolysis, azoturia, paralytic, and myoglobinuria. The causes of these syndromes may be different, but their symptoms are the same and can be similarly treated. Myositis literally means "muscle inflammation" and is a general term for all these syndromes.

Myositis is a painful condition similar to a severe charley horse in a person's leg. The large, fleshy muscles over the rump or along a horse's thigh suddenly spasm and cramp. The horse assumes a stilted gait in the hindquarters, and may eventually refuse to move. The muscles may feel hard as a brick, instead of a normal pliable consistency. There may be tremors or quivers in the muscles. Some

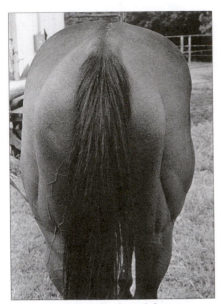

Fig. 3–14. The muscles of the rump and thighs are prone to myositis.

horses seem wobbly and unsteady, while others sweat, act "colicky," and want to lie down and roll. The horse is in obvious distress and in need of immediate veterinary attention. Keep the horse warm with a blanket, and do not move it until professional help arrives.

Normal Muscle Contraction

A normal contraction of a muscle fiber is caused by a series of biochemical events. A muscle fiber is made up of thousands of filaments. There are two types of filaments: *actin* filaments and *myosin* filaments, which partially overlap. The myosin filaments have "heads" which attach to the actin filaments.

A nerve impulse from the brain releases calcium into the muscle cells. Calcium activates sites on the actin filament so that the head of the myosin filament attaches to it. Then the myosin head tilts and swivels to pull the actin filament. The head then detaches and moves to another active site on the actin filament. This cycle of head tilt, filament movement, and head detachment continues to contract the muscle fiber with a ratchet-like movement.

The Role of Calcium

As long as calcium is in the cell, a fiber will continue to contract. A cellular "calcium pump" normally removes calcium from the cell, allowing the muscle fiber to relax. ATP (adenosine triphosphate) energy molecules fuel the pump that removes calcium from the muscle cell.

If calcium channels are blocked due to lack of ATP energy molecules, the muscle cannot relax. Calcium remains in the muscle cells activating the actin filaments, and the heads of the myosin filaments remain attached. This unrelenting contraction, multiplied by many thousands of fibers, causes muscle cramps. With each spasm, more ATP is depleted and the cycle continues.

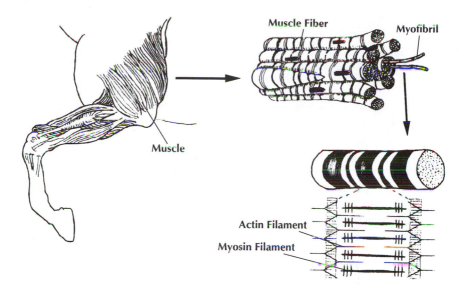

Fig. 3–15. A muscle fiber is made of thousands of filaments.

Muscle and Kidney Damage

As muscle fibers spasm and tear apart, pigment molecules called *myoglobin* are removed by the bloodstream and carried to the kidneys. The kidneys' function is to filter small molecules. The relatively large myoglobin molecules may be trapped inside the kidneys and block them. There, they may interfere with oxygen diffusion to kidney cells, and may cause kidney failure, resulting in shock or death. Kidney damage is proportionate to the amount of myoglobin trapped within the kidneys.

Coffee-colored urine is evidence that myoglobin has reached the kidneys. Intravenous fluid therapy is sometimes necessary to flush the kidneys and improve circulation in the muscles, while anti-inflammatory drugs stop the cycle of muscle damage and pain.

Causes of Myositis

Some horses are taken out to exercise and show signs of discomfort within the first several minutes (Type A myositis), while others develop myositis after several hours of steady exercise (Type B myositis).

Performance can suffer in cases of myositis, even if muscle cramping is not actually seen. The symptoms may be as subtle as poor racing times or a shorter stride than normal.

Type A Myositis

In Type A myositis a horse begins to experience severe muscle cramps after only a few minutes of exercise. This syndrome is caused by stress, hormonal influences, or defects in energy metabolism in the muscle.

Accumulation of lactic acid in the muscles reduces the rate of energy production and the contraction of muscle fibers. Less energy produced means less energy to fuel the calcium pump, and uncontrolled muscle contraction causes the cramping of myositis. A fat or unconditioned horse stores more glycogen in the muscle and metabolizes it less efficiently than a conditioned horse. These factors increase lactic acid production.

Horses that work above the anaerobic threshold at speeds greater than 20 m.p.h. accumulate measurable lactic acid in the tissues and bloodstream. A high concentration of lactic acid in the muscles increases the risk of myositis. Lactic acid does not necessarily cause myositis, but high lactic acid concentrations worsen muscle damage.

Type B Myositis

Electrolyte Loss

Type B myositis develops after long periods of exercise, either during the exertion or within an hour after work has stopped. Endurance horses, such as long distance trail horses and three-day event horses, work mostly at aerobic speeds. Therefore, they develop myositis for different reasons than lactic acid-related myositis in racehorses, jumping horses, or cutting horses. The horse that exercises steadily for long periods can develop electrolyte (body salt) imbalances and dehydration, leading to exhaustion and myositis.

Potassium

Prolonged exercise, especially on an excessively hot and humid day, encourages loss of electrolytes, such as potassium and chloride, in the sweat. Potassium dilates small blood vessels in the muscle during exercise. With low potassium, the blood vessels do not dilate enough to deliver adequate oxygen to the muscles and fuel the slow twitch muscle fibers.

Chloride

A loss of chloride causes *metabolic alkalosis* (increased pH in the bloodstream). An increased pH in the bloodstream directly affects the ability of the muscle cells to extract oxygen from the blood.

Fluid Loss

Fluid loss from sweat dehydrates a horse and decreases the circulating blood volume. Decreasing the amount of blood also limits the amount of oxygen available to muscles.

In sum, the lack of electrolytes and fluids decreases the amount of oxygen available to the muscles. Therefore, aerobic metabolism in the slow twitch fibers cannot continue and the fast twitch fibers are recruited. Lactic acid begins to accumulate, slowing energy production and increasing the risk of myositis.

Also, working muscles generate heat. Heat build-up in the muscles increases the oxygen and energy requirements of muscles, adding to the problems of electrolyte imbalances, dehydration, and energy depletion.

Candidates For Myositis

Horses in Training

A horse in training that is fed rich feed (grain or alfalfa) is a candidate for this syndrome. This is especially true if the horse remains on a generous grain supplement while rested for a day or two, and then is immediately returned to vigorous exercise. When a horse is not active on a particular day, reduce its grain intake. Rapid increases in work difficulty or demands for speed from an unconditioned horse can also cause a crisis.

Myositis is predominantly a disease of the fast twitch muscle fibers. (Slow twitch fibers are surrounded by greater numbers of capillaries, so more oxygen is readily available to them.) FT fibers that receive little or no oxygen are susceptible to impaired blood flow from constriction of blood vessels. FT fibers also produce more lactic acid than ST fibers.

The stress of training can reduce normal thyroid activity and change its control of internal body temperature and oxygen supply to working muscles. A cold day similarly constricts blood vessels in the muscle, so less blood and oxygen are supplied to the fibers. All these factors can lead to excessive lactic acid production.

Genetic Predisposition

Genetic tendencies for myositis have been observed in some breed lines. This tendency may be related to a defect in muscle metabolism in affected individuals. Heavily muscled horses with greater numbers of FT fibers are prone to the disease. Examples of these horses are Quarter Horses, Appaloosas, Paints, and certain draft breeds such as the Clydesdale, Shire, Belgian, and Percheron.

Nervous horses, especially mares and fillies, seem prone to myositis, possibly due to female endocrine influences. Horses that develop myositis may suffer repeated episodes and require careful management and training.

Preventing Myositis

Many factors influencing myositis are out of human control, such as climate, genetics, and skeletal muscle metabolism disorders unique to an individual. Yet, strategies for prevention exist. An educated conditioning program enables a horse to perform the athletic demands with the least stress to body and mind.

Warm-Ups and Cool-Downs

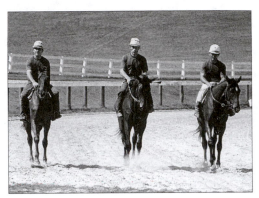

Fig. 3–16. Warming-up is a good preventative measure to help avoid myositis.

Attention to a proper warm-up opens capillary beds in the muscles and activates enzyme systems. A warm-up actually increases muscle temperature by one or two degrees. Warmed muscles are more elastic so they contract and move more efficiently. An adequate cool-down flushes lactic acid from the muscle. A muscle massage loosens fatigued muscles and enhances circulation to the tissues. *(See Chapter 6 for more information on warm-ups and cool-downs.)*

Conditioning

The entire body of a horse benefits from conditioning. It encourages development of the heart and lungs, and of blood vessels and capillaries in the muscles, improving oxygen delivery and toxic by-product removal. Conditioning trains enzyme systems in the muscles to efficiently use energy sources, delays the build-up of lactic acid, and improves muscle tolerance of toxic by-products, to reduce the risk of myositis.

The Sprint Horse

A sprint horse depends on fast twitch muscle fibers to produce acceleration and power. Sprint training increases the anaerobic threshold so lactic acid does not accumulate as quickly and energy production can continue. Sprint training also develops enzymes which buffer the tiring effects of lactic acid.

The Endurance Horse

Training strategies for the long distance performer improve the horse's *aerobic capacity*. Training reduces the cross-sectional area of slow twitch muscle fibers, allowing better diffusion of oxygen into the muscle cells. The longer the slow twitch fibers can function in aerobic metabolism, the longer it takes for recruitment of fast twitch muscle fibers that are more prone to developing myositis. In long distance competitions it is possible to prevent extreme electrolyte imbalances by supplementing a horse with oral electrolytes during the event. A sufficient water supply should always be provided, and the long-distance horse given many opportunities to drink, preventing dehydration. *(See Chapter 6 for more information on dehydration.)*

Other Prevention Methods

Avoid applying water to the large buttock or back muscles of a hot horse that has just stopped working. The cool water causes blood vessels to constrict away from the skin surface, trapping heat and toxic by-products in the muscle. In addition, blood and oxygen circulation in the muscles is diminished, leading to muscle cramping.

To prevent chill and cramping of the working muscles, especially of a long distance competitor, use a rump rug during rainy, cold, or extremely windy conditions. A rump rug covering the haunches keeps the working muscles warm and supple and makes them less likely to cramp.

During periods of inactivity between events, races, or regular training schedules, grain should be reduced. The horse should be turned out for self-exercise to maintain muscle tone.

Anemias caused by intestinal parasitism, or inadequate feed intake or nutrient absorption further reduce oxygen circulation in the blood. Consistent deworming schedules, tooth care, and attention to a horse's overall health and attitude allow it to optimally use nutrients that fuel muscles and help prevent myositis.

HYPERKALEMIC PERIODIC PARALYSIS

Over the last decade, a condition of skeletal muscle weakness has been recognized. This syndrome, *hyperkalemic periodic paralysis* (HYPP) has been genetically linked to a certain line of Quarter Horses.

Clinical Signs

As an episode of HYPP begins, an affected horse experiences persistent muscle twitching over the trunk, hindquarters, flanks, neck, and/or shoulders. Muscles of the face also spasm, causing flared nostrils, and lips that are taut and drawn. In addition, the third eyelid often drops over the eye as the muscles around the orbit spasm.

As the episode progresses, the skeletal muscles become weak, with the horse collapsing to the ground, or sitting on its haunches like a dog. Mild attacks may only elicit signs of muscular weakness such as swaying and staggering, with the horse not going down completely. The horse may buckle at the knees, sag in its hocks, or be unable to raise its head and neck. Throughout a crisis the horse remains alert, although slightly depressed, and is in no pain. The overall relaxed attitude of the animal helps distinguish HYPP from similar-appearing syndromes of colic or myositis. Between episodes of HYPP, the horse appears completely normal.

Cause of HYPP

HYPP occurs due to a defect in the transport system that regulates the movement of potassium and sodium across cell membranes. The problem begins with a protein pore known as a sodium channel. This sodium channel is sensitive to voltage changes within the muscle cell. A horse suffering from HYPP has excess potassium outside the muscle cells, which then creates voltage changes across the cell membrane.

High potassium levels in the blood cause the sodium channels to "leak," and create a hyperexcitable muscle membrane. The muscles begin to contract as seen by muscle twitches and facial spasms. As the muscle tissue repeatedly contracts, additional potassium is transported from inside each cell to the outside, adding to the potassium levels in the bloodstream. This cycle perpetuates the episode.

After several minutes of constant muscle contractions, the muscle membranes can no longer fire. The muscles become paralyzed, and the horse weakens and collapses.

Skeletal muscle stores the greatest amount of body potassium. Horses with HYPP have a lower potassium content in the muscles than normal individuals, possibly due to increased permeability of the muscle membrane to potassium that allows it to accumulate in the bloodstream.

HYPP is potentially fatal due to the adverse effects of high blood potassium levels on the heart. Episodes vary in intensity, and are unpredictable. Most episodes, however, are non-fatal, and last 15 – 90 minutes. Usually an affected horse begins to show signs between the ages of 2 – 4 years.

An attack can be brought on by excess potassium in the diet (for example, alfalfa hay). Also, sudden dietary changes, irregular feeding schedules, or withholding food can cause an attack. Stress from training or transport is also implicated in episodes of HYPP.

Preventing HYPP Episodes

Prevention relies mostly on feeding strategies. Recommendations suggest feeding a diet containing a maximum of 1% potassium, and avoiding alfalfa hay, rich spring pasture, molasses, and sweet feed (which contains molasses). Oats, barley, and corn contain less than 0.4% potassium. Grain portions should be fed in small amounts 2–3 times daily.

Some grass hays contain up to 2.5% potassium so it may be best to have hay analyzed. Dr. Harold Hintz (Cornell University) recommends feeding 50% water-soaked beet pulp with 50% grass hay to meet normal roughage needs while minimizing potassium intake.

Do not supplement affected horses with potassium-containing electrolytes, and read labels carefully on protein and vitamin and mineral supplements to ensure potassium is not included. However, a salt block should be available at all times.

Horses with HYPP should not be confined to stalls, but should be turned into paddocks where they can self-exercise. Preventative medical management of HYPP includes a diuretic (acetazolamide) that stimulates potassium excretion through the urine.

Treatment

If a horse develops beginning signs of an attack, walking or longeing the horse can stimulate the circulation of adrenaline. Adrenaline drives potassium back into the muscle cells. In addition, a small amount of oats or Karo® syrup can be administered to stimulate the release of insulin, which also drives potassium back into the muscle cells. Severe attacks require immediate veterinary attention.

Genetic Test

To detect if a horse may develop HYPP, a blood sample can be evaluated for a specific gene in the DNA. This test is available through the University of California-Davis School of Veterinary Medicine.

Not all horses of the affected lineage have the HYPP gene. If only one parent has the mutant gene, a foal has a 50% chance of being afflicted. If both parents possess the gene, a foal has a 75% chance of developing HYPP. A horse that tests negative for the mutant gene will not pass the syndrome on to future generations, and may confidently be used as breeding stock.

4

PERFORMANCE FEET

Daily care and attention to a horse's feet provide a wealth of information regarding their health. Clean the feet with a hoof pick and examine them for foul odors, stones, nails, or hoof cracks. Watch a horse in motion around the paddock, corral, or pasture so lameness is recognized early.

The size of the feet should be proportionate to the body. Study the feet for balance and symmetry. Note abnormal contours in the hoof wall. Compare the front feet to each other, and back feet to each other. Study other horses' feet and make compari-

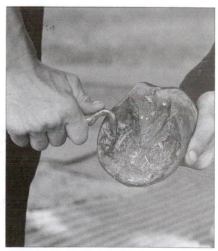

Fig. 4–1. Regular hoof care is essential for good performance.

sons. Develop an eye for the normal; learn to notice oddities. Daily care may prevent a simple problem from developing into a long-term, chronic disease.

FOOT FUNCTION & STRUCTURE

The hoof is the hard outer covering of the foot. Beneath the hoof lies a complex arrangement of bones, cartilage, ligaments, and tendons. The foot is a complex and dynamic structure, elastic and alive.

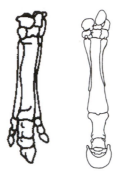

Evolution has developed a horse's front legs from rudimentary fingers. Starting with the tips of a person's middle finger, the fingernail and the small bone up to the first joint corresponds to a horse's front foot. The rest of that finger back to where it joins the hand has developed into the two pastern bones. The cannon and splint bones are similar to the bones in the back of a hand. The other fingers and thumb have disappeared.

Imagine walking on one finger. It is easy to understand why lameness develops when one considers the enormous load per square inch that a 1,000-pound animal places upon each limb during performance.

Fig. 4–2. On the left, ancient horse leg. On the right, modern leg bones and hoof.

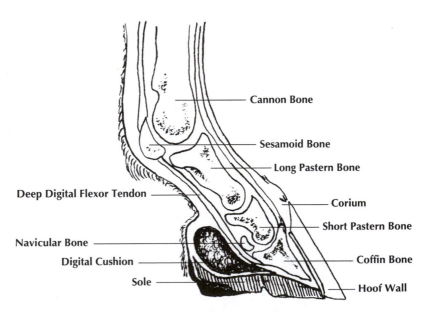

Cannon Bone

Sesamoid Bone

Long Pastern Bone

Deep Digital Flexor Tendon

Corium

Short Pastern Bone

Navicular Bone

Digital Cushion

Coffin Bone

Sole

Hoof Wall

Fig. 4–3. Internal and external structures of the foot.

Circulatory Function

Often a horse is referred to as having five "hearts," each foot contributing to the pumping activities of the heart. As a horse strides forward, the heel contacts the ground before the toe. This impact expands the heel outward, pushing the *digital cushion*, a fibroelastic fatty pad forming the heel bulbs, against the *collateral cartilages*.

As a horse's foot impacts the ground, the frog is compressed while the short pastern bone is forced downwards. Then the digital cushion overlying the internal frog surface is compressed, further expanding the collateral cartilages. This expansion forces the network of blood vessels within the hoof wall to alternately constrict and dilate. In this way, blood and oxygen are moved around the tissues of the foot, and up and down the legs.

The coffin bone lies inside the hoof capsule. A network of blood vessels and nerves holds the bone in position. Seated beneath and behind the coffin bone is the navicular bone. It functionally increases the surface area of the coffin joint, reducing the impact of landing. The deep digital flexor tendon runs behind the navicular bone and attaches to the back of the coffin bone. The position of the navicular bone moves the deep digital flexor tendon away from the center of the coffin joint, creating a larger range of motion of that joint. These internal structures of the foot absorb downward compressive forces by the body and gravity.

Optimal biomechanical function of the foot is determined by the:

- balance of the foot
- conformation
- shoes that are worn
- contour of the terrain
- impact surface of the ground

Any deviation from normal has a pronounced effect on a horse's performance, because all these factors contribute to overall soundness of the limbs.

Health, Genetics, and Performance

The ultimate factor dictating the response of a foot to environmental influences is the genetic predisposition of a horse. It is hard to make an anatomical structure better than its genetic potential. Exercise and good, balanced nutrition maintain foot health and restore diseased feet to normal. The conformational shape, size, and hoof wall thickness are controlled by genetics, but improper shoeing, lack of stable hygiene, and environmental dehydration can adversely alter genetic tendencies.

Hoof Color

Many people claim that hoof color (white versus black) affects the strength and durability of a hoof. Many people believe that white feet are softer, more crumbly, and more predisposed to bruising and injury than black feet. However, a scientific study (1983) on the mechanical properties of equine hooves found *no* difference in the stress and strain behavior or ultimate strength properties between black and white hooves.

Hoof Size

Feet that are too wide are prone to bruising, collapsed heels, and dropped soles. Feet that are contracted with a narrow straight wall do not give under pressure. A small foot or one with poor conformation is prone to problems. Both a too large or too small foot lack shock absorptive ability. Excess concussion is absorbed in the feet and up the limb.

Not all horses have front feet that are exact mates in size and shape, and this may be normal for some individuals. Yet, any difference in size should be viewed with suspicion as a sign of disease.

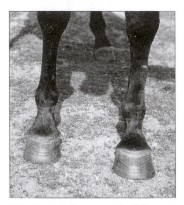

Fig. 4–4. A horse with different sized feet due to disease.

Hoof Structure and Growth

The *coronary corium* underlying the *coronary band* where the hoof meets the skin produces new hoof wall growth. The corium is a layer of connective tissue containing an elaborate blood and nerve supply that nourishes the foot.

Hoof Wall

The hoof wall, composed of *keratin,* is a modified extension of the skin. A continuously growing structure, the hoof grows down from the coronary band. A young horse grows hoof faster than a mature horse. For example, a foal may grow ½ inch of hoof per month, but a mature horse grows hoof at the rate of about ⅜ inch per month.

The hoof also grows at different rates throughout the year, depending on season and climate. It grows fastest during periods of warm temperatures and moisture, corresponding with springtime and lengthening daylight hours.

At the rate of ⅜ of an inch per month, the toe—and any hoof damage—entirely grows out in about a year, while the heels replace themselves every 4 – 5 months.

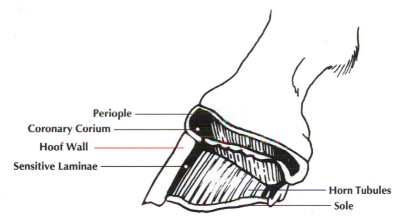

Fig. 4–5. The hoof wall.

Horn Tubules

Elastic *horn tubules* absorb concussion by bending and flexing and by compressing, reducing the impact on other structures in the limbs. Normal moisture content promotes elasticity of the hoof, enabling it to absorb concussion.

By the peculiar anatomy of the hoof, Mother Nature has provided a way of maintaining natural hoof moisture. Moisture in the equine hoof comes from internal water carried through the blood and lymphatic vessels to sensitive structures deep within the foot. From there it is transferred to the horn tubules that make up the hoof wall. Exercise enhances this circulatory process.

Rigid and closely packed horn tubules aligned in a vertical and parallel arrangement in the hoof wall retain moisture much as a sponge holds water. The configuration of the foot dictates the direction in which the horn tubules lay. This factor is important in moisture retention.

For example, one of the problems associated with a long-toe–low-heel configuration is that it loses the neat, parallel alignment of horn tubules. Spacing between tubule cells is spread apart, and moisture is quickly lost from the foot.

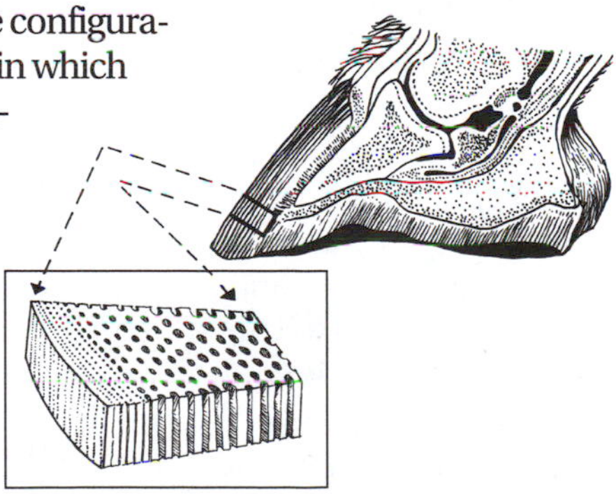

Fig. 4–6. Horn tubules within the hoof.

Periople

A protective, waxy covering called the *periople* delays loss of internal moisture from the hoof. The periople "hoof varnish" is a very thin layer of cells that readily wears off although it continually grows from the coronary band.

Moisture

In an adult horse, the elastic properties of the hoof wall are reduced if normal moisture levels are not maintained at about 25% water. If the

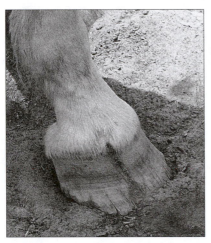

Fig. 4–7. Dry and brittle hoof due to low moisture content.

hoof horn becomes dry and brittle, and is unable to absorb concussion, it will crack in small fissures. Brittle hooves also do not hold nails well so it is difficult to keep shoes on.

Water is Nature's moisturizer, but too much is not good for the feet. Prolonged and excessive moisture from sodden ground or urine-soaked stalls are harmful to hoof moisture. Equally harmful are excessive dryness and abrasion from coarse, sandy soil, or the overzealous use of a farrier's hoof rasp. These situations degrade the thickness and structure of the hoof wall. The hoof then loses its internal moisture retention capabilities and the waxy covering of the hoof wall dissolves.

Hoof Dressings

Hoof dressings of an oil or grease base, especially with the addition of rosin (pine tar) or lanolin, are helpful if the feet experience continuous wet and dry cycles. These dressings act as an artificial periople to reduce evaporation of internal moisture. Daily application is necessary so that the dressing is not worn away as was the original periople.

Some people liberally paint all manners of grease over dry hooves with the mistaken impression that it puts needed moisture back into the foot. This assumption is false because most hoof moisture comes from internal sources, and only a small amount is gradually assimilated by *osmosis* from the environment. Rather than adding moisture to the foot, damp ground slows the evaporation rate of internal moisture from the foot.

Many hoof dressings are astringent and dehydrate the foot. Examples of harsh dressings include those containing turpentine, bleach, formalin, or phenol. Such compounds are useful only if occasionally applied to a moist frog or sole to control bacteria that thrive in wet conditions.

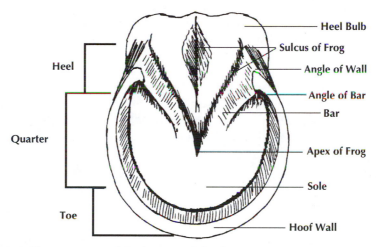

Fig. 4–8. The structures of the bottom of the foot.

Building Strong Feet

The most important ingredients to ensure strong feet are balanced nutrition, exercise, proper trimming and balancing, and basic hygiene.

Balanced nutrition provides energy, protein, vitamins, and minerals for hoof growth. The rate of hoof growth corresponds to a horse's rate of weight gain. Various feed supplements and hoof dressings are also merchandised to strengthen hoof walls.

Supplements
Biotin

Other avenues have been explored to encourage hoof growth. Biotin at doses of 15 – 30 milligrams per day for up to 9 months has been reported to stimulate hoof growth in studies performed on pigs receiving large doses of oral antibiotics. Oral antibiotics kill normal gut flora so the pig is unable to synthesize B-complex vitamins, and subsequently develops cracked hooves. Applying this data to horses suggests that in cases of known B-complex vitamin deficits, biotin may correct cracked hooves.

In many cases of thin, brittle hooves, biotin was added to the diet along with changes in exercise and shoeing. There is no evidence that biotin alone has improved the hooves of these horses, despite related anecdotal experiences. Not only do most foodstuffs, especially corn, provide ample biotin, but a horse normally manufactures the required quantities of biotin in the hindgut every day. However, biotin supplementation is not harmful to a horse, and may be good for a sick or debilitated horse. Biotin is water-soluble and the body rapidly excretes excessive amounts.

DL-methionine

Another supplement said to enhance hoof growth is DL-methionine. It is speculated that the sulfur precursors of DL-methionine contribute to the growth of horn tubules. There is no evidence, however, that this compound speeds hoof growth.

Exercise

The importance of exercise to a horse's feet cannot be overemphasized. Exercise stimulates the expandability of the hoof, increasing the surface area and reducing concussion during a performance effort. It increases blood circulation to the feet, promoting the health and elasticity of the hoof wall, and stimulates new growth of all foot structures. The sole toughens with repeated use, making it less vulnerable to bacteria and bruises. The scrubbing action of soil clods as they are flung from moving feet contributes to foot hygiene by removing dead pieces of sole and frog. Exercise encourages the circulation of tissue nutrients throughout the limbs, and reduces

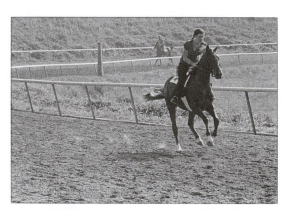

Fig. 4–9. Exercise is an important key for foot health.

the stagnation often seen as "stocked up" legs. It strengthens ligaments and tendons that support the joints and act as shock absorbers to cushion the load on the joints.

Massage of Coronary Band

Massage of the coronary bands stimulates hoof growth. This stimulation is accomplished by applying sheepskin coverings saturated with lanolin over the coronary bands, or by daily massage with vegetable or mineral oil.

Basic Hygiene

Thrush

Reducing equine foot disease depends on care and observation. Thrush *(pododermatitis)* results from moist and unhygienic conditions. Accumulation of manure, rotten straw, or mud on the bottoms of the feet encourages growth of bacteria within the crevices *(sulci)* of the frog. Often, a thrush infection travels deep into the sensitive layers of the frog, causing considerable pain and lameness and adversely affecting the horse's performance.

A foul odor is associated with thrush, and the frog becomes dark and discolored by discharge. The sole should be concave, and the frog firm, but pliable like a rubber eraser. With thrush, the frog feels spongy as it degenerates. Daily foot cleaning removes debris. For most horses, frequent trimming every 6 – 8 weeks removes dead tissue that traps debris. Performance horses may need trimming and shoeing every 4 – 6 weeks. Applying an iodine solution or copper sulfate to the bottom of the foot (frog and sulci) a couple of times each week controls thrush and canker.

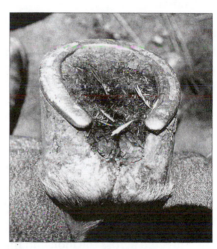

Fig. 4–10. A foot with thrush.

Canker

Canker is a rare occurrence due to modern hygienic practices, but may develop in unusually wet and warm climates. A horse with canker develops a foul smelling, moist infection of the frog and sole. The frog tissues overdevelop *(hypertrophy)*. Affected foot structures are white and have a cottage cheese consistency, in contrast to the black, decaying appearance of thrush. Canker invades deeper into the horny tissues than does thrush, with thrush confined primarily to the frog. Aggressive surgical removal of all affected tissue is required to treat canker.

Abscesses

Watching a horse's movements about the paddock can help an owner or trainer see other causes of lameness such as *subsolar abscesses*. Abscesses result from stone bruises or corns from improperly shod feet. Bruises and corns occur beneath the surface of the sole; they aren't visible with daily cleaning and inspection.

If a shoe is left on a foot for too long (more than 8 weeks), it may pinch the heels. The pinching creates an inflammation near the *angle of the bar* (separating the frog and the sole), producing a corn and possibly an abscess.

Abscesses also occur from nail punctures, or from severe bruising and trauma to the sole. The hoof wall normally diffuses the concussive force from the ground, while the internal structures such as the digital cushion, frog, *laminae*, and coffin bone absorb downward compressive forces by the body and gravity. The ideal weight-bearing surface of the foot is the hoof wall—not the sole. If shoes contact the sole at any point, that pressure will bruise underlying structures. If a hoof is trimmed excessively, or if a foot is worn down by harsh soil conditions, the lack of hoof wall forces a horse to walk on the soles of its feet, setting up conditions for subsolar abscesses, corns, or *laminitis*.

The Hoof as a Visual Record of Stress

Examining the appearance of the hoof tells how concussive forces are directed across the foot, and may indicate illness. Although some changes are internally subtle, over time they will produce a visual record on the face of the hoof. Flares and growth rings in the hoof wall reflect uneven stress. With more impact, the hoof wall steepens; with less, it flares.

Coronary Band Response to Uneven Stresses

A hoof responds to uneven stresses with an increased growth rate at the point of concentrated impact. The less impacted side of the foot experiences a relatively reduced circulation and therefore slower hoof growth.

In a normal foot, the coronary band is a straight line across the front of the hoof, in a plane parallel to the ground. It gradually slopes away to the heels, equally on both sides. Alterations in the circulatory tissue nourishing the foot or uneven stresses on the foot change the alignment of the coronary band. The coronary band re-aligns itself and appears asymmetrical (not properly aligned). This configuration can foretell a lameness problem due to unbalanced feet. Foot imbalances occur from incorrect hoof trimming, or from uneven loading created by poor conformation.

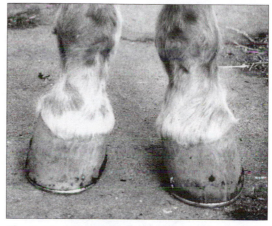

Fig. 4–11. Uneven coronary bands on both feet.

Hoof Wall Response to Uneven Stresses

Abnormal contours and "rings" of the hoof wall provide historical insight into the feet. For example, in chronic laminitis the heels grow faster than the toes. As the toe and heel of the hoof wall are produced at different rates, it assumes a wavy contour. Just like the growth rings of a tree chronicle seasonal and climatic variation in the development of the tree, so does the hoof reflect internal and external stresses on its face.

Ring Development

Fine longitudinal lines in the hoof running from the coronary band to the ground show the position of horn tubules as they grow down from the coronary corium. Anything that interferes with blood flow in the foot directly affects the rate of hoof wall growth. If the growth rate increases or slows in different areas of the foot, a change is visible. Rings develop in the hoof wall as the growth plates diverge between heels and toe.

Improper Shoeing

If a foot is unbalanced, or the shoes fitted improperly, stress lines appear on the hooves as irregularities or ridges at the points of abnormal pressure by the shoe.

Change in Diet

Not all hoof wall rings indicate disease in the foot. A change in diet or quality of nutrition also alters the growth and chemistry of keratin, and may create ridges in the hoof wall. As the hoof grows, an abnormal ring moves toward the ground, followed by healthy and consistent hoof wall.

Seasonal Effects

Seasonal variations produce a similar effect, when the warmth and moisture of lengthening spring days stimulate a surge of hoof growth. Such growth spurts appear as several ridged rings across the hoof wall.

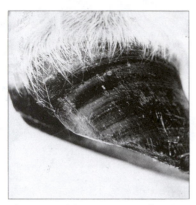

Fever

A fever that lasts for several days also stimulates a growth spurt in the feet, and rings may be evident weeks later. As the heart rate increases, responding to a higher body temperature, circulation to the feet increases.

Inflammation

Any inflammation of the foot or coronary band creates rings in the hoof wall. Increased circulation through the coronary corium causes a rapid growth of the wall, possibly leading to divergent growth planes at the toe and heel.

Fig. 4–12. Divergent growth planes lead to rings in the hoof wall.

Hoof Cracks

An injury or defect in the coronary band often results in a permanent crack in the hoof wall. The permanent crack is due to an interruption of horn tubule growth.

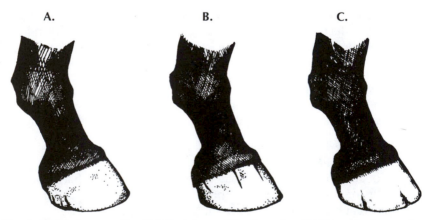

Fig. 4–13. Various cracks. (A.) Quarter and heel cracks. (B.) Toe, quarter, and heel cracks originating at the coronary band. (C.) Toe and quarter cracks.

Another type of hoof crack can start at the bearing surface and work toward the coronary band. Depending on its location it is a toe crack, a quarter crack, or a heel crack, and may indicate an unbalanced foot. Hoof cracks cause pain when the sensitive tissue moves with weight-bearing. Hoof cracks also provide an avenue for infection to invade the inner structures of the foot. Improper trimming and excessively dry or thin walls can contribute to the hoof cracking upon impact. Daily inspection identifies cracks before they become a simmering problem.

Horizontal Grooves and Cracks

Horizontal grooves and cracks across the hoof wall that are parallel to the coronary band may indicate *selenium toxicity*. These cracks usually appear in more than one foot. Because selenium is substituted for sulfur in the amino acids of body proteins, keratinized structures (hair and hoof) are most affected. Hair loss will occur before lameness develops. Eventually, the hoof horn will reflect the internal poisoning of the body by separating from the foot's internal components and sloughing off.

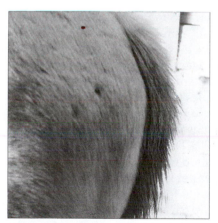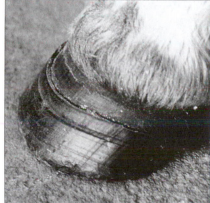

Fig. 4–14. The first symptom of chronic selenium toxicity is loss of tail hair, left. On the right, the same horse with horizontal hoof cracks, which occurs later.

SHOES & PADS
History of the Horseshoe

Since the earliest times that horses have been used as beasts of burden, as transportation, or as war steeds, humans have searched for optimal foot protection to prevent lameness. Foot care for the horse may have begun as long ago as 1600 B.C. Attention to foot care eventually encouraged the development of equine foot gear, with protective shoes dating back at least 2,000 years to the first or second centuries B.C.

Equine hooves did not always benefit from such protection. About 330 B.C., at the time of Alexander the Great, it is reported that cavalry expeditions were interrupted to allow the horses to restore hoof horn to their tender feet. Evidence of the use of horse foot coverings surfaced 200 – 300 years later. A battlepiece mosaic discovered at Pompeii, which fell in 79 A.D., depicts horseshoes fitted to horse feet.

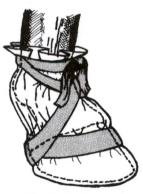

Fig. 4–15. An ancient horseshoe.

Historical predecessors to a modern equine shoe assumed form as very thin plates of gold, silver, or iron that were fastened to leather and then secured by straps attached to the hoof or fetlock. Such "hipposandals" provided some protection from abrasive ground.

A terra cotta Roman tablet illustrates boot-like protective coverings extending up the legs of chariot racing horses to protect them for the brief, but traumatic, period of competition.

Shoes made of durable woven twigs and reeds were used on tender-footed mounts in the days of Julius Augustus Caesar (27 B.C. – 14 A.D.). Another Roman emperor, Nero (56 – 68 A.D.), had his horse shod with silver while his wife, Poppea, protected the feet of her mules with gold.

By the era of the ancient Tartar and Mongolian warriors, at the time of Christ, shoes were more common. Excavation of ancient burial mounds of these warriors unearthed remains of horses still wearing shoes. These "shoes" were circular, nailed only to the outer bearing surface of the hoof, as a "unilateral" shoe.

The nailed horseshoe, as we know it today, was used in Europe by about the fifth century A.D. By the eighth and ninth centuries, lists of cavalry equipment itemized crescent-shaped iron shoes and nails as part of the basic inventory. Until 1000 A.D., shoes were primarily used on war horses or as decorative adornment for nobility. After 1000 A.D., people began to travel farther on newly constructed roads, and horseshoeing became customary.

Historic illustrations describe continual attempts by humans to "defend the hoof" and enhance the usefulness of the horse. Just 100 years ago, the text of Mile's Modern Practical Farriery (1896) commented: "Considering the apparent simplicity of the process to an ordinary observer, the method of fastening a piece of iron to a horse's foot has been the occasion of more dissertations, essays, guides, manuals, "practical" instructions, theories, disputes, and—we sorrow to write it—hard words and abuse, than any other subject we are acquainted with."

Today we take "modern" inventions of horseshoes for granted as these devices allow us to ride our horses over long distances and terrible terrain, to jump and gallop, and to pull heavy loads with a reduced risk of foot injury.

Despite our 20th century technology of rubber, plastic, and metal alloy, the same disputes rage over appropriate methods of horseshoeing. In ancient times the issue was simpler: to shoe or not to shoe, and how to keep a shoe affixed to the foot. Modern civilization has long since overcome such obstacles, offering anything from nails to special glues to affix a plethora of shoe designs to a hoof. Set the traditions aside, and address each horse's feet as a unique case with a unique performance purpose.

Shoeing: Injury Versus Protection

Nobody would argue the intrinsic value of a horseshoe to support the foot off the ground and minimize bruising and *contusion*. Still, a shoe may be a necessary evil: it is protective on one hand, and injurious to the foot on the other.

In an unshod foot the heel impacts the ground slightly before the toe, expanding the heel outward. As a limb bears weight, the short pastern bone compresses against the digital cushion. The digital cushion then pushes against the collateral cartilages, and downward against the frog that absorbs only a small degree of impact shock. Compression of the digital cushion dissipates energy as heat, transferring it to a profuse network of blood vessels in the digital cushion. The bloodstream removes the heat energy up the leg, away from the foot.

When the toe hits, an upward compressive force is relayed through the horn tubules that make up the hoof wall. These cells absorb a great deal of energy by their spiral, spring-like configuration. Laminae that "glue" the coffin bone to the hoof wall further resist the downward forces of limb loading by holding the foot together.

Alterations Caused by Shoeing

- Shoeing adds weight to the limb, which hastens fatigue.
- The hoof wall is weakened by nails.
- The protective periople is often removed with a rasp, interrupting moisture retention properties of the hoof.

A shoe alters the expandability of the entire foot, causing it to absorb concussion rather than dissipate the impact through the limb. Heel bruising, sole bruising, coffin bone inflammation *(pedal osteitis)*, and laminitis can develop.

Because applying a shoe alters the normal biomechanics within the hoof, it is imperative to fit and size a shoe to accommodate the foot. Long-term, improper balancing of a foot or improper fitting of a shoe leads to a sore foot, sprains, tendon injury, or degenerative joint disease.

Shoeing for Protection

Despite the problems mentioned above, unshod horses could not withstand the athletic exertions asked of them. Feet would become too sensitive. The hoof wall would erode so a horse would be weight-bearing on the sole, and stones and rutted ground would severely bruise the feet.

A horse, especially a performance horse, would become crippled. As we ride our horses more rigorously, the foot cannot withstand extended and abrasive wear and tear without a shoe.

Importance of Daily Care

Successful shoeing practices depend on foot care and hygiene by the farrier, and also by the daily caretaker. Picking the hooves daily removes collected wads of manure and pebbles, which may cause sole bruises and lameness. Also, hoof picking prevents overgrowth of bacteria, preventing thrush and canker. During winter in cold climates, remove snowballs from the feet so packed snow and ice won't bruise the sole. During periods of excessive wetness, check that horseshoes are firmly affixed. The sucking action of mud can loosen the nail clinches, twisting the shoe, causing corns, or removing it, causing sole bruises.

Importance of Proper Shoeing

There is no absolute correct angle of the hoof with the ground. The most important rule-of-thumb is that the hoof and pastern are aligned in the same axis angle so they act as a good shock absorber for the limb. If the heel is too low, and the toe too long, the hoof-pastern angle is broken. This configuration places excess stress on the navicular apparatus and heels, and on the ligaments of the coffin joint. If the heel is too high, and the toe too short, a horse may develop a club-footed appearance which can create bruising at the toe.

A shoe limits normal flexibility of the hoof wall and its spread at the ground surface. Heel expansion is possible because the hoof wall is thinner at the heels

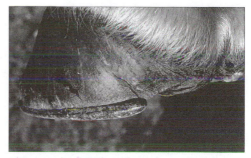

Fig. 4–16. A horizontal crack results from uneven loading across the foot due to a shoe that is too small.

and quarters than at the toe. The heels can expand and rebound with weight-bearing. According to biomechanical stress studies, the *extent* of heel expansion is unaffected by a shoe. However, a shod foot expands *faster* than a barefoot hoof, which changes the shock absorption ability of the foot, especially the horn tubules.

The hoof wall can lose flexibility if:

- a shoe is too small for the foot
- the branches pinch inwards
- the branches do not extend far enough back under the heel to provide weight-bearing support

Stress rings appear at the heels and quarters, or hoof cracks form at the point of compressive loading. Stress rings and cracks are evidence of improper shoeing techniques or poor conformation, resulting in unequal load distribution across the foot.

An appropriately sized shoe applied wide enough at the heels encourages heel expansion. A shoe may also be slippered (beveled) to encourage the heels to expand with impact. Nails should not be placed behind the widest bend in the quarter of the hoof or heel expansion will be limited.

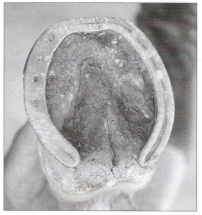

Fig. 4–17. Uneven wear of a shoe due to improper balancing of the foot. This horse also has sheared heels.

Sheared Heels

By studying each foot and its changes over several months, we can appreciate the effects of trimming and shoeing on the hoof. Just as in a barefoot hoof, flares develop on the side of an unbalanced hoof that is least loaded. The heavily loaded side grows hoof wall faster, resulting in a steeper wall. Then the heels may reveal unequal loading stresses, with one heel bulb higher than another. This syndrome is known as *sheared heels*, and can cause lameness if the heel bulbs become unstable.

Corrective Shoeing

Balancing the foot from side to side, and fore and aft corrects many shoeing problems. The goal is to encourage an equal distribution of weight across all weight-bearing surfaces of the foot. With compressive forces evenly loaded across the foot, no one side of the joints or ligaments receives excess strain.

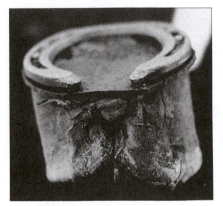
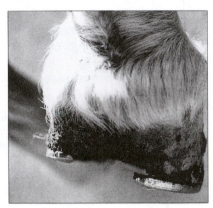

Fig. 4–18. Sheared heels after corrective shoeing.

Fig. 4–19. A poorly balanced foot.

Once a horse has matured in skeletal growth, "corrective shoeing" for poor limb conformation can only attempt to balance and level each foot as best as possible. Filing one side of a foot shorter than the other worsens an already less-than-perfect situation, adding *torque* and strain across the joints.

Padding the Shoe

A still unresolved dilemma exists: to pad or not to pad. There is never *one right way* to approach a problem, so all sides of the argument should be considered. Pads limit normal expandability of the foot by adding rigidity to an already rigid shoe. On the other hand, some horses have naturally tender feet, flat feet, or low pain thresholds.

Pads as Short-Term Treatments

In some cases, it is necessary to do more than just apply a standard shoe to cover the bearing surface of the hoof wall.

Pads may be a necessary therapy for short-term problems, such as healing a:

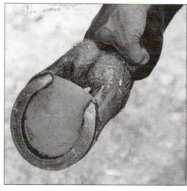

- sole abscess
- nail puncture
- serious bruise
- pedal osteitis
- corn

Fig. 4–20. Shoe with full pad.

Treating Sole Bruises

Sole bruises are frustrating to treat. Most horses respond within a couple of weeks to soaks in warm water and Epsom salt, anti-inflammatory drugs, and rest. Others require 4 – 6 months to recover. Crushing of the *subsolar corium* leaks red blood cells which stain the horn. This stain is later visible as a pinkish area on the underside of the foot. Bruises are not always visible however, at the time of trimming, especially in a black foot. In a thicker-footed horse, bruising may occur deep at the level of the coffin bone so the blood pocket *(hematoma)* is not visible in the thick hoof wall.

Not all sole bruising results in overt lameness; instead, performance may suffer. A horse may race slower, or back off fences. A dressage horse may be unwilling to collect and engage the hindquarters. Or, a horse may be reluctant to make sharp, quick turns if active as a cutting horse, roping horse, barrel racer, or polo pony.

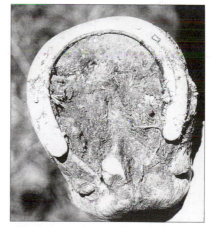

Treating Corns

An improperly fitted or sized shoe, or a foot grown too long between shoeings can result in *corns*. Corns are areas of pressure *necrosis* (tissue death) at the *angle of the wall* and the *bars*. The heel of the shoe applies abnormal pressure to this area if it contacts it. Repeated point loading at the angle of the bar

Fig. 4–21. A twisted shoe can cause corns at the angle of the wall.

85

causes deep bruising and blood or serum pockets beneath the sole. Abscesses may develop, and a fluid pocket in the sensitive tissues can cause lameness.

Fitting a shoe wide at the heels, and long enough in the branches to eliminate pressure at the angle of the bars prevents corns. Schedule appropriate shoeing every 6 – 8 weeks (racehorses and other high level performance horses, every 4 – 6 weeks), and employ a competent farrier who will fit the foot with a properly sized and applied shoe.

Sole bruises or corns can put a horse out of action for a time, and then it may be advantageous to pad, encasing the entire bottom of the foot in a protective capsule. For a normal horse without temporary problems, padding can have some adverse long range effects.

Effects of Long-Term Padding

Weakened Foot

A full pad decreases focal (specific area) bruising of the subsolar corium and sensitive tissues, and slightly reduces concussion to the foot. However, there is a trade off: padded feet become pad-dependent. The foot softens and weakens underneath the pad. If a padded foot loses a shoe, the sole is very soft and vulnerable to injury and deep bruising. Nails tend to loosen easily through a pad, so shoes are lost more often.

Sole Flattening

A padded foot softens and lacks support from the ground surface, promoting sole flattening. A foot that starts out properly cupped and concave may flatten with time under a pad. When the pads are removed, soles are susceptible to repeated trauma.

Thrush Development

Moisture under a pad promotes bacterial growth, resulting in thrush. An inadequate seal of the packing material (commonly used are silicone, oakum/pine tar, or foam) allows dirt to seep in under the pad. Local pressure points of dirt or pebbles create bruises or abscesses, accompanied by lameness.

Special Cases for Padding

A horse with laminitis, navicular disease, chronic heel pain, or a horse that is prone to bruising from genetically flat feet, may need to wear pads continually. In these cases the benefits may outweigh any detriments.

Alternatives to Padding

Consider alternatives before padding a horse's feet. Inactive or stall confined horses develop weak feet that are easily bruised. Turnout and regular exercise strengthen and toughen such feet.

The sole of the foot should be concave, or cupped. Beware the overzealous use of hoof nipper, knife, or rasp that removes too much foot, leaving behind a very thin sole. This man-made insult to the foot is avoided with good common sense and caution by a competent farrier.

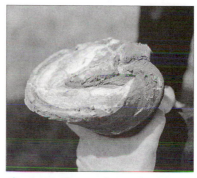

Fig. 4–22. Overzealous trimming causes flat feet where the sole is not concave.

Formulas with phenol, formalin, or Clorox® precipitate sole material and weaken the hoof. Applying a 7% tincture of iodine to the bottom of the sole toughens the foot. A strong iodine solution should not contact the skin as it is irritating. A squeeze bottle allows careful application to the sole and frog.

Wide-Web Shoes

Wide-web shoes increase protection to the bottom of the foot without the ill effects of a pad. Especially with wide-web shoes, the shoe should not contact the sole. The shoe support should rest only on the weight-bearing hoof wall. The sole is meant to bear only *internal* weight as a limb is loaded and advanced along the ground. Whenever the sole contacts the ground, or a shoe rests on the sole instead of the hoof wall, misapplied stresses can damage the foot.

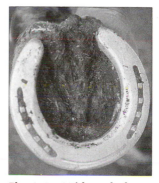

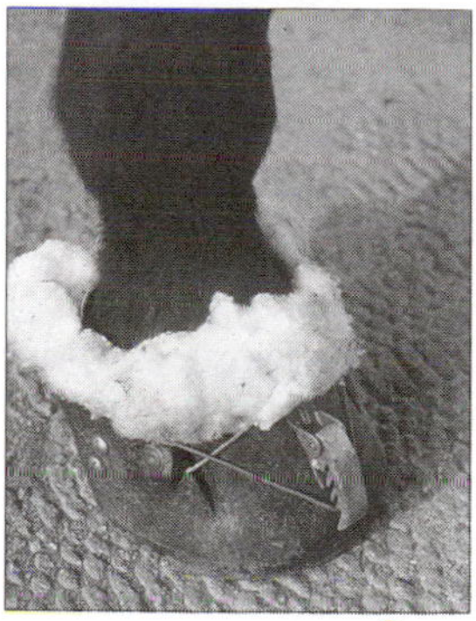

Fig. 4–23. Wide-web shoe.

Easy Boots®

For a long distance trail horse, consider using Easy Boots® over the shoe and foot as added protection. These plastic boots withstand rocky terrain, and have been used successfully on 100-mile endurance competitors. The boot must fit

Fig. 4–24. Easy Boot®.

well and not contact or abrade soft skin tissue such as the coronary band. Cut away the plastic to fit each foot. Cotton packing behind the heel bulbs prevents small stones and dirt from sifting into the boot.

Rim Pads

Some people believe that rim pads minimize the concussion transmitted by a metal shoe up the legs. A pad between the hoof wall and a shoe does not provide the same energy dissipation offered by an unshod foot. A rim pad does provide a lightweight spacer that raises the sole farther from the traumatic ground surface. Rim pads do not exert negative effects on the sole as would a full pad, but remember that nails tend to loosen, and a shoe is more easily lost with any pad. This loss results in trauma and bruising if a shoe is thrown and the foot goes unprotected.

Time and Use

The hoof wall and sole can be strengthened over time. Just as bones in the body strengthen with appropriate stress, the hoof responds to external stimuli. Not only does the foot conform to internal stress, but the hoof also builds stronger horn to accommodate hard ground surfaces. Horses turned out into rocky pastures soon develop tough feet, with stronger soles and hoof walls that are resistant to bruising. These horses are less likely to need pads.

FOOT LAMENESS

Any noticeable lameness or stiffness should receive veterinary attention as soon as possible. Due to the complexity and interaction of the internal structures of the foot, inflammation or trauma of one area can cause a problem in neighboring tissues. Pain in the feet, along with mechanical damage, adversely affects future performance capabilities.

Laminitis

Hoof wall rings can signal a serious insult to the health of the foot in the form of laminitis, where the laminae in the foot die, and the coffin bone detaches from the hoof wall. Equine laminitis, also referred to as *founder*, is a complicated disease with multiple causes. It is a devastating disease deserving immediate veterinary attention. Laminitis varies in degree, from mild to severe, and can seriously jeopardize a horse's productive performance career. A veterinary examination with radiographic evaluation determines whether the source of hoof wall rings is due to laminitis, or simply to uneven concussive stresses, nutrition, fever, or seasonal growth spurts.

Characteristics of Laminitis

An affected horse appears "stiff" in the front end, or shifts its weight from foot to foot. The horse is often reluctant to move, and places both hind legs well under its body to shift weight from the painful front feet to the hind legs. This weight shift is amplified as the horse is asked to turn. A mildly affected horse appears to "walk on eggs." Immediate damage must be attended promptly and the underlying problem corrected.

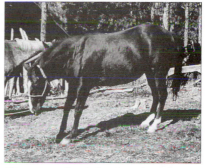

Fig. 4–25. Classic laminitis stance.

Causes of Laminitis

Understanding the anatomical relationships within the foot helps to explain the disease process. Internal parts of a horse's foot receive oxygen through a branching network of blood vessels. The main vessels run down the leg toward the foot. At the coronary band they branch into smaller divisions. The *dorsal laminar arteries* feed the front of the foot as branches of the *circumflex artery* that runs around the bottom of the coffin bone. A latticework of tissue and blood vessels called *laminae* (hence, *laminitis)* support the coffin bone within the hoof wall. For blood to reach sensitive laminae in the front of the foot, it must flow *against* gravity, with blood moving upward from the bottom of the foot.

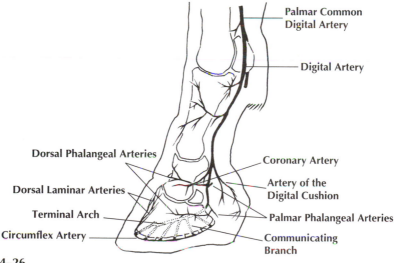

Palmar Common Digital Artery

Digital Artery

Dorsal Phalangeal Arteries

Dorsal Laminar Arteries

Terminal Arch

Circumflex Artery

Coronary Artery

Artery of the Digital Cushion

Palmar Phalangeal Arteries

Communicating Branch

Fig. 4–26.

Any *systemic* disease affecting the entire body that interrupts blood flow to the foot causes an inflammatory crisis within the laminae. Blood and oxygen supplies are reduced to the tissues while blood pressure elevates. A pounding arterial pulse is felt in the lower limb. Constricted vessels shunt blood and oxygen away from the laminar structures in the foot. Decreasing oxygen circulation in the foot causes the laminae to die. Then there is nothing to counteract the weight of the horse and the pull of the deep digital flexor tendon that attaches to the back of the coffin bone. The toe creates a lever effect, further amplifying the pull from the tendon. The coffin bone detaches from the hoof wall.

Without its supportive laminar attachments, the coffin bone can rotate or sink to the bottom of the sole. In a very severe case, the bone may perforate the bottom of the foot. If the laminitic process is halted early, rotation of the coffin bone may be prevented. However, in some cases, it can rotate as soon as 3 hours after the laminae begin to swell.

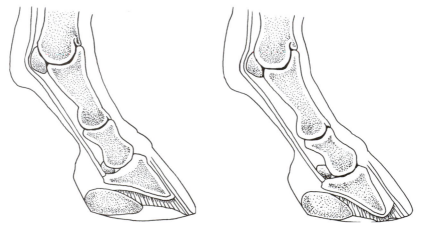

Fig. 4–27. On the left, a normal foot. On the right, a rotated coffin bone.

Metabolic Problems

Whenever normal metabolic functions are altered, laminitis can follow. Stress from transport or disease can cause laminitis. Diarrhea, septicemic infections (overwhelming bacterial infections), kidney, or liver diseases have noticeable effects on the amount of *endotoxin* produced. When excess amounts of this toxin circulate in the bloodstream, the liver is unable to neutralize all of it. A discussion of the gut environment helps to understand endotoxin and its role in laminitis.

Environment of the Gut

Bacterial flora that normally reside in a horse's bowel live in a delicately balanced ecosystem. The food a horse eats influences this environment, with the bacteria slowly adapting to small dietary changes. Rapid overeating of carbohydrate-rich grains promotes overpopulation by *Lactobacillus* organisms. The pH within the intestine changes to an acid environment.

Horses that normally receive grain, such as performance horses, are particularly at risk when suddenly fed an over-generous amount. A normal population of these acid-producing microorganisms already lives in the presence of highly fermentable grain. Grain fed horses typically already have a mild acid environment in their intestines, with conditions primed for impending disaster.

An acid environment disrupts the fragile one-cell barrier between the cavity of the bowel and the blood vessels in the intestinal wall. As the pH continues to decline, other residents of the intestines (the Gram-negative bacteria) die. The cell wall of Gram-negative organisms contains a poisonous component called endotoxin. The death of these microorganisms due to the intestine's acid environment rapidly releases endotoxin into the large intestine where it is absorbed throughout the body.

Role of Endotoxin

The body is consistently exposed to endotoxin as small amounts are released into the bloodstream with the normal, daily death of small numbers of Gram-negative bacteria. Under normal circumstances, the liver detoxifies endotoxin, and local immune responses inactivate it.

Excess endotoxin exerts profound effects. If a horse absorbs an overwhelming amount of endotoxin due to a carbohydrate overload or an underlying metabolic problem, and if the body is previously sensitized to endotoxin as with grain fed horses, a massive immune response results. The immune response creates havoc to the blood supply to the feet and causes founder.

Colic

Colic associated with changes in the normal movement of the intestines also stimulates bacterial overgrowth, and therefore endotoxin production. The harmful effects of endotoxins are felt throughout the horse's body; small blood vessels constrict, including those in the feet.

Occasionally, an overheated or exhausted horse experiences metabolic problems that alter normal blood flow and disrupt the laminar integrity of the foot.

Overweight Horses

Unfortunately, a lot of the horse show world favors overweight horses, and these horses are predisposed to laminitis. Obese horses are prime candidates for founder. These horses suffer from metabolic problems involving a low tolerance for glucose and carbohydrate intake. If a horse consumes a carbohydrate overload in the form of excess grain or rich alfalfa, it is at high risk for founder.

Retained Placenta

A broodmare that has foaled yet retained the placenta for more than 3 – 4 hours after birth is susceptible to laminitis. Endotoxins are absorbed from the uterus into the bloodstream as the placenta decomposes and infection develops.

Pituitary Disorder

Older horses sometimes develop a tumor of the pituitary gland in the brain. *Pituitary adenomas* cause an imbalance in neurotransmitter chemicals and hormones, causing excess production of corticosteroids. Overproduction of steroids, (or too much pharmaceutical steroids) ultimately causes increased glucose in the bloodstream, which can precipitate laminitis. These horses easily go unrecognized. A coarse, shaggy coat that fails to shed out,

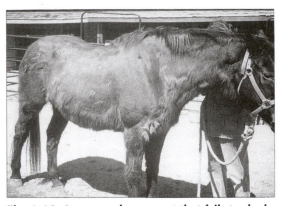

Fig. 4–28. A coarse, shaggy coat that fails to shed out may be a sign of a pituitary adenoma.

or a horse that drinks and urinates excessively may be the only signs of this problem.

Road Founder

Laminitis is also caused by mechanical factors. "Road founder" develops from trauma and bruising of the laminae after vigorous exercise on hard, concussive surfaces. Feet that are excessively trimmed or worn are easily traumatized. Stone bruises or nail punctures that result in infection or foot abscesses can also cause laminitis.

Support Founder

"Support founder" results from an injury, like a fracture, to a leg that renders it inactive for months at a time. Blood flow stagnates in the opposite, uninjured limb, and with excessive weight-bearing, the "good" foot may founder.

Recognizing Chronic Laminitis

A dished contour to the hoof wall, or "laminitic rings" indicate that the horse has experienced prior inflammatory incidents. Horn tubules of the foot normally grow in a straight, nearly vertical line from the coronary band. When the coffin bone is compressed downwards or rotates within the hoof wall during a laminitic crisis, the horn-generating coronary corium is compressed and trapped between the hoof wall and the *extensor process.* The extensor process is a bony protrusion at the top of the coffin bone to which the extensor tendon attaches.

Horn tubules at the top of the hoof wall bend at steep angles, further crushing the sensitive coronary tissue and reducing the blood supply. Once the coronary corium is compressed and its blood supply is limited, oxygen deprivation of the tissues alters growth of the hoof wall in the front third of the foot.

Horn tubules then grow out deformed. Toe growth slows considerably due to misalignment of the horn tubules from the coronary corium. The result is divergent growth planes in the hoof wall.

Extensive collateral circulation in the heels allows them to grow at a normal rate. Unless corrective measures are taken, the front of the hoof wall develops a dish shape, also indicating an internal deformity in the coffin bone.

A horse with chronic laminitis records the decreased circulation to the front of the foot on the hoof wall. The insensitive laminar layer excessively keratinizes as the toe grows out slowly. Thick, irregular ridges form across the wall, parallel to the coronary band. New hoof growth follows these growth planes, maintaining the telltale laminitic rings and dished wall.

Realignment of the horn tubules along this distorted path causes dehydration of the hoof wall, and loss of its elastic properties. With laminitis, circulation to the front of the hoof is reduced.

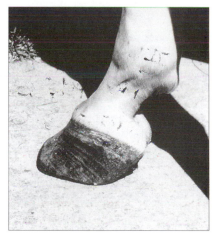

Fig. 4–29. A dished hoof wall is a sign of chronic laminitis.

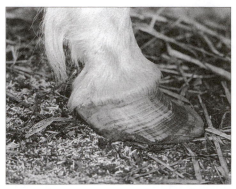

Fig. 4–30. Rings are also a sign of chronic laminitis.

Loss of an internal source of moisture contributes to drying of the hoof wall.

Altered blood flow, dehydration, and reduced weight-bearing due to pain inevitably lead to contraction of the entire foot, as well as a deformed appearance of the wall. The hoof wall tells a story of daily internal and external stresses which shape its strength and outward appearance.

Therapy for Laminitis

There is no single recipe for therapy for laminitis; each case must be tailored to the severity of the crisis and the unique metabolic problem of the horse. Many medical therapies are discussed, and tried with varying success. Basic steps can be taken upon recognition of a crisis:

- Call a veterinarian to attend the cause, e.g., grain overload, retained placenta, concussive trauma.
- Eliminate rich feed (grain, alfalfa, pasture) from the diet to prevent an acidic intestinal environment.
- Put an overweight horse on a diet to reduce metabolic upset, and to reduce weight on the compromised feet.
- Non-steroidal anti-inflammatory drugs (aspirin, Banamine®, phenylbutazone) counteract pain and inflammation, and Banamine® is beneficial against the effect of endotoxins.
- An endotoxin antiserum (by Immvac, Inc.) is available to block release of endotoxins in the horse.
- Provide sandy bedding, as sand provides a cushion under the sole and helps support the foot.
- Apply special pads or wedges under the frog to support the coffin bone.
- Confine the horse so movement does not continue to tear the laminae. Confinement may be necessary for a month or more.
- Warm or cold foot soaks are controversial. While cold soaks reduce pain, they tend to constrict blood vessels. Warm soaks enhance the inflammatory process, yet dilate the capillary beds and vessels within the foot.

• X-ray films are useful after about 24 hours to evaluate the degree of rotation of the coffin bone within the hoof, and to aid corrective hoof trimming to reduce stress on the laminae.

Treating Overconsumption of Grain

Horses that manage to enter a feed room and overindulge in grain can be treated prophylactically (a prevention) against colic or laminitis by a veterinarian if discovered within 8 – 12 hours.

Mineral Oil

Stomach tubing with mineral oil limits fermentation of grain within the intestines and minimizes development of an acid environment. Mineral oil coats the bowel to reduce absorption of endotoxin. An oil coating also protects the fragile intestinal cells from disruption by acids and endotoxin. Its laxative effect aids in rapid elimination of the rich foodstuffs.

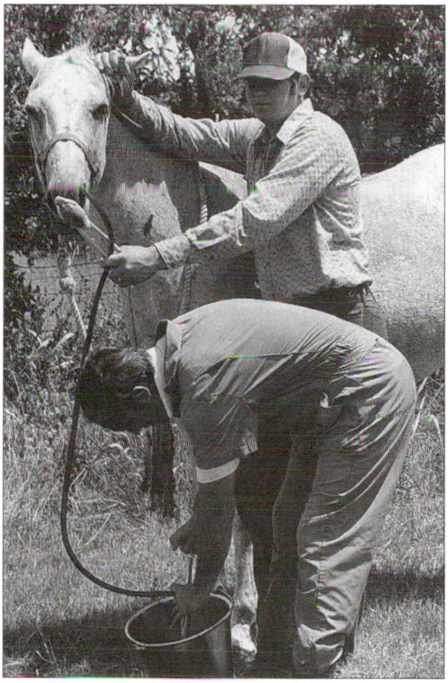

NSAIDs

Non-steroidal anti-inflammatory drugs (NSAIDs) block the progression of the inflammation contributing to the crisis and provide pain relief. Banamine® also counteracts the effects of endotoxin.

Fig. 4–31. Stomach tubing with mineral oil.

Managing Laminitis

Immediate care dramatically affects the outcome and prognosis of the disease. Because the foot grows continually, laminitis is often managed successfully. As a foot grows out, the diseased tissue is removed in successive trimmings.

Preventing Rotation of Coffin Bone

The therapeutic goal is to prevent the bone from rotating or sinking within the hoof wall. This goal is accomplished by:
• vigorous medical management
• corrective trimming and shoeing

- thick wedge pads to relieve the pull from the deep digital flexor tendon
- bar shoes to provide a base of support to the foot

Feet with a rotated coffin bone are frustrating to treat and may never resume normal athletic function.

Preventing Laminitis

An anti-endotoxin vaccine (Endovac-Equi™) is available to immunize a horse against the release of endotoxin before a crisis is precipitated. An antibody response caused by the vaccine neutralizes endotoxin released from dying Gram-negative bacteria. An initial injection is given, followed by a booster about 1 month later. The vaccine is then boosted one or two times each year to protect against the insidious effects of endotoxin.

Research is also underway to produce a vaccine which forms antibodies against *equine tumor necrosis factor* (TNF), a by-product of the inflammation caused by endotoxins.

Because endotoxin comes from many different Gram-negative bacteria, it is difficult to make a vaccine to stimulate an antibody response that is cross protective against all varieties. However, only one type of antibody must develop against equine tumor necrosis factor so this vaccine holds promise for the future.

A horse's feet are sensitive indicators of its overall well-being. A well-balanced ration and consistent exercise and turnout are key ingredients to a horse's health. Consult with a veterinarian about dietary management, weight control, foot hygiene, and health. Good management and a general physical exam can deter many of the causes of founder.

Navicular Disease

Any interference with normal limb function impairs a horse's performance. The athletic horse is subject to a variety of lameness problems. One disease that can develop in the actively working horse involves the *navicular apparatus* of the foot: the *navicular bone*, *navicular bursa*, and the deep digital flexor tendon. Conformation and the type of athletic endeavor equally contribute, but there is strong evidence that improper shoeing predisposes a horse to navicular disease. Horses that perform rigorous, concussive activities such as racing, jumping, roping, or polo absorb considerable impact in their feet. It is essential that their feet be balanced and appropriately shod.

Structure of Navicular Apparatus

The navicular bone is a shuttle shaped bone wedged between the coffin bone and the deep digital flexor tendon in the foot. The flexor tendon passes behind the navicular bone, attaching to the back of the coffin bone. Between the navicular bone and the tendon is a bursa that provides a smooth gliding surface for the tendon. The bottom *(flexor)* surface of the navicular bone is also smooth, and enhances the gliding effect.

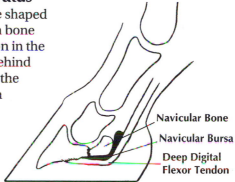

Navicular Bone

Navicular Bursa

Deep Digital Flexor Tendon

Fig. 4–32. The navicular apparatus.

The top *(articular)* surface of the navicular bone increases the surface area of the coffin joint. Increasing the surface area of this joint decreases the concussive load on it as the limb impacts the ground. The top of the coffin bone is supported by ligaments that anchor to the wings of the navicular bone. These ligamentous supports, along with the deep digital flexor tendon below, maintain the position of the navicular bone within the foot.

Inflammatory changes involving the navicular apparatus, including the bone, bursa, tendons, and ligaments damage the surface of the flexor tendon that contacts the navicular bursa. Navicular disease develops from increased pressure between the bone and the tendon, or from local tendon strain. Tendon fibers may rupture and roughen. The roughened tendon erodes the flexor surface of the navicular bone, compromising the smooth gliding motion of the tendon and causing pain and lameness.

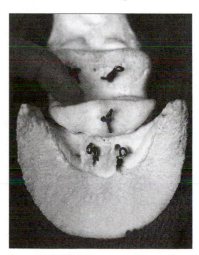

Fig. 4–33. The finger points to the navicular bone.

Characteristics of Navicular

Navicular disease commonly occurs in Thoroughbred, Standardbred, Quarter Horses, and Warmblood breeds, although no breed is immune to the disease. It is not a genetically transmissible disease, but certain conformational traits predispose to it and bone and conformational structure are heritable traits. A horse with a straight shoulder, upright pasterns, and small feet is prone to develop the disease. Similarly, a flatfooted horse with a low heel is also at risk.

The disease usually surfaces between 4 and 9 years of age, but can occur in any age horse. Navicular disease typically affects both front feet, although one may be more painful than the other. Lameness may be intermittent, and may appear at different times in each foot. It develops slowly over time, and is aggravated by hard work, while rest alleviates the symptoms. An affected horse may point an aching foot in front of it, with the heel elevated slightly off the ground. It may shift its weight back and forth between sore feet. Lameness is exaggerated on hard packed surfaces or hills, and eased by soft, level ground.

Navicular Stride

The typical stride of a "navicular horse" is short and choppy to reduce the impact upon the sore heels. The horse stumbles frequently. Some horses try to land toe first, instead of landing with the normal placement of heel first. These individuals are prone to bruised toes, and a sole abscess can develop with severe bruising.

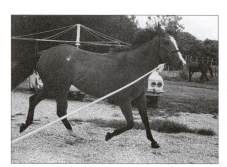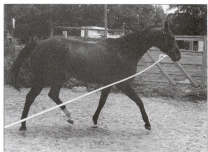

Fig. 4–34. On the left, a normal horse lands heel first. On the right, the navicular horse tries to land toe first.

Change in Foot Size

As the disease progresses, one or both forefeet may appear noticeably smaller, with the heel contracted and drawn in. The frog appears shrunken and diseased. It is sometimes hard to tell if a foot is contracted if both forefeet are affected. A contracted heel represents underlying pain in the foot that forces a horse to reduce the normal weight-bearing load on that foot.

Theories on Navicular Development

Concussion Theory

One explanation speculates that excess concussion between the navicular bone and the deep digital flexor tendon results in inflammation of the bursa, coffin joint, and associated structures. Inflammation stimulates demineralization and thinning of the navicular bone. Normally, concussion is not a problem because structures like the horn tubules, frog, and collateral cartilages dissipate energy from the foot.

The concussion theory also suggests that poor hoof conformation or trimming creates vibrations and oscillations within the structures of the foot. Friction produced between the bone and the tendon cause fraying and degeneration of both structures.

Impaired Blood Supply

A second, but unsubstantiated theory, blames an impaired blood supply to the navicular bone as a prime factor in navicular disease. Damage to the ligaments attached to the navicular bone may interfere with blood supply, as blood vessels enter through this region. Lack of oxygen from a reduced blood flow creates pain and furthers the disease process in the navicular bone. Experiments have attempted to prove this theory, with no success.

A Current Theory

Dr. Roy Pool (University of California at Davis) has developed a "unifying" theory that unifies several previous theories to explain the events leading to navicular disease. Bone is a dynamic organ, continually remodeling in response to exercise and stress. When excess pressure is placed on the navicular bone, inflammation and microscopic swelling in the bone amplify the remodeling process.

Compression between the bone and the deep digital flexor tendon stimulates remodeling activity. Cells that demineralize the bone outstrip the ability of bone builders to produce new bone. "Holes" form in areas where the tendon has compressed the navicular bone, and the defect is filled in with granulation tissue. Scar tissue forming between the tendon and the bone is called an *adhesion*. Adhesions limit the mechanical efficiency of the limb and create pain as they continually tear when the horse moves.

Damage to the deep digital flexor tendon where it contacts the navicular bursa develops from increased pressure between the bone and the tendon, or from local tendon strain. Some tendon fibers may tear and roughen. Roughened tendon erodes the flexor surface of the navicular bone, and compromises the smooth gliding motion of the tendon.

Joint Inflammation Theory

A further clarification of the disease progression has been proposed by Dr. Paul W. Poulos (University of Florida). He suggests that vigorous work and poor shoeing lead to inflammation of the joints next to the navicular bone. Joint inflammation causes the *synovial membrane* (the lining of the joint) to swell and infiltrate the navicular bone. The membrane remains permanently embedded in the navicular bone. Eventually, the bone and flexor tendon adhere to one another, spurs develop on the bone, and ligamentous attachments lose their flexibility. Deterioration progresses, as does lameness.

Improper Shoeing

Excess concussion and trauma to the heel occur as a result of shoeing in a long-toe – low-heel (LTLH) configuration, which works to a mechanical disadvantage for a horse. Of horses with navicular disease, 77% have a low, under-run heel. A low heel increases the pressure between the navicular bone and the deep digital flexor tendon.

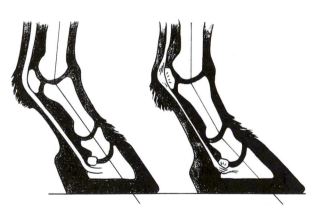

It reduces the weight-bearing surface area, therefore the foot is less able to absorb impact. The horn tubules grow horizontally which lessens their ability to absorb energy. The center of gravity of the foot is moved forward, shifting an excessive amount of concussion to the heels. A low heel also places extra strain on the other ligaments and tendons in the back of the leg and foot.

Fig. 4–35. On the left, a normal foot. On the right, a LTLH foot configuration strains the flexor tendons.

A long toe lengthens the lever arm, making it more difficult for a horse to move the foot. The limb fatigues faster. Tendinitis develops from strain of the flexor support structures, especiallyof the deep digital flexor tendon.

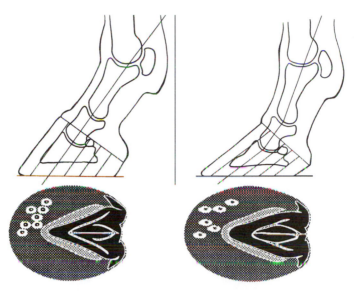

Fig. 4–36. On the left, a properly trimmed foot and horn tubules. On the right, a LTLH foot and elongated horn tubules.

In an LTLH foot, the hoof-pastern axis angle is broken. This places excess tension on the deep digital flexor tendon, further compressing the navicular bone. An unbalanced foot forces uneven stress on the joints and all internal structures of the foot. The difference between a correct angle and an incorrect angle can be subtle to the untrained eye, but over time the incorrectly shod horse will develop lameness problems. Increased and

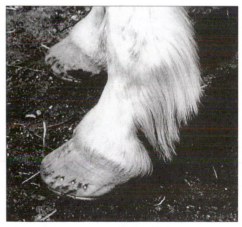

Fig. 4–37. An LTLH configuration.

uneven loading on an unbalanced foot predisposes to navicular disease, or it worsens an already existing condition.

Diagnostic Tests for Navicular

Diagnosis of navicular disease is not a clear cut issue. To classify a horse as truly "navicular," an obvious lameness or stilted gait should be apparent.

Many criteria are used to diagnose the disease and make a prognosis for continued athletic function. Gathering all diagnostic information enables a veterinarian to make a clinical diagnosis. A horse may be diagnosed with true navicular disease if it demonstrates some of the following symptoms:

- lameness
- sensitivity to hoof testers over the heel
- trotting off lame after flexion of the foot
- lameness improves with palmar digital nerve blocks, but switches to the opposite foot

A veterinarian's clinical experience may support a judgment despite lack of fulfillment of all criteria.

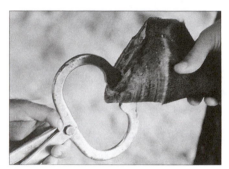

Fig. 4–38. Hoof testers help locate the source of pain.

Hoof Tester

Hoof testers are specially shaped "pliers" that pinch specific areas of the foot. A horse's response to the testers allows a veterinarian to localize the source of pain, and to suggest appropriate therapy. A hoof tester applied across the heels, or between the center of the frog and the hoof wall often elicits pain from a diseased horse, but not always.

Flexion Test

Another diagnostic test is called a "flexion test." The coffin and pastern joints are tightly flexed for 1–2 minutes, and the horse is trotted off. In a navicular horse, flexion of the coffin joint exaggerates lameness by increasing the tension on the deep digital flexor tendon and compressing the navicular bursa and bone. A similarly effective method asks a horse to stand on a block to elevate only its heel, and then the horse is trotted off the block to evaluate change in lameness.

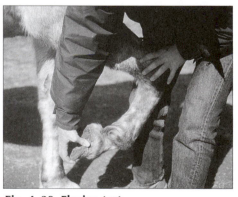

Fig. 4–39. Flexion test.

Nerve Block

As a diagnostic workup continues, local anesthetic is injected into the *palmar digital nerves* on both sides of the lower pastern to create a *nerve block*. If a lame horse improves from this particular nerve block, then the source of pain is the back one-third of the foot. However, other structures are present there besides the navicular apparatus.

For example, disease of the digital cushion, heel bulbs, collateral cartilages, presence of an abscess or corn, or thrush must be ruled out before claiming disease of the navicular apparatus. With navicular disease, a nerve block of one foot often improves the gait in that limb, only to accentuate lameness in the opposite limb.

The Role of X-Ray Films in Navicular Diagnosis

Once the source of pain is localized to the navicular region, a veterinarian may pursue radiographic analysis. Multiple views of x-ray films show all contours of the navicular bone. Irregular and rough contours may support evidence for disease of the navicular apparatus. A fracture of the navicular bone can also be identified on x-ray film.

X-ray films do not always show symptoms of navicular disease. The reverse is also true: many horses show radiographic "lesions," only to be totally sound and free of navicular disease. For example, normal wear and tear lesions show up on x-ray films in an aging horse. These lesions must be distinguished from a disease process, so a horse is not unnecessarily condemned.

Too often navicular x-ray films are used to determine a "no or go" on the purchase of a potential athlete. Keep in mind that some horses may have sore heels due to incorrect shoeing. X-ray films are used only to corroborate the clinical picture. Occasionally, a horse meets the clinical criteria, but shows no radiographic changes despite obvious evidence of navicular or coffin joint disease. Only 60% of cases with clinical lameness correlate with radiographic evidence.

Lollipop Lesions

Changes in the size, number, and configuration of the blood vessel channels on the flexor surface of the navicular bone indicate disease of the coffin joint. Mushroom-shaped holes in the bone are called "lollipop lesions" where synovial tissue (resulting from coffin joint inflammation) has infiltrated the navicular bone. Like an old scar, these lesions may reflect a current or a resolved problem. Although coffin joint disease and navicular disease are related, lollipop lesions do not necessarily indicate navicular disease.

Cystic Lesions

Cystic lesions in the navicular bone represent severe inflammatory disease accompanied by demineralization of the bone, and adhesions resulting from coffin joint inflammation. The presence of large cysts in the navicular bone indicates an active degenerative process.

Bone Spurring

Spurring on the wings of the navicular bone as seen on x-ray film represents damage to ligaments due to the stress of exercise, abnormal foot conformation, or fatigue. This change is seen in older horses with many years and miles of exercise, without accompanying lameness or navicular disease. However, in a young horse bone spurring may indicate navicular disease.

Navicular Bone Thinning

Thinning of the flexor surface of the navicular bone reveals tendinous adhesions and erosion of the cartilage. This radiographic change is seen with 80% of horses with navicular disease and may be the only radiographic image that corresponds to damage from the navicular disease.

All horses respond to pain differently. Some may experience navicular disease, yet have too much heart to quit. Other individuals cannot tolerate even small degrees of pain, and their usefulness for performance is limited.

Management Techniques for Navicular Disease

Therapy for a horse with navicular disease is aimed at *reducing pain,* and should not be misconstrued as a *cure.* The disease is a degenerative process, and will progress over time.

Corrective Shoeing

Corrective shoeing improves over 50% of affected horses, but it may take up to 4 months for results to be appreciated. Balance of the foot is essential to therapy. The foot should land flat, with a horse's weight distributed equally over all weight-bearing structures of the foot. A properly balanced foot not only relieves pain, but prevents development or progression of navicular disease.

If a rod is dropped perpendicularly through the center of the cannon bone, it should drop just behind the heel bulbs. This area is where a horse needs the base of support. The ends of the shoe should extend past the heels of the foot, ending approximately ⅝ of an inch in front of the heel bulb, at most.

Many shoes are incorrectly affixed with the branches ending 2 or more inches before the back of the heel bulbs. Affixing a shoe this way creates a long-toe–low-heel effect and a broken hoof-pastern axis angle, which amplifies heel concussion. If a shoe is too small for the foot, as the foot hits the ground it will drop backwards with the body weight behind it, increasing tension on the deep digital flexor tendon, and compressing the tendon and bone.

An appropriately sized large shoe provides ample heel extension. The shoe can be applied wide enough at the heels to encourage heel expansion. A shoe may also be slippered (beveled) to encourage the heels to expand with impact.

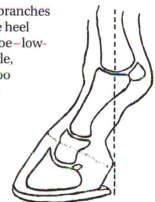

Fig. 4–40. A perpendicular line lands behind the heel.

Consistent trimming is important. As a foot grows, the toe lengthens faster than the heels, placing additional stress on the deep digital flexor tendon. Excess toe must be removed every 5 – 8 weeks to remove its lever arm effect.

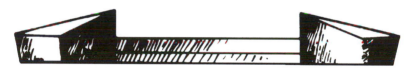

Fig. 4–41. Rear view of a slippered shoe, which encourages heel expansion.

Rolled Toe and Raised Heel

To move the center of gravity back in line with the skeletal column, the toe is shortened and rolled to "shorten the wheelbarrow." Allowing the force to pass through the bony skeletal column decreases the load on the deep digital flexor tendon, and more quickly "dumps the load" by making it easier for the foot to lift and breakover.

Bar Shoe

A bar shoe stabilizes the heel region and reduces trauma. Bone demineralization is reduced fivefold by applying bar shoes to a navicular horse. The shoe should be long and wide at the heels to increase the surface area of contact with the ground, and to encourage hoof expansion for enhanced circulation in the foot. A wedge pad, which is a full pad that is thicker at the heel than at the toe, reduces heel concussion, and relieves tension on the deep digital flexor tendon.

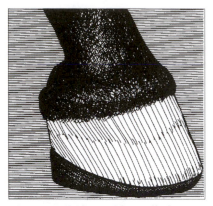

Fig. 4–42. A shoe with a rolled toe and raised heel.

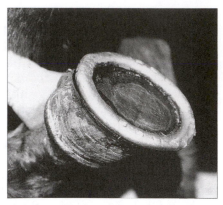

Fig. 4–43. Egg-bar shoe with full pad.

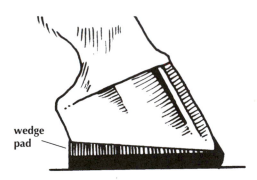

wedge
pad

Fig. 4–44. A wedge pad reduces heel concussion.

The equine foot is a sensitive gauge for exactness of technique. A slight deviation in the balance of the foot or shoe causes corrective shoeing to fail as a therapeutic aid.

Exercise Program

Another important aspect in managing horses with navicular disease is an exercise program of at least 2–4 miles a day, or 30 minutes a day, rather than applying the old theory of stall rest and confinement. Rest seems to aggravate the problem. Daily exercise reduces the formation of scar tissue and adhesions of the flexor tendon, while a horse maintains fitness, flexibility, and ample foot circulation. Confinement causes affected horses to move stiffly despite efforts of corrective shoeing.

NSAIDs

Non-steroidal anti-inflammatory drugs relieve both pain and the inflammatory process. Low levels of phenylbutazone, Banamine®, or aspirin may allow a horse to work comfortably and relatively pain-free. These medications also temporarily arrest the deterioration process.

Vasodilatory Drugs

A peripheral vasodilatory drug called *isoxsuprine hydrochloride* has been used with varying success. It appears to be most effective if administered early in the disease. This drug promotes blood supply in the lower limb to improve the blood flow in the foot, and it has mild anti-inflammatory effects. Isoxsuprine is relatively free of side effects, but it should not be used for pregnant mares. In addition, the drug is still not approved by the American Horse Shows Association, so a withdrawal time of up to 4 days is necessary to comply with regulations before showing or racing.

Neurectomy

Some horses do not respond to any of the above mentioned therapies. These horses may be candidates for a *neurectomy* if they are to resume athletic function. A neurectomy involves cutting the palmar digital nerves on both sides of the pastern. Cutting the nerve prevents the transmission of pain from the foot to the brain. The palmar digital nerve is the same nerve that is injected with local anesthetic to arrive at a diagnosis. Whatever the degree of gait improvement achieved by the nerve block will be the maximum improvement gained by a neurectomy.

Neurectomies are not without complications, and should be seriously considered. Possible problems include:

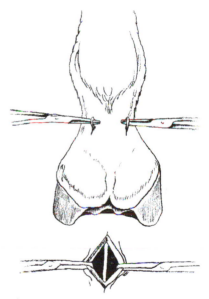

Fig. 4–45. Nerving incision site.

- A *neuroma* can form at the surgical site, causing a painful lump of nerve tissue, again resulting in lameness.
- The palmar digital nerve can regenerate over time and defeat the surgery.
- Occasionally, stray nerve branches of the palmar digital nerve provide enough sensation to the heel to prevent a complete return to soundness.
- Rarely, the deep digital flexor tendon ruptures, or circulation to the entire foot may be disrupted, causing the hoof to slough off.

A neurectomized horse cannot feel the back third of its foot, but it retains complete sensitivity in the other two-thirds. The owner of a neurectomized horse should recognize that if the horse steps on a nail in the heel, it will be unaware of it. It will not feel abscesses in the back third of its foot, and a fracture of the navicular bone will go unnoticed. These are the risks taken with a "nerved" horse, but the possible return to athletic function may outweigh any disadvantages. Almost 60% of neurectomized horses remain sound for 1 – 3 years.

Navicular disease continues to be one of the more frustrating lameness problems to manage. Time, cost, and emotional involvement in training a performance horse are major investments. A veterinary prepurchase exam can steer a prospective buyer away from identifiable problem horses or conformational predispositions to foot disease.

5

PROTECTING
THE RESPIRATORY
SYSTEM

The unique anatomy of the equine nasal cavity, pharynx, and larynx is an evolutionary structure of sophisticated aerodynamic design. With each breath, a horse fuels its body with vital oxygen, "feeding" the muscles, brain, and heart so it can perform to its optimum athletic capabilities.

The overall health of the equine respiratory system is as essential to optimal performance as a sound set of legs. Respiratory health dictates stamina, and contributes to mental willingness. The lungs must pull in oxygen to fuel the musculoskeletal tissues, heart, liver, kidneys, and intestinal tract. These parts of the equine machine are interdependent, each part depending on the others for optimal performance.

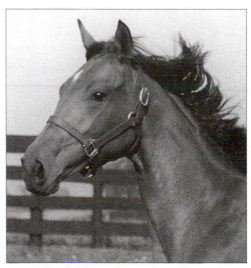

Fig. 5–1. Much of the space in a horse's head is dedicated to respiration.

Man-made impositions of hardware in the mouth, head carriage, and weight-carrying also change normal breathing functions. To understand the dramatic effect that human demands have upon the equine respiratory tract, we must first examine how it works.

The respiratory tract, or airway, is a two-part system. The upper airways include all structures from the nostrils to the *thorax*. (The thorax is the part of the body between the neck and the abdomen.) These structures are the nasal passages, pharynx, larynx, and trachea. The lower airways resemble a tree, as larger *bronchi* branch over and over again into smaller *bronchioles*, ending in air saccules *(alveoli)* within the lungs.

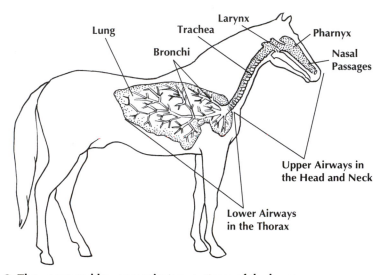

Fig. 5–2. The upper and lower respiratory systems of the horse.

ACCOMMODATING AIR FLOW

The equine body has developed special adaptations to best accommodate air flow. Air is a mixture of gases, the most important of which is oxygen. As a horse inhales, its rib cage and thorax expand to create a negative pressure, or vacuum, within the thorax. Air then flows into the nostrils, along the nasal passages, over the soft palate and through the pharynx, through the larynx, down the trachea, and into the lungs, sucked in to fill this void.

Due to differences between the relatively positive atmospheric pressure outside and the negative pressure inside the thorax, twice as much energy is required for the horse to inhale as to exhale. With any suction force, structures surrounding the airway would tend to collapse. Yet the equine respiratory tract is protected from such dynamic collapse in many ways. For example, the nasal cavity is supported largely by bone. Special dilating muscles in the nostrils, the nasopharynx above the soft palate, and the larynx also help to overcome the suction force of inhalation. The larynx is suspended from the base of the skull by a rigid bony scaffold called the *hyoid apparatus.*

The trachea is kept spread and open by reinforcement with rings of cartilage. A strap muscle *(sternothyrohyoideus)* extends from under the sternum (the breastbone in the chest, running between the forelegs), up the chest and along the underside of the neck to attach onto the hyoid apparatus. Contractions of this muscle bundle keep the trachea and larynx open under athletic demand. This muscle group is visible as a bulging strap along the underside of the neck in the horse that travels with head up and back hollowed. Contractions of the diaphragm, which is a dome-shaped muscle behind and beneath the lungs, additionally enlarge the

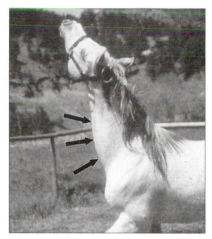

Fig. 5–3. The strap muscle is visible when the horse throws its head back.

airways and keep the trachea open. The airway's interconnected tissue framework enables it to operate in response to oxygen demand.

Size of the Airways

The size of the air passages directly influences the efficiency of air flow. According to the laws of physics, air flows best down a straight, circular tube with smooth, rigid, and preferably parallel walls.

Resistance to air flow is dramatically affected by the diameter of the tube. For example, if the diameter of the tube is increased to twice its original size, air flow is *sixteen times* as efficient. Therefore, if the horse's airways are as straight and smooth as possible, with minimal bends or obstructions, air flow is optimized, the oxygen demand is met, and performance is enhanced.

Inflammation of the airway with swelling or mucus, any mechanical obstruction (such as roaring, chronic pharyngitis, soft palate hypertrophy, nasal polyps, etc.), or any bend in the airway functionally creates a smaller diameter and therefore greater air flow resistance.

In a normal horse that does not suffer from respiratory disease or mechanical obstructions of the airways, the upper airway still creates more than half of the total air flow resistance.

Air Flow and Exercise

The mechanics of breathing in the exercising horse are quite different from the resting horse, because more oxygen is needed to metabolically support the body in exertion. The anatomy of the pharynx, larynx, and trachea require the exercising horse to stretch out its neck and head. For example, a horse at play that is running in the field, or a determined racehorse as it speeds down the track, extends the head and neck forward. This position streamlines the airway, minimizing air flow resistance.

Streamlining the Airways

Certain anatomical events occur for an exercising horse to maximize air flow. The nostrils dilate to improve air intake. Erectile tissue in the nose is abundant in blood vessels that constrict, further widening the nasal passages and limiting air flow resistance down the airway.

When the horse extends its head and neck, the airway is straightened out, eliminating bends and turbulence. Also, the elastic mucosa lining the top and bottom walls of the nasopharynx and larynx is stretched, providing a smoother surface and reducing air flow resistance.

Small muscles hold the soft palate down and the roof of the nasopharynx up, but these muscles are somewhat weak and need head and neck extension to prevent fatigue.

As the larynx outwardly expands and opens, the airway into the trachea is smoothed to limit resistance. During exercise, a normal larynx expands its cross-sectional area three times wider than at rest.

Flexion at the Poll and Neck

Partial flexion of the head and neck, required by show jumping and dressage, restricts this airway streamlining by creating a bend in the airway. When a horse is asked to flex at the poll and neck to improve its balance and impulsion, it is no wonder that the horse reacts with mental resistance and evasion as it struggles to optimize its air flow. The horse attempts to maintain air flow by carrying itself "upside down" with the neck arched towards the ground and the back hollowed. This upside-down carriage allows it to extend the head and neck, opening the airways.

When a horse is trained to go on the bit, it loses some of its airway freedom. The upper and lower walls of the nasopharynx are relaxed and flaccid. (This causes air to vibrate in the pharynx and results in noise.) If the head is maintained in this flexed position while faster and more difficult demands are asked of the horse, it may not be able to perform to its utmost due to lack of oxygen.

Meeting the Air Demand

Because the horse is strictly a nose-breathing animal, physical adaptations accommodate the demand for air at speed. In the back of the mouth, a sheet of tissue arises from the bottom of the hard palate and extends backwards and up across the nasopharynx. This sheet of tissue is called the *soft palate*, and a hole *(ostium)* at the back of it provides a "buttonhole" through which the larynx fits.

For normal respiration, there must be a perfect air-tight fit between the soft palate and the larynx so the "button" (larynx) fits snugly against the "buttonhole" (ostium of the soft palate). The tongue is connected to the larynx so when one moves the other must move. Swallowing, hanging the tongue out of the mouth, or pulling the tongue behind the bit causes the larynx to move in relation to tongue position. When the larynx or soft palate moves, the seal between them is broken *(laryngo-palatal dislocation)*, which creates an obstruction with partial closure of the airway.

Bit Evasion

A horse may evade a bit in the mouth by moving its tongue around. The larynx may slide backwards and separate from its snug fit with the soft palate. If the tongue is pulled over the bit, swallowing returns it to normal. Swallowing requires a complete disconnection of the larynx from the ostium of the soft palate. It closes the airway so food or saliva are not drawn into the lungs.

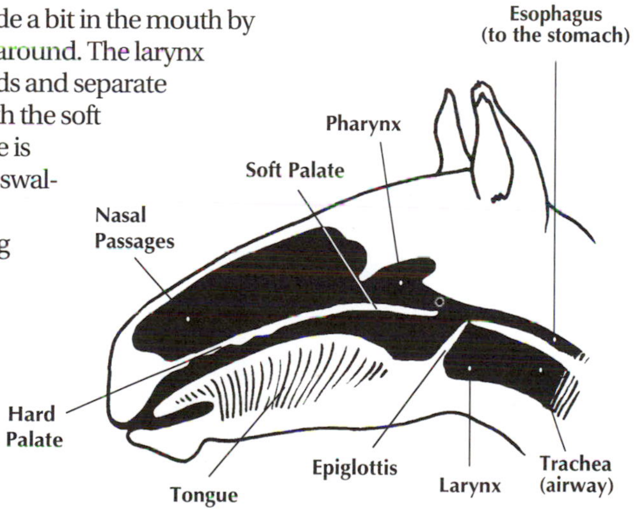

Fig. 5–4. Swallowing breaks the seal between the soft palate and the larynx.

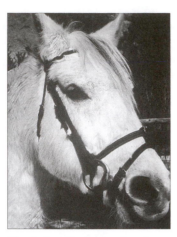

Fig. 5–5. A flash noseband keeps the mouth shut.

Other bit evasion tactics include opening the mouth. This action breaks the airtight seal of the lips. Air entering the mouth causes the soft palate to vibrate or lift up. Laryngo-palatal dislocation may result. Use of a dropped noseband, a flash, or figure-eight noseband keeps the mouth shut and deters these evasion tactics. However, nostrils should not be pinched by snugging the noseband down too tightly.

A bit that fits properly and is comfortable encourages a horse to accept it, and reduces the horse's tendency to spit out the bit. If a performance horse is ridden "onto the bit," a goal is to achieve jaw flexibility and softness. Bit acceptance is often accompanied by excessive salivation, which may stimulate swallowing with a brief laryngo-palatal dislocation.

Roaring

To increase the cross-sectional area of the larynx during exercise, the two arytenoid cartilages on either side of the larynx must be opened. Opening of the arytenoid cartilages is regulated by the recurrent laryngeal nerves. Damage to one or both of these nerves or their loss of function results in a syndrome called *laryngeal hemiplegia*, which is a paralysis usually of the left side of the larynx. Air flow resistance through the greatly diminished airway results in a "roaring" sound in an exercising horse. Such horses are subject to "choking down" or suffocation, followed by abrupt halt of exercise. A milder form of this syndrome contributes to exercise intolerance, because the horse is unable to breathe in enough oxygen to fuel the body.

Roaring is diagnosed by passing an endoscope into the nose to the back of the throat. It may be necessary to examine the horse while it is working on a treadmill.

Surgery may return the horse to athletic performance. The most common surgical procedure to correct roaring is called a tie-back, where the cartilage is actually tied open. There are other, more controversial methods, for example, nerve implants. After roaring surgery, a course of antibiotics helps prevent infection, and the horse should be stalled for 6 weeks. Then, it can be gradually reintroduced to exercise.

Not all roaring and gurgling sounds are caused by laryngeal paralysis. Some horses just like the noise that resonates in the nostrils and purposefully allow them to flap with inhalation.

Bleeding

Another syndrome which causes exercise intolerance is exercise in-duced pulmonary hemorrhage (EIPH), or "bleeding." One theory states that respiratory disease weakens some areas of lung tissue, causing bleeding. Another theory holds that conditions of recurrent laryngeal neuropathy (RLN), including roaring, cause bleeding. RLN causes an upper airway obstruction which may exert enough pressure changes in the lungs to cause rupture of capillaries and bleeding. *(See Chapters 5 & 6 for more information on roaring, RLN, and EIPH.)*

Performance and Air Flow

Exercises requiring optimal respi-ration are more affected by laryngo-palatal dislocation or loss of streamlining of the airways. For example, steeplechasing and cross-country events exert dramatic de-mands on the respiratory system.

The jumper that is lifting its body while weight-carrying needs all the oxygen it can get to fuel the muscles. An endurance horse oper-ates best aerobically (with oxygen), and any limitation to air intake can severely compromise performance. Polo ponies and dressage horses rely on both aerobic and anaerobic (without oxygen) fueling systems, but again, the more oxygen pro-vided to the system, the greater the stamina. *(See Chapter 3 for more information.)* Likewise, a racehorse cannot sacrifice even the smallest amount of incoming air as it races down the track with its head and neck stretched forward to improve airway efficiency.

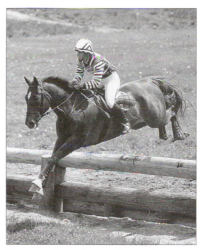

Fig. 5–6. Eventing and steeplechas-ing require a very hardy respiratory system.

Other less challenging athletics do not require the horse to operate at maximal exertion. The horse can therefore compensate for a slight loss in respiratory efficiency.

Keep the need for airway efficiency in mind when the horse seems to pull excessively on the reins while galloping. Sometimes the pulling is a credit to the horse's willingness and desire to run, but it may indicate that the horse cannot get enough air. By relaxing a little and letting go of its head and allow-ing it be comfortable, both rider and horse will have a better ride.

Respiration at Speed

At a gallop, respiratory rates run as high as 150 – 200 breaths per minute. The respiratory rate is directly synchronized with the stride frequency in a canter or gallop (unlike the walk or trot). When the forelimbs are forward and not weight-bearing, the rib cage is also pulled forward and expanded outwards, and the neck is up, allowing the horse to inhale. Inertia moves the internal organs backwards, further expanding the thoracic space. As the forelimbs impact the ground, the rib cage absorbs the force and compresses inward. Like a piston, the internal organs move forward, the neck is down, and air is forcefully exhaled.

RESPIRATORY ILLNESS

Just as good quality nutrition gives a horse the resources to build healthy tissue, so does the quality of the air around the horse determine the health of the respiratory system, and entire body.

Management greatly influences a horse's respiratory health. During winter, many horses are confined inside a stable, rather than turned out into the cold, wet, or snow-laden air. The atmosphere of the barn must be evaluated. Are there noxious fumes or dust? Is there a damp, musty odor, or ammonia fumes? Are there dust particles floating in the air? Are the horses coughing?

The result of poor management is a heavily polluted environment. A stabled horse breathes this environment around the clock. It is important to understand the effects that a contained, polluted atmosphere has on the respiratory system.

Defense Against Foreign Particles

Upper Airways

Nasal Passages

During inhalation, the horse's airways filter a large percentage of particles in the air. Nasal passages filter the largest particles. Humidity in the air increases a particle's size and density, because water condenses on it. These large particles are easily trapped by the nasal passages, preventing entry to the respiratory tree. However, some large particles are so heavy that they fall out of the nasal filtration trap and are inhaled into the upper airways.

Mucociliary Apparatus

The upper airways have a clearance mechanism is called the

mucociliary apparatus (MCA). Particles deposited in the upper airways are cleared away from the lungs by a one-way flow of mucus that lies on top of the *epithelial cells* lining the airways. These are specialized cells with beating cilia that propel the mucous layer, with attached particles, outwards towards the throat, where it is swallowed or coughed away. The epithelial cells are damaged by infectious agents, noxious gases (ammonia or carbon monoxide), or extremes in temperature or humidity. Interference in their function severely reduces the efficiency of the MCA.

Coughing

Another airway clearance mechanism is coughing. Certain nerves in the upper airways respond to dust, ammonia, and other irritants. These nerves stimulate a cough reflex to forcefully expel mucus and particles from the airways.

Excessive inflammation caused by irritants also stimulates a reflex constriction of the bronchioles in the lungs. This constricted diameter of air passages diminishes the efficiency of the coughing clearance mechanism.

Lower Airways

Combined with an effective mucociliary apparatus, specialized white blood cells called *alveolar macrophages* provide a primary line of defense against infection of the lower respiratory tract. An alveolar macrophage binds microorganisms, such as bacteria and viruses, to its cell membrane, and internalizes and inactivates each organism.

Smaller particles, and droplets of water containing bacteria and viruses *(droplet nuclei),* may remain suspended in the inhaled air, not dropping out until they reach the bottom of the lungs. Normally, any particles that descend past the mucociliary apparatus are removed from the lungs by a fluid layer that slowly moves outward until it reaches the MCA. Or, the particles may penetrate through the mucous layer to be consumed and destroyed by alveolar macrophages, or they are circulated with the alveolar macrophages to the MCA. Nerve endings in the smaller airways do not elicit coughing, but they will stimulate airway constriction. Interference in any of these events results in inadequate control of infection. Both the macrophage and the MCA are adversely affected by poor air quality.

Hay and Bedding Dust

Many barns have overhead hay storage that can compromise the respiratory system. As hay is thrown from the loft above, a large quantity of dust and mold spores are cast out to sift down through the atmosphere.

It may take several hours for small fungal spores to settle out of the air. Also, horses moving around in their stalls kick up bedding and dust. Dust concentrations in the air can increase up to threefold, further irritating the respiratory tract.

Fungal Spores

Damp, decomposing bedding generates ammonia fumes, and promotes development of fungal spores. Warm temperatures, coupled with a high relative humidity caused by inadequate ventilation, encourage fungal growth. Fungal growth is greater in straw than in wood shavings. Horses lying in straw and moldy bedding are subjected to massive numbers of mold spores even in the best ventilated stable.

The "hay dust," fungal spores, and other irritants start a degenerative process in the airways by causing a hypersensitivity reaction similar to allergies in people. Horses continually exposed to these air contaminants may develop *chronic obstructive pulmonary disease* (COPD). Studies show that feed and bedding are the main sources of stable dust.

Riding Arena Dust

Many exercise and riding arenas connect to the stabling area, providing a warm enclosed space to ride during bad weather. Unfortunately, this practice complicates the problem of confinement in the barn. As horses and people move around these arenas, stirred dust mixes with the still air inside the barn. Not only are working horses exposed to this polluted air, but so are stalled horses.

Attempts to water the arena to hold down the dust increase the humidity in the barn. If an arena is "moistened" with an oil mixture instead, oil particles in the air have toxic effects on the respiratory tract.

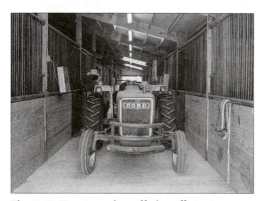

Fig. 5–7. Tractors give off air pollutants.

Humidity

High humidity levels contribute to respiratory infection. Adequate and effective floor drainage of water or urine is essential to limit humidity in the barn, and to remove moisture from bedding.

Carbon Monoxide

Machinery, such as tractors, are driven in and out of some

barns to assist with stall cleaning or raking of the arena. Machinery contributes to build-up of carbon monoxide fumes within the stable. Appropriate ventilation is important when this equipment is in operation.

Respiratory Viruses

One often hears the axiom: "No legs, no wind, no horse." All too frequently the emphasis is placed upon the "no legs" portion of this statement, and the health of the equine respiratory tract is taken for granted. A mild bout of influenza is explained away as "...something it will get over." Ironically, a respiratory infection may require 3 weeks for a return to health.

Urbanized living congregates horses together in big barns and stables, increasing the opportunity for viral respiratory illness. More horses are housed under one roof, and are stressed by training and competition. A viral respiratory outbreak can easily grab hold and maintain itself in a concentrated equine population. Transcontinental and intercontinental transport of competition and breeding horses increases possibilities for spreading viruses on a global scale.

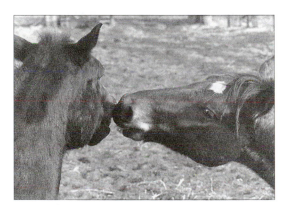

Fig. 5–8. Nose to nose contact is one method of spreading viruses.

Spread of infectious respiratory viruses occurs by droplet nuclei in the air, or directly from nose-to-nose contact. Viruses are also spread by indirect contact with tack, stable personnel, or in a contaminated grooming or wash stall common to all horse traffic.

Replication of a Virus

Unlike bacteria, viruses cannot duplicate themselves without inserting themselves into a host cell. There, they command the cell's replication mechanisms to reproduce the virus. Eventually, the cell is so full of new viral particles that it bursts. The cell is killed and viral particles are released to infect other cells.

The horse's immune system recognizes the viral proteins as foreign, and begins to produce antibodies. Specifically, antibodies recognize *hemagglutinin (HA) spikes* on the surface of viral particles. They attach to the virus and neutralize it. Each HA spike is made of a specific sequence of amino acids (components of proteins). Recognition of these specific amino acids on the spike is essential for the antibody to attach to it, with subsequent neutralization of the virus. In this way, antibodies disrupt viral replication by preventing them from entering the host cells.

Effects of Vaccination

On the Immune System

Vaccines train a horse's immune system to respond to viral particles. The initial vaccination, called *primary immunization,* primes the cells which produce antibodies. Subsequent boosters stimulate actual antibody production. A booster vaccine stimulates a rapid immune response, and the antibodies rise to high levels due to antibody "memory," or *anamnestic response.* "Anamnestic" is the Greek word for recollection. To invoke the anamnestic response, it is necessary to wait 4 – 6 weeks for the second booster.

Vaccination stimulates the immune system to make specialized antibodies against a specific strain of virus. Vaccine also stimulates cross-protective antibodies against variations of a strain. Antibodies developed against a specific strain are better at neutralizing that particular virus than are cross-protective antibodies. Yet, cross-protective antibodies rally when a horse is exposed to a similar, but unfamiliar virus.

Because antibodies prevent the virus from invading respiratory cells, an immunized horse does not develop clinical symptoms of disease. Vaccinations are *not* completely protective, but they reduce the risk of contracting disease, while minimizing symptoms. Both illness time and recovery time are shortened dramatically in a vaccinated horse.

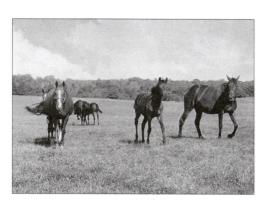

Fig. 5–9. Serious epidemics may be prevented if at least 70% of a herd has been vaccinated.

On Herd Health

Vaccinating a herd or a large population of horses reduces the number of susceptible horses. Antibody levels are present in the entire group, preventing a viral infection from gaining a foothold. Assume, for example, that only 10% of a herd has been vaccinated. During an outbreak, the virus carried by the other 90% is an overwhelming challenge to the immune systems of the vaccinated horses. Vaccination is therefore not enough to protect the vaccinated 10% against an overwhelming insult. A vaccine breakdown results, with clinical disease in epidemic proportions.

To prevent serious epidemics, at least 70% of a population should be vaccinated. When an outbreak does occur, all as yet unaffected individuals should be vaccinated to limit the spread of disease. Vaccinated horses develop a high level immune response that "blocks" further transmission of virus from horse to horse. There is no point in vaccinating already-sick animals.

Factors Affecting a Vaccination Program

Aggressive immunization programs help ensure respiratory health. However, the most aggressive vaccination program will not entirely eliminate disease if horses are stressed, overcrowded, or faced with poor stable hygiene, inadequate nutrition, or parasitism.

Age of the Horse

Each horse's immune system is unique in its ability to respond to vaccines. The age of a horse determines how frequently it should be boostered. Young horses under 2 years old are most susceptible to respiratory viruses. Because a youngster has not encountered a full spectrum of viruses or bacteria, its immune system is not fully competent to ward off all infections.

Occupation

The occupation of a horse is critical in determining a vaccination schedule. A highly competitive and mobile horse is frequently exposed to respiratory viruses, and should be vaccinated every 2 – 3 months. Although a horse may not be clinically ill, it can carry a virus home and spread it to others. Horses in boarding stables,

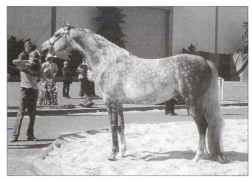

Fig. 5–10. A competitive and mobile horse is frequently exposed to viruses.

121

or in barns with these transient individuals, have a high risk of exposure.

A horse that rarely socializes with strange horses may only need boosters twice a year. This program may be sufficient to maintain a protective antibody level. In 6 months, antibodies do not decline so low as to prevent an anamnestic response to a booster vaccine.

Previous Vaccinations

The number of previous vaccinations an individual has received should be considered in planning vaccination frequency. As the number of booster injections that a horse receives in its lifetime increases, the duration of an antibody response also increases. However, the level of antibody response can only increase up to a certain point.

Vaccine Types

Finally, the type of vaccine used determines booster frequency. *Inactivated* or *killed* vaccines protect for barely up to 3 months, whereas a *modified live* vaccine protects for 4 – 6 months, depending on the product. Some killed vaccines use carrier agents, called *adjuvants*, that affect how well immunity is stimulated. (The adjuvant is the liquid carrier which contains the virus.) A "depot" adjuvant enhances both the level and duration of antibody response by slowly releasing the vaccine over several weeks. As the foreign protein is presented to the immune system over a prolonged period, it continually stimulates antibody production.

Respiratory Virus Modification

Viruses can modify themselves so they are no longer recognized by the immune system. There are various strains or subtypes of viruses, and it is necessary to immunize against viruses that are currently prevalent, and are not out-dated. Use of vaccines with "current reference viruses" is important for effective immunization.

Viral Shift

Viruses modify themselves in two ways. The first, called *viral shift*, is the appearance of an entirely new strain of virus due to a combination of two different strains. For example, the last major shift of equine influenza virus in the U.S. occurred in 1963 with the outbreak of the Miami/63 strain. In the past few years, new subtypes of equine influenza virus have appeared in Europe and China. With intercontinental movement of horses, there is an increased possibility for exposure to new subtypes that horses are immunologically ill-equipped to combat.

Antigenic Drift

The second method by which a virus alters itself is *antigenic drift*. An antigen is any foreign protein presented to the immune system to stimulate antibody production. Drift is a minor change in the viral antigenic structure and makeup. If viral proteins are changed in a process of *mutation*, antigenic drift results and a horse's immune system cannot defend against it. Neutralization by antibodies is prevented, and viral infection and clinical disease develop.

Viral Duplication

Whenever a virus successfully infects a horse and begins to duplicate itself, there is an opportunity for mutation and drift. The rate of drift is relative to the number of passages through horses, so the more horses infected in a population, the greater likelihood of antigenic drift.

Antibodies are less effective at neutralizing these different "looking" viruses created by antigenic drift. Disease produced by a viral mutant is not necessarily more severe, but a horse's immune system is less able to defeat a mutant virus. Unvaccinated and immunologically naive horses are susceptible to illness. Sick horses are reservoirs for disease.

Reporting outbreaks of respiratory disease in a horse or herd to a veterinarian tracks epidemics, shifts in viral subtypes, and antibody response to various vaccines. This practice ensures that vaccines are up-to-date with the current reference viruses.

Telling others about the need and frequency of immunizations against respiratory viruses benefits the entire horse population. Limiting the number of susceptible animals that could carry viral respiratory disease promotes health within a population. Keeping current with an aggressive immunization programs prevents loss of valuable training, conditioning, and competition time.

Influenza Virus

The "flu" can strike rapidly and unexpectedly, usually requiring an incubation time of only 1 – 5 days. An affected horse is lethargic, depressed, unresponsive, and often is disinterested in food. Rectal temperature may reach 103° – 106° F. The respiratory rate increases to 60 breaths per minute. A sick horse moves with deliberate concentration, indicating aching muscles *(myalgia)* or head. Often, a watery, nasal discharge is observed, and a dry hacking cough is heard in about 40% of affected horses.

Some horses' immune response is effective enough so they are not apparently ill, but they may still have a *subclinical infection* that allows shedding of viral particles.

Coughing is a principal means of spreading the virus from horse to horse. Respiratory secretions ejected from a coughing horse into the air contain infective doses of viral particles. If viral particles are coughed into a moist environment, such as a damp barn or shipping van, the influenza virus remains alive and infective for several days.

Infectious secretions are passed by direct nose-to-nose contact, and from contaminated housing, food, water, human hands, or clothing.

The First Line of Defense

Secretory antibodies in the nasal passages are the first line of defense against influenza virus. Secretory antibodies respond to influenza virus only if previously "trained" to do so either by a prior infection or by vaccination. If the virus is inhaled, and not neutralized by secretory antibodies, it colonizes the mucous membrane lining of the upper respiratory tissues and trachea.

Circulating Antibodies

If the flu virus penetrates this first line of defense, antibodies circulating throughout the body limit the infection. Circulating antibodies also develop in response to prior infection or vaccination.

Damage to Airways

The flu virus invades and kills the ciliated epithelial cells lining the respiratory tract. Cilia are tiny hair-like structures protruding from the cells which trap debris. At 4 days after successful invasion by an influenza virus, there is a significant degeneration of these cells. By 6 days after infection, the cells are almost entirely denuded of cilia, and the respiratory tract cannot adequately clear debris, dust, viruses, or bacteria from the lungs.

The mucociliary apparatus that normally moves debris out of the airways no longer functions properly. Depending on the infection's severity, it takes 3 – 6 weeks to repair once the virus is defeated and healing begins. Even in an uncomplicated case of influenza, a minimum of 3 weeks is necessary for functional recovery of the respiratory epithelium.

Because the denuded respiratory tract epithelium cannot respond to further insult, opportunistic bacterial infections can develop, possibly leading to pneumonia, long-term damage to the lungs, or death.

Resuming Exercise

Exercise can resume 7 – 10 days after body temperature returns to normal and coughing altogether stops. (Once clinical symptoms have abated, a horse is still infectious to others for 3 – 6 days.) If exercise causes coughing, wait another 4 or 5 days before resuming a training program. To ensure full recovery, a horse with a mild illness and a cough should not return to full training for 3 – 5 weeks.

Recovery Period

Having a horse removed from training and competition for a month or more for full recovery is an emotional and economic cost to a horse owner. However, if a horse is prematurely returned to work, a relapse is possible. In rare instances, the heart is affected by the influenza virus and develops an arrhythmia. In general, the mortality rate from an influenza infection is remarkably low in uncomplicated cases.

An adult horse receiving adequate supportive care, rest, and protection from secondary complications usually recovers uneventfully with no permanent problems. Careful monitoring during both sickness and recovery are essential to success.

Only 5% of foal deaths are caused by respiratory viral infection. However, a common cause of foal death (up to 6 months of age) is bacterial pneumonia. This pneumonia is a secondary infection to a viral respiratory infections. Once the protective defense of the respiratory lining is breached, a young horse can rapidly deteriorate in as quickly as 48 hours.

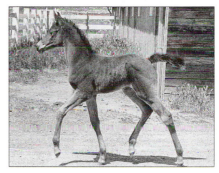

Fig. 5–11. Foals are particularly susceptible to bacterial pneumonia.

Prevention

It is best to avoid equine influenza viral infection if possible. The protective antibody response to an influenza virus infection is rapid, but short-lived. By about 100 days, circulating antibodies have diminished and a horse is again susceptible to illness. (A human influenza antibody response lasts for 6 months up to years.)

New arrivals to a herd or barn should be quarantined for 2 – 3 weeks. This practice isolates horses that are incubating disease or are shedding viral particles.

Equine influenza was first identified as a subtype-A1 virus, but a more virulent form appeared in an epidemic in 1963 called the subtype-A2 flu strain, also known as the Miami/63 influenza strain. The outbreak in Europe in the late 1980s involved a drifted form of subtype-A2 virus. It is important to use a current vaccine to ensure the horse is protected against the current strain of influenza virus.

An active performance horse is frequently exposed to respiratory viruses, and can carry these viruses home to other animals. Such horses should be vaccinated often, preferably every 3 – 4 months.

Equine Herpes Virus

Another respiratory virus for which a vaccine is available is the Equine Herpes Virus (EHV), or *rhinopneumonitis*. Often referred to as "Rhino," the virus has different subtypes. EHV-1 causes viral abortion, a neurological form of this disease, and also takes a respiratory form. EHV-4 primarily takes a respiratory form.

Abortion occurs from 14 – 120 days after exposure to the virus. A mare may show no signs of disease, but the placenta and fetus are invaded by the virus. Most EHV-1 abortions occur in the last half of pregnancy, particularly the last trimester.

EHV-4 must replicate before clinical signs appear. It has a longer incubation time than the influenza virus, taking as long as 3 weeks. An infection may not be as severe as that seen with the flu because the horse's defense mechanisms begin to respond to EHV during the incubation period.

Symptoms

Fevers can run as high as 106° F with this virus. Early in the course of disease, a watery, nasal discharge develops. This discharge often progresses to a mucopurulent discharge, which contains both mucus and pus, due to secondary bacterial infection. For this reason, rhinopneumonitis is nicknamed the "snots."

Vaccination Schedule

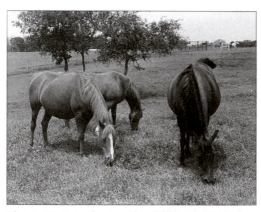

Fig. 5–12. Broodmares should be vaccinated for Rhino infection, which can cause abortion.

Horses less than 2 years old are most susceptible to EHV-4, yet any stressed, mobile, or competitive horse, and any pregnant mare should be vaccinated against this respiratory virus. The length of EHV vaccination protection is limited to less than 3 months, so pregnant mares should receive EHV-1 vaccines at 5, 7, and 9 months of pregnancy. For respiratory protection only, in non-pregnant horses boosters every 3 months will suffice. (There is currently no vaccine to protect against the neurologic form of EHV.)

EHV may not be a problem in some areas, but horses that travel may contact it. Although they may show no outward clinical signs, they bring it home with them.

Rhinovirus

The rhinopneumonitis virus (EHV) should not be confused with the Rhinovirus (ERV) for which there is no vaccine. ERV is associated with a fever lasting 1 or 2 days, swelling of the pharyngeal lymph nodes accompanied by a sore throat, and a watery to gray-green nasal discharge due to inflammation of the trachea and lower airways, or *tracheobronchitis*. Frequently, horses are infected without producing clinical signs, and serve as carriers to other, less durable individuals.

Heaves (COPD)

Chronic obstructive pulmonary disease (heaves) is a respiratory syndrome in horses similar to asthma or emphysema in humans. It is sometimes referred to as "heaves" or "broken wind." COPD often occurs in stabled horses. An overwhelming concentration of organic dust allergens in the environment, particularly molds and mold spores, initiates a hypersensitivity reaction. Some horses become allergic to alfalfa hay and exhibit a similar clinical response.

Viral invasion of the respiratory tract lining can also stimulate the development of COPD. The airways become hyperirritable, leading to spasms in the airway. Also, the destroyed ciliated epithelium lining the respiratory tract regenerates with thickened or altered cells, causing excess mucus production.

Symptoms of COPD

Large amounts of mucus or pus accumulate in the air passages. Constriction and spasm of these small airways *(bronchoconstriction)* results in their narrowing, causing obstruction. A horse has difficulty exhaling or properly ventilating the lungs. It stands depressed, with nostrils flared, with an increased

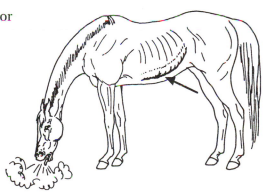

Fig. 5–13. A heave line between the flank and the thorax.

respiratory rate (greater than 20 – 24 per minute). Occasionally, a wet or pus-filled nasal discharge is present. Wheezing may be audible. An increased exhaling effort is obvious with each breath. Forceful exhaling over time overdevelops abdominal muscles that labor to push air out of the lungs. This overdevelopment is visible as a *heave line* between the flank and the thorax. A severely affected horse loses its appetite, loses weight, and appears unthrifty. Chronic coughing is a key symptom of this disease, particularly if a cough persists for several weeks.

The Disease Process

The sequence of events that stimulate this condition begin with an inhaled allergen, such as mold. If hay is baled with a high moisture content, heat generated in the bale encourages the growth of mold. A horse with no symptoms may develop them within 1 or 2 hours and up to 10 hours after exposure. An allergic response proceeds rapidly, calling in specific inflammatory cells.

Mast cells release substances, such as histamines, that cause spasms and constriction of the smooth muscles of the airways, and an increase in mucus production. A type of white blood cell, *neutrophils*, release substances that also constrict the airways and enhance mucus production. Normal airflow is interrupted by all these changes:

- thickening of epithelial cells lining the airways
- bronchoconstriction
- excess mucous congestion
- inflammatory cell infiltration

The mucociliary apparatus clearance mechanism is seriously impaired. Bronchial nerve reflexes become hyper-reactive and result in coughing.

Managing COPD

The goal for managing COPD is to reduce allergen levels below a threshold that causes clinical disease in the individual. It is not possible to remove all allergens from the environment. Each horse responds differently to similar allergens, just as do people. What may be below threshold level for one horse, may still be allergenic for another.

Drugs

Many pharmacological drugs are available to deal with COPD, but have temporary effects unless management is altered. These drugs include prednisone, terbutaline, and aminophylline. Clenbutenol is a very effective drug, but it has not yet been approved by the FDA.

Housing

A horse should be moved to open air, if possible, with constant fresh air flow into the environment. Bedding should be wood shavings, peat moss, or shredded paper, but *not* straw. Housing should be located at least 50 yards upwind of any hay supply.

Feeding

The horse should be fed off the ground, not out of racks or raised feeders. By keeping its head down as it eats, normal blowing ejects particles from the nasal passages. Never feed moldy hay, and remove alfalfa from the diet if a horse seems at all sensitive to it.

A cubed or pelleted diet is preferable, or at least wet grass hay. Even good quality grass hay contains a large amount of fungal spores. Wetting the hay may not completely prevent allergic effects due to continued exposure to the offending antigen. A pasture situation is ideal, particularly if plants are not in bloom. Tree and grass pollen have been implicated as allergens, as have straw mites.

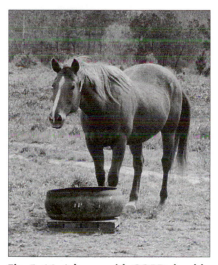

Fig. 5–14. A horse with COPD should be fed off the ground.

Vaccinations

A viral respiratory infection weakens a horse's resistance to other disease, and renders a horse more susceptible to COPD. Once a horse has developed COPD, its respiratory immune system is weakened against further viral and bacterial insult.

A horse afflicted with COPD should be kept in as dust-free an environment as possible. To successfully manage a horse with compromised respiratory health is frustrating and requires diligent attention to detail. Prevention of the problem requires unpolluted open air, and good clean living.

Bacterial Infection
Secondary Infections

During a viral infection, bacteria that normally inhabit the upper airways may colonize, infect, and inflame the lower airways. Normally, the mucociliary apparatus and macrophage systems clear bacteria, but viruses destroy the ciliated epithelial cells of the MCA, and reduce the ability of macrophages to attach to, digest, and kill bacteria.

Strangles

Strangles is a bacterial infection not associated with a viral infection. It is a bacterial respiratory disease, also called *equine distemper*. This disease is caused by *Streptococcus equi*. Normally the bacteria invade the upper respiratory tract, multiplying in the lymph nodes of the head.

Symptoms

Affected horses have a fever and a mucopurulent nasal discharge often accompanied by a cough. Other signs are similar to viral respiratory infections: the horse is depressed and off feed, and reluctant to swallow due to a painful throat. The most telling indication of a strangles infection is the enlargement of the lymph nodes under the jaw *(submandibular lymph nodes)* or in the throatlatch *(retropharyngeal lymph nodes)*. If the lymph nodes swell to grotesque proportions, the windpipe is so obstructed as to make breathing difficult — a horse can then "strangle" to death for lack of air.

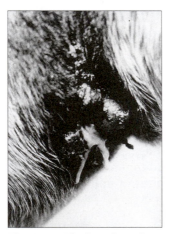

Fig. 5–15. The lymph node eventually breaks open.

Lymph Node Action

An abscessed lymph node eventually breaks open and drains a thick creamy pus, contaminating the environment and other horses with highly infectious material. Even before the lymph node breaks, sick horses pass the infection to others through nasal discharge or coughing. Communal feeders and waterers, and nose-to-nose contact also spread the disease.

Any horse showing the slightest hint of impending sickness should be isolated as far from other horses as possible. An infected horse continues to shed bacteria for up to 6 weeks, despite appearing fully recovered.

Complications

Occasional complications from a strangles infection can be serious, including:

- a bacterial pneumonia as the infection invades the lower respiratory tract
- a guttural pouch infection leading to a chronic nasal discharge
- purpura hemorrhagica
- bastard strangles, where the infection travels to the lymph nodes of the intestinal tract, abdominal organs, or the brain

Young horses less than 3 years of age have a difficult time coping with infection. Mature horses usually have sufficient immunity to prevent the disease from turning into life-threatening pneumonia.

Vaccines

Once the Strep bacteria has contaminated a property, it survives for months in the environment, in carrier horses that harbor the bacteria without showing clinical signs of illness. The carrier horses provide a reservoir for cyclical infection. Horses moved to that location, or horses that have not yet become sick can be vaccinated against strangles. Vaccination is only about 60% – 75% effective in preventing disease, because the intramuscular injection stimulates a systemic immunity in the bloodstream rather than a strong local immunity in the upper respiratory tract, where the bacteria first invades.

Currently, efforts are directed towards an effective strangles vaccine that would be administered as an oral or nasal spray. This method would stimulate secretory antibodies in the horse's nasal and oral passages. These locally stimulated antibodies would prevent invasion of the bacteria in the upper respiratory tract.

Preventing Respiratory Illness

Maintaining excellent hygiene and minimizing the horse's stress are key elements in preventing respiratory illness. To significantly reduce shedding of bacteria and viruses in the environment, aggressive respiratory vaccine programs should be implemented. A virally-infected, coughing horse sprays millions of viral particles into the air. Horses protected by vaccines are less likely to develop clinical viral disease or associated bacterial infections; subsequently, they are less likely to shed these organisms in epidemic or infectious doses.

By keeping accurate records and a calendar, it is easy to implement an effective vaccine schedule to avoid respiratory illness. Respiratory vaccines are extremely cost-effective as insurance that a horse can train and deliver an optimal athletic performance.

Pregnant Mares

To start a vaccination program, a pregnant mare is vaccinated about 1 month before foaling. This practice allows enough time to develop antibodies, which will secrete into the mammary glands where they are available to the foal in the *colostrum* (the first milk).

Any mare that receives a vaccination booster every 3 months before foaling will provide plenty of antibodies to the foal through the colostrum. Colostral antibodies provide passive protection to a foal until it is about 3 months of age. Until then, maternal antibodies from the colostrum block a foal's active immune response to a vaccine, so a foal is unlikely to benefit from vaccination until it is 3 – 4 months old.

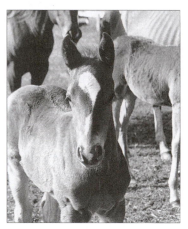

Fig. 5–16. Foals should begin vaccinations at 2 – 3 months.

Foals

The age at which foals are started on a vaccination program depends on the vaccination status of the mare. If a mare has a cloudy history or is not current on her vaccines, it is better to start vaccination of a foal between 2 – 3 months.

The first vaccine given primes the immune system, and turns on the cells which produce protective antibodies. Then, it is necessary to wait 4 – 6 weeks to booster a second time and invoke the anamnestic response. After that, an optimal schedule includes respiratory vaccine boosters every 3 – 4 months to all horses over 2 years of age.

Respiratory Vaccine Schedule

If a horse is less than 2 years old, highly stressed, highly mobile, or at risk of exposure to a transient population, vaccinating every 2 – 3 months may be necessary.

An effective respiratory vaccine schedule is as follows:

- Vaccinate pregnant mares at 5, 7, and 9 months of pregnancy against rhinopneumonitis viral abortions. Use approved products for pregnant mares.
- Immunize pregnant mares every 3 – 4 months with influenza vaccines.
- Vaccinate pregnant mares 1 month before foaling, using encephalitis - tetanus - influenza (EWTF) vaccine.

- Vaccinate foals at 3 months with encephalitis - tetanus - influenza and rhinopneumonitis vaccines. If an adult horse has not received vaccinations before, begin immunization as for foals.
- Booster foals, or horses started on a vaccine program for the first time, 4 – 6 weeks later with EWTF and rhinopneumonitis vaccines.
- Vaccinate any age horse every 3 months with influenza and rhinopneumonitis vaccines once a primary immunization program has been initiated as above.
- Vaccinate at least 2 weeks before anticipated exposure, travel, or stress, if possible.

If it is uncertain whether a horse will develop a vaccination reaction, vaccinate at least 2 weeks before a competitive event or transport so muscle soreness is resolved and a horse can compete to potential. The immune system will have developed heightened antibody protection against viruses by then.

Vaccination Reaction

Some individuals develop adverse reactions to injections. Mild influenza-like symptoms, such as fever, depression, or a lack of appetite may occur. Lower leg swelling, or muscle soreness at the injection site are common vaccination reactions. Uncommonly, a localized abscess develops at an injection site.

Some horses react adversely to a specific adjuvant (the liquid carrier which contains the virus). Switching products and manufacturers periodically may prevent these reactions. Other horses benefit from an intravenous injection of a non-steroidal anti-inflammatory drug when vaccinated to prevent ill-effects. Rarely, an adverse reaction is severe enough to preclude use of a specific vaccine. An owner or trainer must weigh the benefits versus the risk of foregoing a vaccine.

New Vaccine Developments

Temperature-Sensitive Vaccine

To develop an influenza vaccine without adverse side effects, researchers are developing a temperature-sensitive vaccine given as an intranasal spray. The vaccine virus can replicate at the lower temperatures of the nostrils, but cannot migrate further into the warmer respiratory tract. Replication in the nasal passages stimulates development of secretory antibodies that are the primary line of defense against upper respiratory infections. Developing an intranasal spray inoculation against the subtype-A2 influenza is still in the research stages.

Genetic Engineering Research

A variety of other genetic engineering efforts are also in the infant stages of research. One such effort involves developing recombinant strains of viral vaccine by reassorting and combining genetic material from two different strains of influenza virus. Such a mutant would stimulate antibody production, yet would not produce illness or cause a horse to be infective.

Maintaining Air Quality

Poor ventilation in a barn creates an inadequate air exchange, and promotes a build-up of humidity, irritants (dust, allergens, and gases), and an increase in numbers of airborne, disease-causing agents *(pathogens)* in the environment. Dust not only irritates the respiratory lining, but it also provides a vehicle for particles, increasing the *dose* of pathogens introduced into the airways.

Ammonia fumes degenerate the ciliary epithelial cells, in essence paralyzing them, as well as decreasing the secretion of the mucous layer. Ammonia suppresses the ability of macrophages to kill bacteria. If a person can smell the ammonia fumes, the levels are too high.

An increase in humidity forms aerosolized droplet nuclei. These droplets enclose the bacteria or viruses, protecting them from the lethal effects of drying or temperature extremes. Protection from the elements enhances the spread of respiratory pathogens.

Benefits of Ventilation

An increase in numbers of circulating pathogens in the air presents an increased dose to a horse's respiratory tract. Under normal circumstances, the immune system may be able to inactivate a low dose level, whereas a greater dose can overwhelm and infect a horse with disease. Most infections are dose-dependent, meaning that exposure to a small quantity of a pathogen results in a milder disease or one that passes unrecognized. Frequent and rapid air turnover by a good ventilation system reduces the concentration of particles in the air (and dose).

Natural Ventilation

A natural ventilation system is achieved by holes in the walls and/or under the eaves of the roof, or by cross-ventilation created by doors open at opposite ends of the barn. Wind forces air through the building, but can create drafts if openings are inappropriately placed.

An example of good ventilation is stalls with ventilation openings with dimentions of 2 feet by 2 feet in the walls, and 1 foot by 1 foot near the roof. Larger wall openings allow a horse to put its head outside, giving it fresh air, and relieving mental boredom.

Convection

If the air is still, or the holes are baffled to prevent drafts, the only means for air movement is by natural convection. Convection results from a temperature difference between the warmer air inside the stable (generated by the horses) and the cooler air outside. Hot air rises to exit from the upper holes, while cool, fresh air enters lower holes.

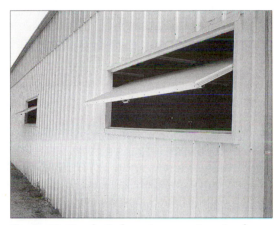

Fig. 5–17. Good windows to promote natural ventilation.

Effective insulation of a building increases the temperature differences between the inside and outside of the barn, maximizing natural convection. Roof insulation reduces radiant heat loss during cold winter nights, decreasing condensation (and resultant humidity) in the building.

In a very large horse barn (twenty or more horses) it is difficult to maintain precise mixing of the air masses. Barns that are shut up tightly in the winter, with all doors and windows closed, have still air conditions with inadequate ventilation. Auxiliary ventilation openings along the roof allow entry of air into and out of the building, or specialized air flow systems should be installed.

Mechanical Air Flow Systems

Mechanical air flow systems should be exhaustive rather than recirculating, with a minimum air exchange of four times every hour. Anything less than two air exchanges per

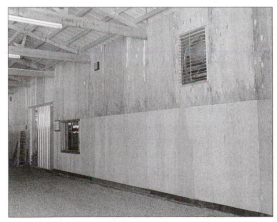

Fig. 5–18. Exhaust fans placed away from air inlets allow air turnover.

hour results in a dangerous build-up of mold spores. Exhaust units should be placed at a sufficient distance from the air inlets for adequate air turnover.

Ideal Management Practices

Optimal air quality in a barn to promote respiratory health depends on specific measures:

- Institute an ideal ventilation system in the barn to bring in fresh air, and to exhaust the old air.
- Separate riding and exercise areas from the stabling section.
- Store hay in another building. This practice reduces air pollutants, and decreases a fire hazard. Hay stored under cover from the weather develops less mold.
- Use good quality, dust-free bedding.
- Ensure adequate drainage for water and urine.
- Clean stalls frequently to reduce ammonia levels. Apply 1 or 2 pounds of hydrated lime to the stall floors after cleaning to reduce ammonia levels. A product called clinoptilolite (Sweet PDZ /Stall Fresh®: Temeco Comp) reduces ammonia levels if applied to floors after cleaning. It works particularly well with sawdust bedding, rather than straw.

By following these practices, not only will the air quality and health of the horses improve, but humans will directly benefit from these good management procedures. The air quality will be healthful, and the horse will feel better, look better, and perform better.

Stress Factors

Training and Exercise

Stress increases the risk of respiratory infections. Routine training and strenuous exercise are frequent stresses to a horse. This stress results in increased *cortisol* secretion by the body, coupled with exercise-related inflammation of the lung tissues. Cortisol is a steroid hormone that inhibits the immune function of the alveolar macrophages and other white blood cells.

Cortisol depletes the number of immunoglobulins in respiratory secretions. Immunoglobulins are specialized proteins that decrease the ability of bacteria and viruses to attach to and infect epithelial cells. They also coat the organisms with a substance to enhance uptake by white blood cells. Immunoglobulins chemically attract other white blood cells to the area to help clean up infection.

Transportation

Transportation over long distances is a stressful condition that increases a horse's susceptibility to viral or bacterial infection, particularly 1 week after the trip. Horses subjected to stresses such as hard training, competition, and travel benefit from optimal air quality. Other significant stresses that adversely affect a horse's immune response include overcrowding, poor quality nutrition, fatigue, and rapid changes in temperature.

Rapid Temperature Changes

It is preferable to maintain a constant temperature within a barn rather than having extreme fluctuations between hot and cold temperatures. Many stalled horses are blanketed and often are body clipped. The only insulating layer of protection against cold for a clipped horse is the blanket. If a horse is blanketed at the beginning of the winter season, or clipped to prevent growing a winter hair coat, it is necessary to consistently blanket it throughout the cold season. If the horse has a fur coat and is not used to being blanketed, be careful of overheating it by blanketing on a sporadic basis. Chills and drafts, or improper cooling out of an overheated horse further compromise the immune response.

6

CONDITIONING FOR PERFORMANCE

MAXIMIZING POTENTIAL

An elite equine athlete is born with a potential to excel, and an intelligent conditioning program maximizes that potential. Different breeds and individual horses excel in endurance type or sprint type sports depending on their conformation and the inherited composition of their muscle fibers. Muscles, the cardiovascular system, the respiratory system, and neuromuscular coordination respond favorably to conditioning programs. The most effective conditioning program carefully strengthens ligaments, tendons, bones, joints, and muscles to avoid injury, while also developing the cardiovascular system to full capacity.

Competitive Edge

A primary goal of training is to improve a horse's *aerobic capacity*. The aerobic capacity is the ability of the horse to exercise longer and farther without using anaerobic metabolism. Anaerobic metabolism produces energy without using oxygen. A more efficient method of energy production is aerobic metabolism, which produces energy using oxygen.

Unlike anaerobic metabolism, aerobic metabolism does not generate toxic by-products which can cause muscle fatigue and soreness. A horse that is conditioned to perform for long periods using aerobic metabolism, where fuels (glycogen and fatty acids) are converted to energy with oxygen, often has the competitive advantage.

When either the oxygen or the fuels are depleted, the horse begins to rely on anaerobic metabolism of glycogen. At this point, the horse has reached the anaerobic threshold. Lactic acid, which is a toxic by-product of anaerobic metabolism, begins to accumulate in the muscles and bloodstream. Eventually, this accumulation results in fatigue, which is the limiting factor in performance. (See *Chapter 3 for more information on metabolism.*)

Submaximal Exercise (Endurance)

Most horses work at aerobic levels if their *heart rate* remains under 150 beats per minute (bpm). This exercise is called submaximal, or endurance exercise. Examples of this level of activity include pleasure riding, competitive trail events, endurance racing, dressage, and the roads and tracks phase of three-day eventing. At or below this heart rate, lactic acid does not accumulate in the muscles. Any small amount of lactic acid that forms is flushed from the muscles by the circulation or is aerobically metabolized.

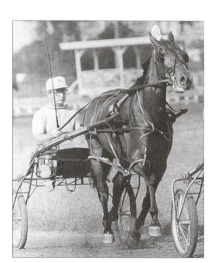

Fig. 6–1. Standardbred racing uses anaerobic and aerobic metabolism.

Maximal Exercise (Sprint)

Sprint sports require maximal exercise which in most horses occurs at heart rates above 180 – 200 bpm. These sports depend almost exclusively on anaerobic energy metabolism. Quarter Horse racing and barrel racing are good examples of such athletic efforts.

Combination Exercise

Examples of activities that depend on both aerobic and anaerobic metabolism are Thoroughbred and Standardbred racing, jumping, polo, cutting, reining, ranch work, and three-day eventing.

EFFECTS OF CONDITIONING
Conditioning Muscles Aerobically

The longer a horse can exercise using oxygen to produce energy, the longer fatigue is delayed. The body adapts to aerobic conditioning by improving the muscle systems that use oxygen to produce energy. These systems include improving blood circulation, improving metabolism, and converting some FTb (fast twitch low oxidative) muscle fibers to FTa (fast twitch high oxidative) muscle fibers. *(See Chapter 3 for more information on muscle fiber types.)*

Blood Circulation

Aerobic conditioning develops extensive capillary beds in the muscles and decreases the cross-sectional area of the ST (slow twitch) muscle fibers. Both factors improve blood circulation, which supplies more oxygen and helps remove toxic by-products like lactic acid. More oxygen and less lactic acid in the muscles reduces fatigue.

Metabolism

Increasing the length of time during which muscles are fueled by glycogen and fatty acids improves the aerobic capacity. Glycogen is a connected chain of glucose sugar molecules, and is a carbohydrate obtained from grain and forage. Fatty acids are produced by carbohydrate fermentation in the large intestine, or from fats in the feed.

With the blood circulation increased, the increased availability of oxygen promotes the use of fatty acids as a fuel rather than glycogen. The glycogen in the muscles and liver is spared, leaving more fuel in reserve for later use. Prolonging the time until glycogen reserves are depleted also delays the onset of fatigue, and reduces muscle soreness.

Each muscle cell that uses oxygen to convert fuel to energy has energy factories within it called mitochondria. The number of mitochondria increases with aerobic conditioning, improving oxygen use and energy production in the muscle cells.

Converting FTb to FTa

Aerobic conditioning improves a horse's aerobic capacity by converting up to 7% of FTb muscle fibers (low oxidative) into FTa muscle fibers (high oxidative). These FTa fibers can use oxygen to produce energy. Thoroughbreds and Standardbreds are able to compete at speed for longer distances than the Quarter Horse types (Quarter Horse, Paint, and Appaloosa) because they are genetically endowed with more FTa

141

than FTb fibers.

Improving the blood circulation, improving metabolism, and increasing the number of FTa muscle fibers improve the horse's ability to exercise longer, faster, and farther without the effects of lactic acid build-up in the muscles. However, with faster or longer exercise, the horse's aerobic capacity is exceeded and all three types of muscle fibers (FTa, FTb, and ST) are depleted of fuel. Therefore, improving the anaerobic method of energy production is also essential.

Conditioning Muscles Anaerobically

Over a period of months, sprint conditioning repetitively depletes these fuel stores. In response, the muscles "learn" to store more fuel.

Anaerobic metabolism requires specific enzymes to convert fuel into

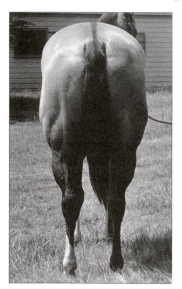

energy without oxygen. Sprint conditioning improves anaerobic metabolism by developing the cellular systems which produce these enzymes. Body systems which remove lactic acid from the working muscles, including the cardiovascular system, also improve through sprint conditioning.

Increasing Muscle Mass

Sprint conditioning increases the cross-sectional area of muscle fibers. An increase in the area of each individual fiber increases muscle mass as a whole. Most affected are the gluteal and thigh muscles, the chest, and the forearm muscles. Increased cross-sectional area of muscle fibers creates strength for the fast, explosive acceleration so vital to a successful sprint horse.

Fig. 6–2. Sprint conditioning strengthens gluteal and thigh muscles.

Buffering Lactic Acid

Anaerobic metabolism during sprint conditioning produces lactic acid, which causes fatigue. Muscle tissue normally contains protein buffers that neutralize lactic acid. Sprint conditioning stimulates the production of these proteins, which increases the buffering capacity of muscle cells, and therefore delays fatigue. *(See Chapter 3 for more information.)*

Using Lactic Acid as Fuel

The stamina of the sprint type horse also depends on the availability of glycogen supplies. If glycogen is depleted, the muscles run out of fuel, and muscle contractions weaken. A sprint horse works so quickly and for such a brief duration that lactic acid cannot be immediately flushed from the muscles. Some of this lactic acid can be metabolized by FTa muscle fibers that use oxygen to produce energy. Any lactic acid that can be converted to energy by FTa fibers improves a sprint horse's stamina.

Anaerobic training helps a horse's muscles learn to tolerate the anaerobic state. They learn to store more glycogen, increase in mass, develop enzyme systems to neutralize lactic acid, and can even produce energy from lactic acid to a small degree.

General Muscle Conditioning

Some conditioning effects do not depend on the type of metabolism occurring in a muscle fiber. Efficient heat dissipation and improved neuromuscular coordination are examples of general conditioning benefits.

Improving Heat Dissipation

The biochemical reactions that burn fuels for energy also produce heat as a by-product. Conditioning improves a horse's sweating mechanisms to efficiently dissipate heat from the working muscles. Reducing heat build-up further delays the onset of fatigue. *(See Chapter 8 for more information.)*

Improving Neuromuscular Reflexes

Conditioning improves neuromuscular reflexes, which in turn improves muscle coordination and efficiency of motion. Muscles work together to prevent straining a muscle, or damaging a joint. To prevent excessive exertion and damage in early stages of conditioning, *agonist* muscles have opposing *antagonist* muscles to counteract them. For example, an agonist flexor muscle that flexes a joint is opposed by an antagonist extensor muscle. This system limits muscle action to a safe degree.

A young, awkward horse does not have fine tuned coordination of the agonists working in concert with the antagonist muscles. If too much demand is placed on an undeveloped musculoskeletal system in the form of speed or distance, the unfit horse becomes muscle sore and is at risk of ligament or tendon damage as the muscle groups work against each other. Over time, reasonable repetitive exercises coordinate movement and improve neural signals to the muscles.

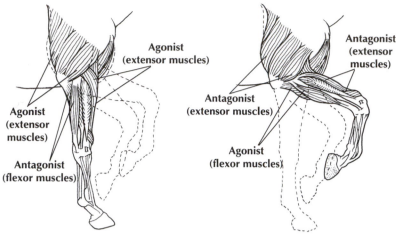

Fig. 6–3. Agonist and antagonist muscles work together to move a joint, each limiting the others' range of movement to prevent muscle and joint damage.

Conditioning the Respiratory System

The parts of the respiratory system include the larynx, trachea (windpipe), lungs, and diaphragm. The respiratory system does not directly adapt to conditioning. However, as other body systems (such as the circulatory system) become stronger, the respiratory system must maintain its efficiency of oxygen intake.

The relationship of the respiratory system to the abdominal cavity helps maintain breathing efficiency at speed. At the canter and gallop, each stride is accompanied by a breath. The synchronization of breathing with the stride prevents motion from interfering with air intake.

Synchronization of Stride and Breath

When the forelegs are off the ground in the canter or gallop, they are reaching forward. The head and neck swing upward, and pull on connecting muscles that attach to the thorax. This action pulls the rib cage forward and expands it outward. The body accelerates forward as the hind legs push off the ground. At the same time, the internal organs are displaced to the rear, making more room in the chest. The combination of rib movement and internal organ displacement allows efficient inhalation.

When the leading foreleg hits the ground, the rib cage is compressed as it absorbs some of the force of impact. The fast-moving horse slightly decelerates and, like a piston, the internal organs slide forward to

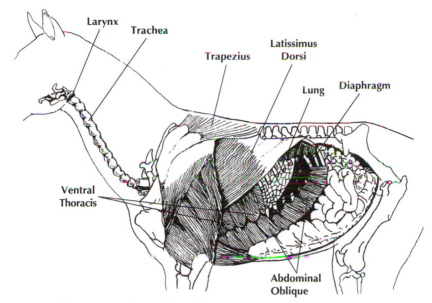

Fig. 6–4. The organs and muscles of the respiratory system.

squeeze air from the lungs. The compression of the rib cage and forward movement of the intestines promote exhalation.

As the number of strides increases with speed, each inhalation and exhalation must move as much air as possible to fuel the tissues with oxygen. Muscles that work the respiratory system (the diaphragm, abdominal, and thoracic muscles) become stronger with conditioning.

Conditioning the Cardiovascular System

If a horse is to use the aerobic method of energy production, it must have adequate oxygen. Improving a horse's aerobic capacity in the skeletal muscles, therefore, requires similar development of the cardiovascular system. Conditioning strengthens the heart to contract with increased power. At rest, a horse's skeletal muscles receive only 15% of the total blood flow in the body, but during rigorous exercise, 70% of the blood is circulated to the muscles, carrying oxygen to support aerobic metabolism. Blood flow to the skeletal and cardiac muscles and to the lungs increases 20-fold with conditioning.

Increased Red Blood Cells

During intense exercise, a horse increases its oxygen consumption

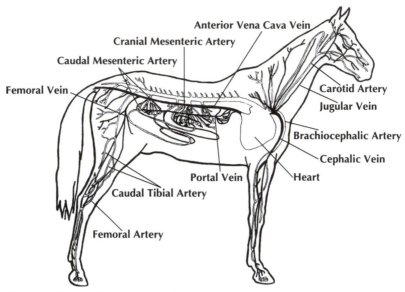

Fig. 6–5. The cardiovascular system.

36-fold. Red blood cells contain *hemoglobin* which binds oxygen and carries it through the bloodstream to the organs and tissues. To accommodate the huge demand for oxygen, the bloodstream is flooded with a reserve of red blood cells. These cells are stored in the spleen for times more oxygen is required in the muscle tissues. With conditioning, the number of hemoglobin molecules in the body increases up to 50%. At high altitudes, a horse's body similarly compensates for the reduced oxygen by manufacturing more hemoglobin, increasing the oxygen-carrying capacity of the blood. More oxygen in the blood means more oxygen available in the muscles for aerobic metabolism.

Heart Rate
Resting Heart Rate
A horse's heart rate increases sixfold during exercise to further improve the circulation of blood and oxygen to the tissues. A horse's normal resting heart rate is between 30 and 40 bpm, but some horses may have resting heart rates in the low 20s. At maximal exertion the heart rate may be as high as 240 bpm.

Conditioning does not necessarily lower a horse's resting heart rate. The resting heart rate seems to be genetically determined. However, conditioning will lower the horse's working heart rate at a specific effort. Lowering the working heart rate decreases the energy consumption of the heart, and gives the heart more time between beats to fill with the maximum volume of blood possible. When the heart is pumping more blood per contraction, blood flow to the tissues is optimized, therefore ample oxygen reaches the muscles.

Heart Rate Recovery

Conditioning improves a horse's heart rate recovery so that when exercise stops, the heart rate quickly returns to the resting rate. The heart rate of a well-conditioned endurance horse should drop to 100 bpm within 1 minute, and to less than 60 – 70 bpm within 10 minutes of rest. A sprint horse should recover to 150 – 180 bpm after 30 seconds, and to a rate between 100 – 140 bpm after 1 minute.

If recovery exceeds the recommended time, the horse's speed should be decreased or the distance shortened. Evaluating the heart rate provides detailed information about when to push to the next level of fitness without injury.

Heart Rate Variables

Heart rate is a measure of work output and is affected by many variables. The hotter and more humid the day, the more effort is required of the horse. The difficulty of terrain and footing affect a horse's heart rate, as do distance and fatigue, fear and excitement, and the genetic predisposition of a horse's muscle fiber type. An illness like a fever or colic will also raise the heart rate.

VALUE OF A HEART RATE MONITOR

One way to consistently evaluate the horse's working heart rate is by using a heart rate monitor. A heart rate monitor is a pocket-sized digital computer that is plugged into electrodes. These electrodes are placed on the horse's withers and beneath the girth. It is a handy, inexpensive device that enables a scientific training program to achieve maximum results.

The monitor allows the athlete's work effort to be measured by the working heart rate while it is still exercising. Without the use of a heart rate monitor, by the time a rider stops the horse, dismounts, and counts the heart rate for 15 seconds, it has dropped 50 – 100 bpm.

Monitoring Working Heart Rate

With a heart rate monitor a horse can be ridden within its abilities while its level of fitness is systematically evaluated. For example, a horse in endurance type training moves at paces of walk, trot, and slow canter

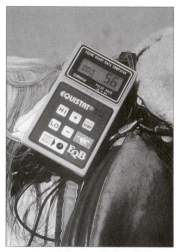
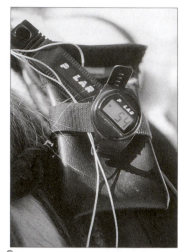

Fig. 6–6. On the left, an EqB Equistat® heart rate monitor. On the right, a V-Max heart rate monitor with wrist watch receiver. Both types are valuable conditioning tools.

with a heart rate between 124 – 150 bpm. To develop the aerobic capacity, work the horse just below the level of lactic acid accumulation. (Lactic acid accumulation begins at heart rates above 150 – 160 bpm.) The time necessary to develop the aerobic capacity will vary with the individual. As the aerobic capacity improves, work the horse at 200 bpm for short periods. This training effect further improves a horse's aerobic capacity while minimizing the risk of musculoskeletal injury.

A heart rate monitor also enables the rider to gradually increase the distance at a specified heart rate, incrementally and safely stressing the cardiovascular and musculoskeletal systems. Each progressive level of challenge created by an increase in speed *or* distance stimulates the body's adaptive response.

For example, hill

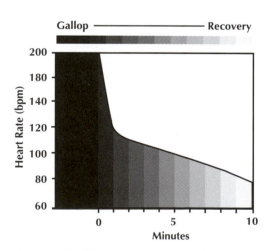

Fig. 6–7. Ideal heart rate recovery after a 1 – 2 mile gallop.

climbs elevate the heart rate and lactic acid production, but once at the top of the hill, the heart rate should decrease to less than 150 bpm for muscle recovery and removal of excess lactic acid. Within 1 minute of downhill, the heart rate should be less than 110 bpm.

Another example of the use of a heart rate monitor in conditioning is the training of a racehorse. After a 1 or 2-mile gallop at 200 bpm, the heart rate should recover to less than 120 within 2 minutes, and to less than 80 within 10 minutes.

Detecting Fatigue

A monitor accurately gauges a horse's work effort to indicate the onset of fatigue. The heart rate elevates as fuel reserves are depleted. If the heart rate increases at a constant work effort, the pace should be reduced to avoid metabolic or musculoskeletal problems.

Detecting Injury

Not only does a heart rate monitor fine tune a horse's conditioning program, but it is acutely sensitive to subtle pain created by a beginning musculoskeletal injury. If a horse's normal working heart rate at a specific task is known, and there is a rise of 10 bpm over normal while the horse is attempting that task, work can be stopped immediately before a mild injury is aggravated.

Performing a Field Fitness Test

A heart rate monitor is useful to perform a *field fitness test* to evaluate a horse's aerobic capacity. This test is done by measuring the velocity at 200 bpm (V_{200}) after a warm-up period. Velocity is the distance per unit of time (miles per hour, for example). To perform the field test, measure and mark off a set distance of ¾ – 1 mile, and then record the time it takes for the horse to cover that distance with the heart rate maintained as close to 200 bpm as possible. The fitter the horse, the faster it must go to achieve a heart rate of 200 bpm, and the greater its aerobic capacity. V_{200} can be compared every month, determining improvements in fitness. Heart rate measurements only evaluate aerobic capacity, however, not structural strength.

If a horse is unfit initially, then evaluate it at 160 bpm (V_{160}). This is the rate at which lactic acid accumulates faster than it can be metabolized. The speed it can go at this heart rate while lactic acid is being formed defines the horse's aerobic capacity. V_{160} is not a perfectly accurate indicator of fitness because pain or excitement can artificially drive the heart rate up to 160 bpm without muscular work being performed. However, it is a useful rate to start with for a horse re-entering training after a long layoff, or for an older or young horse at risk of musculoskeletal injury at fast speeds.

CONDITIONING PREPARATION

Conditioning a horse does not just apply to exercise programs. It is important to also "condition" a horse's overall health to provide it with a solid metabolic and structural foundation.

Veterinary Evaluation

Before beginning an intensive training schedule, arrange an appointment with a veterinarian for an evaluation. A veterinarian can assess the horse's general physical condition, with nutritional planning to accommodate the level of work the horse currently sustains and the rigorous level of athletics it should reach in the months ahead.

Feet

The feet should be balanced and shod before beginning a consistent exercise schedule. As workouts accelerate, healthy feet are imperative to ensure continued soundness. Conscientious maintenance prevents bruises, torn hooves, or hoof cracks. A properly balanced foot best absorbs concussion and deters lameness. *(For more information, see Chapter 4.)*

Diet

Rigorous exercise requires more food. However, be careful not to feed too much rich spring grasses, alfalfa hay, or grain as these feeds can lead to gas colic or laminitis. Horses need ample roughage in the diet to maintain a healthy intestinal tract. *(For more information, see Chapter 7.)* Check stored hay supplies to ensure that they have not become dusty and are free of mold. Dust and mold are harmful to the lungs, and can result in chronic respiratory disease.

Teeth

Only a well-nourished athlete can perform to potential. A horse's teeth should be examined and floated, if necessary, to encourage efficient digestion of food. Teeth should be in good condition so feed is adequately ground and can be processed by the digestive tract, decreasing the possibility of gaseous or impaction colics.

Floating the teeth also eliminates sharp edges, preventing painful ulcers in the mouth that might interfere with bitting or response to bit contact. If *wolf teeth* are present, remove them before beginning the conditioning schedule so healing can proceed with minimal interference to performance.

Immunizations

The athlete should be on a thorough immunization program before and during a conditioning regimen. Protection against viral respiratory diseases is critical because a performance horse is exposed to other horses as it campaigns. The body is mildly stressed by exercise workouts, and the immune system is further challenged by contact with other horses and new areas. "Spring" shots consist of a booster vaccine for Eastern and Western encephalomyelitis (sleeping sickness), tetanus, influenza, and rhinopneumonitis. Plan to boost respiratory vaccines (influenza and rhinopneumonitis) every 3 months.

In areas where diseases such as strangles, Venezuelan Encephalitis, Potomac Horse Fever, *equine viral arteritis*, or rabies are prevalent, include vaccines to build immunity to these threats. *(For more information, see Chapter 5.)*

Deworming

An aggressive deworming schedule every 6 – 8 weeks reduces the damage caused by intestinal parasites. Intestinal worms also cause colic by interrupting normal intestinal movement and altering the blood supply to the intestines. Clean the manure from the paddock twice a week to limit reinfection with parasite eggs. *(For more information, see Chapter 14.)*

Stall Hygiene

If a horse is confined to a stall, careful attention should be paid to daily stall cleaning and hygiene. Removing fecal matter and soiled bedding prevents reinfection by parasite eggs, and controls the conditions that favor thrush. Removing urine-soaked bedding also reduces ammonia fumes, promoting respiratory health.

TRAINING METHODS

Ultimately each athlete is trained for a specific task. However, the performance horse must have a strong foundation on which to build for each phase of the conditioning process. A strategically planned conditioning program means a commitment to pursue it for many months.

Consistency of workouts is an important ingredient to increasing biomechanical strength. "Progressive training" methods include a recovery period for the body to adapt to training and stress. In this way, a horse continues to build strength with less risk of strain or fatigue, and develops into a fit athlete.

Humans typically require about 10 weeks to increase muscular strength by 50%, because neuromuscular coordination is required for "neural learning" and control. Similar biophysical processes occur in horses, and all body tissues must respond to incremental challenges. Tissue with a generous blood supply responds quickest: muscle tissue is the fastest to respond (about 3 – 6 months), ligaments and tendons take longer to condition (6 – 12 months), and bone takes the longest time to fully condition (1 – 2 years). To advance a horse to absolute peak condition may require as long as **2 years**.

Once a horse has been well-conditioned, it does not rapidly lose fitness. While people lose fitness in only 2 weeks, a horse retains condition for a month or more, and is able to return quickly to previous levels of conditioning. Once a foundation has been built, only 3 – 6 months is necessary to return a horse to peak condition after a long layoff.

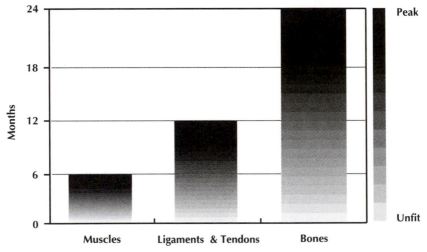

Fig. 6–8. Conditioning times of body structures.

Value of Repetition

Progressive increases in speed or distance over time (conditioning) enhance strength and durability. Once a conditioning program is begun, commit to it. To condition a horse, it must be *repeatedly and consistently* stressed before the tissues have a chance to fully recover from a prior workout. This method promotes adaptation and strengthening of body structures to build a solid foundation. Bone, cartilage, ligaments, and tendons must be slowly trained over time to meet the demands of added exertion. Sudden speed bursts on unconditioned support structures in the limbs can overload these living components, resulting in damage and lameness. Progressive stresses, however, challenge the tissues and result in *strength* training of muscles, ligaments, and bone.

Value of Walking

Do not underestimate the value of walking. Walking improves condition by slowly stimulating ligaments, tendons, and muscles to accept a slight increase in load. Walking loads a horse's ankle with 2½ times its weight. The stifle and hip are loaded

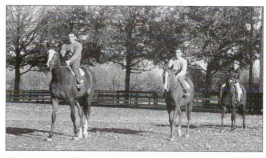

Fig. 6–9. Walking is important for conditioning.

with 1½ times the horse's weight. Walking increases the heart rate to 90 bpm. Blood vessels dilate and become elastic, allowing blood to flow with less resistance. An adequate warm-up of 10 minutes of walking enhances delivery of blood and oxygen to working muscles. Only a small percentage of muscle fibers are recruited at a walk, primarily the slow twitch and a few of the fast twitch high oxidative muscle fibers. These muscle tissues learn to improve oxygen delivery and removal of toxic by-products. Walking alone does not adequately stress the tissues to train them to higher levels of effort. However, it is an excellent starting point to build on, and is useful for a relaxed exercise.

Value of Swimming

Swimming can be added to a routine conditioning program of flat and hill work to provide cardiovascular and respiratory conditioning without concussive stress on the limbs. It is also a useful form of training that

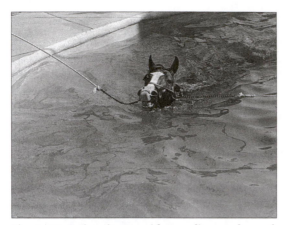

Fig. 6–10. Swimming provides cardiovascular and respiratory conditioning without weight-bearing.

can be applied to a young horse or while rehabilitating an injured horse. For the young horse, swimming strengthens the cardiovascular system without straining growing bone, and develops joints, tendons, and ligaments. The exercise of swimming maintains cardiovascular and respiratory fitness of an injured horse without any loading stress placed on the injured limb. The movement of the limbs through the water passively stretches healing joints and tendons, and the water massages the tissue to improve circulation.

However, using swimming as the sole means of exercise while rehabilitating a horse will not provide the cyclic loading stress on bones, joints, tendons, ligaments, and hooves that is part of a normal conditioning process. The horse will also require the weight-bearing stresses of adequate land preparation before beginning or returning to competitive athletics.

Phase 1: Long Slow Distance Training

Long Slow Distance (LSD) is used to build a foundation for further training for any equine sport. As an initial conditioning technique it slowly develops the structural strength of bone, muscle, ligaments, joint cartilage, and hooves with minimum risk of injury. All LSD work is performed below the anaerobic threshold so minimum lactic acid accumulates. LSD develops muscle fibers that use oxygen to burn fuel for maximum stamina.

An intelligent conditioning program starts with long, slow mileage, and speed is then increased gradually as the months go by. As a horse is incrementally challenged, speed and distance are *never* increased at once. One or the other is increased, but never both together.

The first month of conditioning is different for a young horse or for a horse recovering from an injury or illness than for a mature and sound horse. Young or injured horses need a lower intensity schedule so as not to overtax their systems. The second and third month of conditioning is the same for either level of fitness; however, these exercises are recommendations only. Every horse is different and trainers or owners will need to make adjustments. Tailor the conditioning program to the athlete. Veterinary advice is recommended for all phases of conditioning.

LSD Training for the Young or Injured Horse

During the first month of LSD training for the young or injured horse, it is best to start working on flat, even, and forgiving footing, preferably in straight lines. Longeing strains underconditioned joints and tendons.

PHASE I — YOUNG OR INJURED HORSE	
Long Slow Distance Training	
FIRST MONTH **Week 1**	**15 – 20 minutes, every other day or 3 days per week** **Alternate between ⅔ walk and ⅓ trot**
Week 2	**30 minutes, 3 – 4 days per week** **Alternate between walk and trot**
Week 3	**30 – 60 minutes, 4 – 5 days per week** **Increase distance but keep speed same as first two weeks** **Lengthen trot duration** **Mild inclines at the walk**
Week 4	**Add canter intervals for 1 – 2 minutes** **Change leads intermittently**
SECOND MONTH (Same as Mature, Sound Horse)	**Build to 10 miles per day at walk and trot, 3 – 4 days per week** **Increase mileage not speed**
THIRD MONTH (Same as Mature, Sound Horse)	**Add speed for HR 120 – 150 bpm for 1 hour:** **4 – 7 m.p.h. in hilly terrain *or*** **8 – 12 m.p.h. on level ground**

Fig. 6–11.

The First Month

Spend the first 2 weeks of the program alternating between the walk and trot, while spending two-thirds of the overall time at a walk. Start with 15 – 20 minutes for each exercise period, working up to an hour by the end of 2 weeks. Initially, it is best to exercise a horse every other day, or 3 – 4 days a week, as this schedule allows time for some tissue recovery and adaptation between stress efforts.

The third week, add a day of exercise and increase the distance but work at speeds similar to the first 2 weeks. The duration of trot intervals can be lengthened to several minutes at a time. Very mild inclines can be added for the walk interval.

The fourth week, add canter intervals of 1 – 2 minutes, but don't forget to ask intermittently for both leads, so both sides of the body are exercised equally. Within a month, the horse should be consistently working for 60 minutes, 5 days a week, at an average of 4 – 5 m.p.h.

LSD Training For the Mature and Sound Horse

The First Month

LSD training for a mature, uninjured horse can be slightly more demanding than the program outlined above. Initial workouts can begin with 20 – 30 minutes of walking and slow trotting. After 1 week, workouts should last a minimum of 30 minutes, 4 days a week. By the end of the second week, the horse can work for 30 – 60 minutes to stimulate an aerobic training effect. During the third and fourth weeks, a horse can walk and slow trot 4 – 6 miles a day, about 5 days a week. Several minutes of canter intervals can be introduced at the beginning of the fourth week.

Vary the types of exercise performed, not only to supple and strengthen different muscle groups, but to keep a horse's mind interested and active. Variety can include arena work, cavalletti poles, and trail rides. Race training could include off-track walking, or riding, and hand-grazing when *(and where)* possible provides a change of scene on a scheduled rest day.

The Next Two Months

During the second month of workouts increase mileage, not speed, building to 10 miles a day of walk and trot, 3 – 4 days a week. The third month add speed. The conditioning goal is to work at a heart rate of 120 – 150 bpm for at least 1 hour. To achieve this goal, work the horse at 4 – 7 m.p.h. in hilly terrain, or 8 – 12 m.p.h. on level ground such as a track.

PHASE I — MATURE AND SOUND HORSE	
Long Slow Distance Training	
FIRST MONTH **Week 1**	**20 – 30 minutes, 3 days per week** **Alternate between walk and slow trot**
Week 2	**30 – 60 minutes, 4 days per week**
Week 3	**60 – 90 minutes, 5 days per week** **Walk and slow trot 4 – 6 miles per day**
Week 4	**Add canter intervals for 3 – 5 minutes**
SECOND MONTH	**Build to 10 miles per day, at walk and trot,** **3 – 4 days per week** **Increase mileage not speed**
THIRD MONTH	**Add speed for HR 120 – 150 bpm for 1 hour:** **4 – 7 m.p.h. in hilly terrain** *or* **8 – 12 m.p.h. on level ground**

Fig. 6–12.

Phase 2: Cardiovascular Conditioning
The Fourth Month

The second phase of conditioning improves a horse's cardiovascular fitness to increase oxygen delivery to the tissues and delay the onset of fatigue. Hill training is an excellent way to improve both the musculoskeletal and cardiovascular systems. Working a horse on hills is similar to weightlifting; it develops shoulder muscles, hip extensors, and the quadriceps muscles which swing the hind leg forward. As muscles become more powerful, locomotion is less tiring and the whole body operates more efficiently. Perform downhill work slowly to reduce wear and tear on the forelegs. A slow downhill trot helps a horse learn balance, but it should not be overdone.

Once the horse has successfully come through the first 3 months of LSD, 20 – 30 minutes of extended trot on flat ground warms the muscles and increases circulation, preparing the horse for a slightly greater intensity of exercise. Then a gradual increase in duration or speed of hill work can be incorporated into the training periods.

During the fourth month, add speed workouts once or twice a week to stimulate the fast twitch high oxidative muscle fibers. *Fartleks*, or speed plays, include short, fast gallops or uphill canters interspersed between walk, trot, and canter paces. Both high intensity, short duration exercises and low intensity, long duration exercises improve a horse's aerobic capacity.

Once the musculoskeletal system is strengthened through LSD, and the cardiovascular system is similarly strengthened, customize the training program towards the specific tasks of the intended competitive athletics through *interval training*.

PHASE II — ALL HORSES
Cardiovascular Training

FOURTH MONTH	• **Warm up 20 – 30 minutes at an extended trot on flat ground** • **Add speed play workouts including short, fast gallops or uphill canters once or twice per week** • **Increase duration *or* speed of hill work** • **Slow downhill work at the walk and some trot**

Fig. 6–13.

Phase 3: Interval Training for Speed and Anaerobic Tolerance

Interval training teaches a horse's body to tolerate the anaerobic state, and it develops a horse's inborn potential for speed. These goals are accomplished by performing repeated bouts of high intensity exercise for a set distance or time, followed by a walk or trot recovery period between each high intensity effort. This technique conditions horses for maximal exertions up to 3 minutes without risking structural damage.

Training Effects

The effects of interval training (IT) include:

• strengthening of the heart, with increased blood pumped with each contraction
• expansion of blood vessels
• increased blood vessel elasticity to improve blood flow

Optimizing Oxygen Use

With interval training, fast twitch high oxidative muscle cells produce mitochondria. More mitochondria increases the use of available oxygen and produces more energy.

Interval training also encourages the spleen to increase the storage capacity for red blood cells. These red cells should enter the circulation about twice a week by sprinting the horse about ¼mile. If this does not occur, inactive red blood cells are destroyed by the spleen because they distort with age and lose their oxygen carrying capacity.

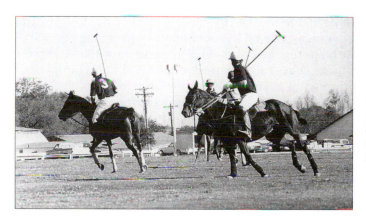

Fig. 6–14. Polo ponies benefit from interval training.

Reduced Lactic Acid

Interval training creates less lactic acid, delaying fatigue. Lactic acid fatigues muscles because it generates an acid environment (low pH) in the muscles. It takes about 30 minutes to clear lactic acid from the muscles and bloodstream after hard or prolonged exercise. Walking or slow trotting maintains blood flow to the muscles and flushes away lactic acid.

The intermittent recovery periods during IT promote *partial* lactic acid clearance from the muscles. Initially, recovery periods of 5 – 10 minutes flush enough lactic acid from the muscles to prevent rapid fatigue. Yet the fast intervals of IT challenge muscle cells to adapt to a low oxygen environment and to increase the anaerobic threshold. Eventually with improved condition, the recovery periods can be shortened to 5 minutes, and the high intensity work can be sustained for slightly longer.

The Fifth Month

By the fifth month, add interval training to the conditioning program about twice a week. IT is particularly useful for the racehorse, event horse, or polo pony because it improves lactic acid tolerance. It enables a horse's heart, lungs, and muscles to accommodate speed work for a competitive advantage. An endurance horse can also benefit from sessions of interval training. IT provides resources for when the endurance athlete lapses into anaerobic work due to difficult mountainous climbs, an excessively fast pace, or the onset of fatigue.

Challenge Without Risk

Over each exercise session of interval training the horse is cumulatively worked at greater distances and higher speeds than it would normally encounter if it were asked to gallop continuously. A horse can tolerate such training stress if it is not maintained for long periods. For example, the horse may be exercised at a heart rate of 180 – 200 bpm for at least 2 minutes. A trot recovery period of 4 – 5 minutes brings the heart rate down toward 100 bpm. Because the high intensity periods are of limited duration, musculoskeletal injury is reduced, yet the horse is challenged at intense conditions similar to or greater than competition.

It is necessary to incrementally challenge the equine athlete. Without some "moderate" stress to the system, the system will remain at current strength. A heart rate monitor enables the trainer to find a level of safe stress by working the horse between 180 – 200 bpm. The heart rate should drop to 110 bpm or below before embarking on the next high intensity interval. The heart rate recovery takes up to 10 minutes in an unfit horse and 4 – 5 minutes in a fit horse.

PHASE III — ALL HORSES	
Interval Training	
FIFTH MONTH	**Twice a week, repeated sets of high intensity work with walk or trot recovery between:** **Exercise at HR of 180 – 200 bpm for 2 min.** **Trot recovery period:** • **4 – 5 min. for a fit horse** • **Up to 10 min. for an unfit horse *or* until HR drops to 110 bpm or below**

Fig. 6–15.

Long Fast Distance Training

Long, fast distance training methods often lead to failure. Prolonged speed creates breakdown injuries or exhaustion. This training method does not allow the body to repair, much less strengthen, between efforts. The horse continually disintegrates and cannot improve past a certain performance level.

CAUSES OF POOR PERFORMANCE

To have the winning edge, an equine athlete must be able to summon all its resources to maximize performance. Some days everything clicks into place, and the horse just cannot be beat. But occasionally a horse reaches a period of crisis where performance begins to wane, imperceptibly at first, and then more consistently with each workout.

Overtraining

A common reason for poor performance is a phenomenon known as *overtraining*. A horse is ridden too often at too high a level of demand without a sufficient recovery period. Muscles exhaust their energy supplies during strenuous exercise, and they need time to restore energy and enzymes to drive biochemical reactions. Usually complete recovery only takes 12 – 24 hours. After extreme exertion, such as a competition or hours of very hard work, several days of rest may be necessary to replenish the stores. If a horse is continually pushed past the body's limit, all its reserves are depleted. The horse cannot compensate for the lack of muscle fuel needed to drive performance, and fatigue results.

Without rest and replenishment of carbohydrates, the depleted muscle cells of the overtrained horse will consume each other in an attempt to metabolize protein into glycogen. The bright bursts of brilliant performance typical of that individual fail to appear.

Initial Indications

Initial indications that a horse is stressed from an excessively intense training schedule include:

- elevated resting pulse
- abnormal sweating
- muscle tremors
- elevated working pulse
- poor heart rate recovery
- diarrhea

Symptoms of Overtraining

The overtrained horse is recognized by:

- failure to gain weight
- stiff and sore muscles
- stance becoming less alert
- weight loss
- dull eyes
- picking at food

Rest and Relaxation

If a horse starts to fail in performance, try backing off to an every other day training schedule rather than a daily workout, or consider walking for an hour on one of the days scheduled for a rigorous training period. Once the horse's fatigued body starts to recuperate, appetite will improve. The horse will facilitate its own rehabilitation by consuming needed nutrients and energy. Often trainers and riders attempt to supplement a horse with food additives and vitamins to restore luster, when what it really needs is rest and relaxation. To determine whether a horse is suffering from muscle damage or nutritional deficiencies, blood chemistry profiles can be analyzed before and after exercise.

Inability to Perform

Not all horses have the ability to be a premier athlete. It is sometimes puzzling that a horse that has everything in its favor is unable to meet an expected level of performance, especially when compared to other similarly endowed horses. Sometimes a horse does not have the combination of attributes to drive it to a pinnacle of excellence. Many times a horse's genetic capabilities are not properly suited to the assigned career. In other instances there is a physiologic reason for failure to perform to expectations.

Exercise Intolerance: Musculoskeletal Pain

A primary cause of exercise intolerance is injury or pain in the musculoskeletal system. If a horse hurts while exercising, it will try to avoid any movement that stimulates pain. Behavioral changes are a tip-off that something is wrong. The horse may swish its tail, pull its ears back, menace when saddled, or refuse the task at hand.

A practical and inexpensive method of detecting very subtle pain is to consistently ride the horse with a heart rate monitor. After many readings of the normal heart rate response to a given exertion, it is possible to identify beginning signs of discomfort. The heart rate rises during exercise that normally would not cause heart rate elevation.

Examples of Musculoskeletal Pain

Back pain results from improper conditioning, overexertion, forced head sets, or poor saddle fit. A heavy rider mismatched to a small horse also causes the horse back pain, as does an unbalanced or inexperienced rider. Poor conformation in the form of a long back exaggerates all of these factors. A horse with a sore back communicates displeasure by humping the back, kicking, bucking, wringing the tail, or gnashing the teeth.

A jumping horse with back pain may refuse or rush a jump, jump too flat, or twist the hind legs when clearing the jump. An event horse may demonstrate similar problems: the horse's speed may slow, and enthusiasm wanes as it fatigues faster than normal. Standardbred racehorses are also prone to back pain, as are dres-

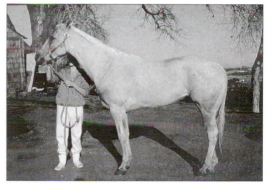

Fig. 6–16. A horse with a long back is predisposed to chronic back pain.

sage horses that are asked for continuous efforts of collection and engagement of the hindquarters.

A horse with muscle problems in any part of the body quickly stiffens and tires with exertion, leading to poor performance. Tying-up *(myositis)* can cause a horse to stop work because of severe pain. *(See Chapter 3 for more information.)*

A horse with chronic arthritis often experiences days when the pain is aggravating enough that performance suffers. A horse with sore feet is especially prone to poor performance as its stride shortens, and muscles become restricted and tight as the horse tries to guard against the pain.

Hoof Imbalance

A frequent reason for musculoskeletal pain is hoof imbalance. Because the lower joints of the limb primarily move in flexion and extension with little rotation or sideways motion, defects in conformation or unbalanced shoeing create abnormal sideways stress on the lower joints. One side of the hoof contacts the ground before the other, placing strain on joint ligaments and cartilage. The hoof records this stress with an uneven coronary band, along with flares and ridges in the hoof wall.

A long-toe – low-heel foot configuration creates extreme and prolonged fetlock drop, resulting in excessive pull on the deep digital flexor tendon and coffin joint. This poor type of foot alignment creates low grade chronic pain which reduces performance. A treadmill gait analysis effectively analyzes dynamic placement of the foot in motion. This analysis may be important because "balance" of the static foot does not always produce optimal results for the moving limb.

Diagnostic Lameness Exam

A veterinarian can identify the source of the pain with a lameness workup. A diagnostic lameness exam includes:

- careful evaluation of the horse at the trot on different ground surfaces (hard or soft), with or without a rider's weight, and on different inclined planes
- hoof testers to check for a specific painful area
- careful palpation and manipulation of all structures in the limb to test for a pained response
- flexion tests of the affected limb to stress different joints
- diagnostic nerve blocks to anesthetize parts of the limb starting from the ground and working up the limb in a process of elimination
- radiographic evaluation of the painful area that has been isolated through the clinical exam and the above described diagnostic procedures

New Techniques

Sophisticated technology is also incorporated into an exam of the musculoskeletal system if the source of the problem is not readily apparent. Video technology enables the veterinarian to analyze a horse's gait in slow motion for an accurate measure of foot fall, stride length, and imbalance to diagnose an obscure lameness. Detailed gait analysis on a treadmill helps a veterinarian recommend shoeing changes that might improve the horse's movement.

Diagnostic ultrasound is useful for assessing the health and integrity of tendons and ligaments. *(See Chapter 9 for more information.)*

Nuclear scintigraphy is a technique that involves injecting a radio-opaque dye into the bloodstream. Then a computer-generated gamma scan of the bones, muscles, and joints identifies areas of inflammation where the dye concentrates. These areas of increased circulation are called "hot spots."

Infrared thermography is a tool to measure the temperature differences within tissues to similarly identify pockets of inflammation.

Lameness Classification

To facilitate communication with a veterinarian when discussing an injury, the American Association of Equine Practitioners (AAEP) provides terminology classifying lameness relative to the degree of severity. Lameness is best seen at the two-beat gait of a trot. As the affected limb hits the ground, the horse lifts the head in an effort to quickly remove the weight off that leg. As the sound limb hits the ground, the head drops because the horse is willing to assume weight on the good leg.

Grade 1 lameness is difficult to observe because it is inconsistent, but may appear while circling, weight-bearing, or on hard surfaces. A visually apparent head nod or bob occurs with each stride in a circle in a Grade 2 or greater lameness. Any lameness that persists as a Grade 3 (visible at every stride) or more should quickly receive veterinary care.

LAMENESS CLASSIFICATION	
Grade	**Observable Signs**
Grade 1	Difficult to observe, not consistently apparent with weight-bearing, circling, inclines, or hard surfaces.
Grade 2	Difficult to observe at walk or trot in straight line. Apparent with weight-bearing, circling, inclines, and hard surfaces.
Grade 3	Consistent at trot under all circumstances.
Grade 4	Obvious lameness with marked head nodding, hitching, or a shortened stride. Visible at walk.
Grade 5	Minimal weight-bearing in motion and/or at rest, or the inability to move.

Fig. 6–17.

Exercise Intolerance: Respiratory Problems

Another common cause of exercise intolerance is a failure of the respiratory tract to meet the demands of performance. The respiratory tract is divided into two sections: upper and lower.

Upper Respiratory System

The upper respiratory system includes the nostrils, nasal passages, pharynx, larynx, and trachea up to the thorax.

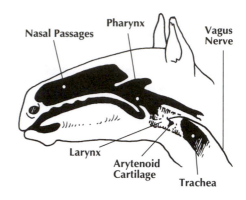

Fig. 6–18. The upper respiratory system.

Roaring

Racehorses, steeplechasers, eventers, and jumpers are often asked to perform at peak speeds, and the tiniest impairment to respiratory ability can quickly turn a potential winner into a loser. At least 5% of Thoroughbred racehorses suffer from *laryngeal hemiplegia* (also called recurrent laryngeal neuropathy, or RLN) which causes a *roaring* condition.

The muscle which opens the arytenoid cartilage of the larynx is stimulated by the recurrent laryngeal nerve (a branch of the vagus nerve). If the nerve is damaged, the muscle is paralyzed. The cartilage then collapses into the airway. As air passes through the diminished opening, air turbulence creates a roaring noise with each breath. A horse with this condition is unable to breathe enough oxygen to fuel the demanding muscles, therefore speed and performance are severely compromised.

Dr. W. Robert Cook has linked a narrow jaw width with RLN. The average Thoroughbred has a normal jaw width equivalent to at least 4 fingers (7.2 centimeters). To measure the jaw width, fold the fingers at the joint below the knuckles with the back of the hand resting against the underside of the horse's neck. The fingers are placed between the lower jaw bones at the level of the throatlatch. The narrower this measurement, the greater the likelihood the horse will be afflicted with some degree of RLN.

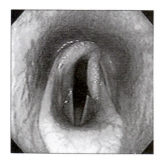
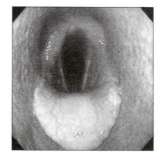

Fig. 6–19. On the left, the arytenoid cartilage before surgery, seen through an endoscope. On the right, the airway after surgery.

Roaring is also diagnosed by passing an *endoscope* into the horse's nose to the back of the throat. To determine the extent of the laryngeal paralysis, it is sometimes necessary to examine the horse while it is working on a treadmill. Surgery is moderately successful in returning affected horses to top performance.

Other Throat Problems

Other throat problems can lead to a diminished opening of the larynx and airway obstruction and can be identified with an endoscope. These problems include:

- *dorsal displacement of the soft palate*
- *epiglottic entrapment*
- *pharyngeal lymphoid hyperplasia*
- *arytenoid chondritis*

The first two syndromes interfere with the seal created by the soft palate and the larynx that maintains air pressure in the airways. The other two syndromes involve inflammation and distortion of the back of the throat that may obstruct normal air flow.

Lower Respiratory System

The lower respiratory organs include the branches of the trachea, bronchi, and the left and right lungs. Problems relating to the lower respiratory system usually result from viral or bacterial infection, or allergic reactions. Viral respiratory infections can predispose to:

- bacterial pneumonia or pleuropneumonia
- lung abscesses
- chronic obstructive pulmonary disease (COPD, or heaves)

These problems may produce lasting conditions that permanently interfere with a horse's respiratory capacity and performance. On rare occasions, cancer in the thorax may slowly compromise a horse's lung capacity.

Bleeding

Exercise-induced pulmonary hemorrhage (EIPH) is primarily a condition seen in racehorses; affected animals are called *bleeders*. Blood accumulates in the airways, and occasionally flows from the nose. It is not always easy to diagnose a horse affected by EIPH. Sometimes the horse coughs, or swallows excessively. On occasion, a horse may have trouble breathing. Difficulty in breathing may cause it to pull up suddenly during a race. The best way to identify a bleeder is to examine a suspect horse with an endoscope within 2 hours after exercise.

Vigorous Activity

Researchers are still trying to understand what actually causes EIPH. It seems to be a syndrome of horses that exercise strenuously, as with racing or steeplechasing. As many as 50% – 70% of horses participating in these sports have some degree of EIPH.

Lung Damage

EIPH may be the result of altered blood flow in areas of the lungs that have suffered previous inflammation. Inflammation in the airways increases blood flow in the walls of small airways, making them susceptible to rupture.

With maximal exertion, the lungs are inflated to full capacity at rates greater than 150 breaths per minute. If a previously damaged region of the lung fails to inflate, the adjacent good lung tissue that has inflated may distort the diseased area. Altered pressure differences develop between the good and bad lung tissue. Pressure changes and tissue tearing may rupture fragile capillary walls in the diseased lung area, causing bleeding.

The uninflatable area of the diseased lung can be a result of:

- prior infection or inflammation that has grown scar tissue
- mucus or debris in the airways following an attack of influenza or pneumonia, which reduces the opening of the airway, creating uneven pressures in the lungs
- allergies which constrict the airways with spasms, and functionally reduce the opening of the small airways

Upper Airway Obstruction

Although lower airway disease is the currently accepted theory to explain EIPH, Dr. W. Robert Cook maintains that RLN creates pressure changes in the lungs by obstructing airflow through the upper respiratory tract. As a horse with RLN inhales, the collapsed arytenoid cartilage obstructs airflow. This obstruction creates above normal pressure changes in the lungs that are strong enough to damage blood vessels in the lungs and cause bleeding.

Predisposition to EIPH

In summary, a horse may be predisposed to EIPH because of the following conditions:

- lung tissue has been damaged from inflammation due to viral, bacterial, parasitic infection, or allergic reactions
- blood pressure increases due to tremendous heart pumping during strenuous exertions
- a genetic predisposition to weak blood vessels lining the lungs
- recurrent laryngeal neuropathy

Lasix®

The impact of isolated incidents of EIPH on performance is not very well understood. Pre-race prevention using a diuretic called furosemide (Lasix®) has improved racing times in horses afflicted with EIPH. Because it is a diuretic, Lasix® causes urination within minutes. There is no doubt that chronic bleeding permanently alters lung tissue with an adverse affect on performance.

Prevention of EIPH

Prevention is difficult to define for a disease which is not entirely understood. However, any management procedures that can be used to minimize disease of the small airways may prevent EIPH. These techniques include:

- improved ventilation in barns
- relatively dust-free bedding
- high quality, dust-free, and mold-free hay
- ample recovery time (3 weeks) for respiratory infections
- an aggressive viral vaccination program of 4 times per year against influenza and rhinopneumonitis
- deworming at 6 – 8 week intervals to minimize damage from worms migrating through the lungs

Horses should be screened for RLN by an endoscopic exam, and the jaw width evaluated using techniques developed by Dr. W. Robert Cook.

Exercise Intolerance: Cardiac Problems
Heart Irregularities

Heart disease is uncommon in horses, but heart murmurs or irregularities in heart rate (arrhythmias) can be evaluated by ultrasound and an ECG (electrocardiogram). *Degenerative myocardial disease* is unusual, but does occur. Chronic respiratory disease places strain on the heart, and can create arrhythmias. Viral, bacterial, or protozoal infections can injure the heart valves. Electrolyte imbalances in the exercising horse have profound effects on heart contraction and cardiac output. Any condition that creates anemia or interferes with blood flow to the heart muscle also compromises the heart's effectiveness as a pump to supply blood and oxygen to the tissues. Certain drugs, toxins, or electrolyte imbalances can mimic heart disease symptoms, including:

- rapid heart rates   • irregular heart rates
- poor recovery rates   • acute fatigue   • fainting

Anemia

Red blood cells (RBCs) contain hemoglobin, which carries oxygen to the tissues as the blood circulates through the body. Any condition that results in blood loss or a failure of the body to manufacture red blood cells leads to *anemia.* A large intestinal parasite load can consume blood. A chronic infection or inflammatory condition consumes both white and red blood cells resulting in a net loss of RBCs. Nutrient deficiencies of iron, copper, protein, and B vitamins can impair the body's ability to manufacture sufficient RBCs. A blood sample can be evaluated for anemia, along with the body's ability to produce RBCs.

Packed Cell Volume

The *packed cell volume* (PCV) measures the percentage of circulating red blood cells in the bloodstream. Normally a horse has a PCV of around 40%. A highly fit individual may store up to one-third of its RBCs in the spleen. Because the RBCs are present but hiding in the spleen, a fit horse may have a PCV about 30%. A horse with a PCV of less than 30% is considered anemic, and efforts should be made to identify the source of the lack of RBC.

Ulcers

A competitive horse is a stressed horse and is therefore prone to bleeding gastric ulcers. Often a horse with stomach ulcers has episodes of colic. If this condition is suspect, the stomach can be examined with an endoscope. Feces can be evaluated in the lab for the presence of digested blood that may indicate a bleeding intestinal ulcer.

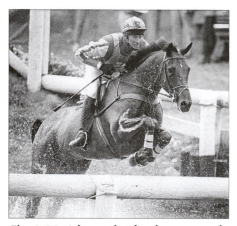

Fig. 6–20. A horse that has been properly warmed up before competition performs better and more safely.

WARM-UPS & COOL-DOWNS

The horse is naturally designed for short bursts of speed to flee predators. In the wild, it does not have to sustain this flight or fight response for more than a few moments. Today, horses are asked to perform for extended periods at a maximal level of work. Many equine sports require fast bursts of speed combined with abrupt stops and turns, or jumping over obstacles while carrying a rider.

Other sports involve long hours of steady work under saddle with infrequent rest periods. Just as with human athletes, a horse needs to limber up and stretch before beginning a workout.

To prevent injury, each workout should include a routine of warm-ups and cool-downs before and after exercise. Muscles, ligaments, and tendons should be properly prepared for the demands of athletic exertion. This preparation involves at least 15 – 20 minutes of warm-up to stimulate blood circulation to the tissues, and to slightly raise body temperature a few degrees. Warmth and circulation improve the flexibility of the musculoskeletal system, improving efficiency of muscle work and reducing the risk of injury to ligaments, tendons, and joints.

Warm-Up Exercises

Walking

Walking is a preliminary exercise to gradually increase the respiratory rate and heart rate, flushing the muscles with blood and oxygen. Walking lightly stretches tendons and ligaments to improve their elasticity as the tissues heat up from movement. Joints are also warmed and lubricated.

Walking can be done under saddle, in hand, on a longe line, or by using a hot-walker. Brisk walking for 5 – 10 minutes sufficiently prepares the musculoskeletal system for more work.

Trotting

After walking, the horse can then be trotted for another 5 – 10 minutes to further warm the muscles, and to stretch tendons and ligaments. Urge the horse forward at a vigorous pace, which further improves the respiratory intake of oxygen and accelerates the heart rate. These physiologic changes allow the musculoskeletal system to handle increased stress.

Manual Stretching Exercises

Once the muscles, tendons, and ligaments are warm, manual stretching exercises add flexibility. If a muscle is stretched 100% of its functional length before contraction, the strength of the muscle contraction works at maximum efficiency. Most horses are trained at a muscle exertion of only 60% of maximum contraction length, leading to tight, unsupple muscle with a diminished range of motion. Sudden loading of a short, tight, and inelastic musculotendinous unit may tear muscle or tendon fibers. To maximize muscle and tendon elasticity, apply stretching exercises in both warm-ups and cool-downs.

During a stretch, maintain each limb in a slightly flexed position to avoid strain to the tendons and ligaments of the lower leg. Grasp the limb above the knee or just below the hock. Each pull should be concentrated above the knee or hock for a greater range of motion in the shoulder or hip joints and their associated muscles.

Hold each stretch for 15 or 20 seconds. It may take several days of practice for a horse to become accustomed to the strange feel of these stretches without resisting. Do not force the stretch. Ask the horse to passively "let go" in response to a gentle tug.

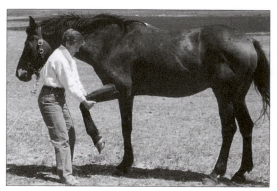

Fig. 6–21. Foreleg stretch.

Forelegs

Pick up each front leg individually and gently pull it forward to stretch the shoulder and forearm muscles. Then ease the limb forward and across the body toward the other foreleg. Also pull the leg gently to the outside, and then backward toward the hind legs.

Hind Legs

Hind leg stretches are similar to foreleg stretches. Each hind leg is first stretched directly behind the horse, then toward the opposite hind leg. The hip and upper leg are then stretched forward toward the front legs, and finally gently tugged out to the side.

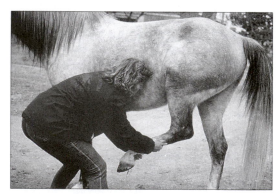

Fig. 6–22. Hind leg stretch.

Suppling Exercises

While mounted, relax the horse's neck and back muscles by bending the head and neck to the side (toward the rider's leg) with a slight jiggle of the rein. This technique softens the poll and jaw as the horse gives to the rein.

A long, downward stretch of the head and neck can be accomplished by making the horse reach down for a carrot or other treat. This stretch loosens the back and loins, while the horse also relaxes mentally.

Moving in circles, figure eight patterns, and serpentine patterns asks the horse to step under the body with the inside rear leg, stretching the back and haunches.

Lateral exercises, such as leg yields or side-passes supple the poll, neck, shoulders, back, and haunches. The horse gradually begins to actively carry itself by using muscle groups in concert.

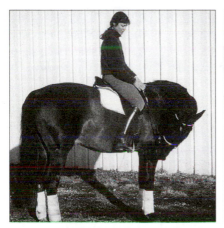 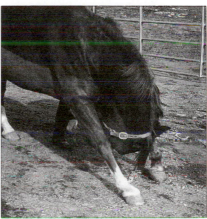

Fig. 6–23. Bending the head to the side softens the poll and jaw.

Fig. 6–24. Bending for a carrot stretches the back and loins.

Long-Term Benefits

Stretching and suppling exercises have more long-term benefits than just the immediate improvement of tissue elasticity. Daily application of stretching exercises both before and after exercise ultimately:

- develops a longer stride as shoulders move with greater freedom
- improves the range of motion in both shoulder and hip muscles to facilitate lateral movements
- improves flexibility in the upper limbs, reducing the risk of injury during stressful demands
- causes less fatigue because muscles and joints are pliable
- improves circulation to all the tissues, requiring less effort during a warm-up and conserving energy for the athletic exertion

Specific Sports Warm-up

The entire warm-up process, exploring all varieties of stretching and suppling exercises, can take as long as 30 minutes. As the warm-up intensifies after the first 20 minutes, a jumping horse might be asked to trot cavalettis, or jump several small obstacles (less than 2 feet high). A western performance horse would be worked at intervals of trot and canter in figures using the entire arena. A trail horse could gradually begin a mild incline after 10 or 15 minutes of trotting. A racehorse would be breezed at a slow canter after the initial warm-up to gradually increase cardiac output and blood flow to the muscles.

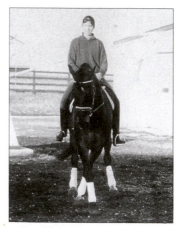

Fig. 6–25. Side-passes supple the poll, neck, shoulders, back, and haunches.

Cool-Down Exercises

After a horse has finished a workout, devote 15 – 30 minutes to cooling down at a walk or slow trot. It is best to keep a horse moving during a cool-down to dissipate heat generated by working muscles. Dissipating heat will cause muscle and body temperature to slowly decline. Blood that was routed to the muscles is gradually redirected back to internal organs. Oxygen is replenished to muscles that reached an oxygen debt, and accumulated lactic acid is flushed from the muscles. Removal of lactic acid from the muscles is important for alleviating muscle soreness that can occur after exercise.

Post Exercise Stretches

While walking, a loose rein encourages the horse to stretch its own neck and back, relieving tension on overworked muscles that might begin to tighten. Once dismounted, the same manual stretches that were used during warm-up can also be used in a cool-down. Stretching reduces post exercise muscle soreness.

Muscle Massage

Muscle massage relaxes tight muscles, improving oxygen circulation in the muscles, and removing toxic by-products. The large muscles over the hip, neck, back, and thighs particularly benefit from 20 – 30 minutes of massage.

With firm pressure, use the heel of the hand or the fingertips to create a circular massaging motion over each muscle group. The horse will relax and most likely will lean into the pressure. As a finishing touch, apply a thick rubber curry comb in a circular motion to stimulate the skin and superficial muscles, while removing sweat and dirt from the coat.

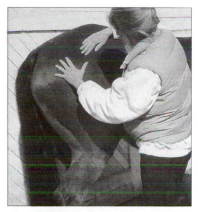

Fig. 6–26. Massaging relaxes tight muscles after exercise.

Food and Water

Once the horse's chest is cool to the touch, offer it hay and water. Wait about half an hour after the horse is *fully* cooled down before offering grain. Then blood flow is restored to the intestines, and the horse is less likely to develop gaseous colic.

Warm Weather Cool-Downs

During hot and humid weather, a horse may need additional help cooling down. Sponging the head, neck, chest, and legs helps remove body heat by improving evaporative cooling. Soak the large blood vessels along the neck and legs for maximum cooling, but stay away from the large muscle groups over the back and hindquarters. Sponging water on overheated, large muscle masses can cause them to spasm, and the horse then ties-up. After a pleasure ride that stimulated only a light sweat, the horse can be bathed following 15 – 30 minutes of cool-down.

Besides soaking the neck and chest, place the horse in an area shaded from the sun. If the air is particularly still, improve heat dissipation by directing a fan on the horse to push cool air past the skin.

For a horse that exercises during warm weather, it is best to maintain as lean a body weight as possible. Extra body fat delays heat dissipation from the muscles, and dramatically increases the cooling period.

Cool Weather Cool-Downs

It is important to cool down the working muscles adequately after a hard workout any time of the year, but it is essential during the cooler seasons. Working skeletal muscle generates a large amount of heat, and if insufficiently cooled down, or if exposed to cold rain or water directly after a workout, muscle tissue may begin to spasm and cramp.

Insulation Delays Cool-Down

Fat Insulation

Fat is an insulating layer that acts as a "cushion" against climatic elements. A thin horse has fewer fat reserves against chills than an individual with a healthy covering of flesh.

On the other hand, an overweight horse has the opposite problem from a thin horse. Heat dissipates slowly from an overweight or underconditioned horse. An overweight horse may finish exercising with only a slight dampness around the neck. Then, 2 hours later, it may be soaked in the neck, chest, and girth areas because heat loss through the skin continues after exercise.

Hair Coat Insulation

When dry, the horse's hair coat provides insulating protection from chills and damp. A dense winter hair coat protects a horse from the elements, but its length makes it difficult to cool down the horse.

The shortened daylight hours of winter stimulate hairs to grow longer due to the effect of reduced light on the brain's *pineal gland.* A horse with a thick, heavy coat experiences the same phenomenon as a fat horse because the hair layer insulates against cooling. Delayed sweating is a natural occurrence, yet steps must be taken to protect damp horses from drafts and chills.

Horse hairs are evenly distributed on the body, rather than in clusters, as in dogs or cats. The loft in a horse's hair coat insulates it and retains body heat.

Cool-Down Methods

An adequate cool-down permits the circulation to flush away toxic by-products and heat, and prevents tying-up. Consider special cool-down procedures during winter weather such as walking, drying the hair coat, cover-ups, and body clipping.

Walking

Walking for 15 – 30 minutes cools muscles after an exertion, releasing much of the heat that contributes to sweating. Walking is the best way to cool down a horse in cold weather. Either hand walking or mechanical "hot-walkers" are useful. Walking maintains good circulation to the muscles, which dissipates heat.

Many people mistakenly believe that walking a horse after exercise will dry a damp hair coat. If the sun is shining, it dries a wet coat as the horse walks. However, a dry coat does not mean the horse is fully cool, and a cool horse may also be wet.

As muscles cool down, so do ligaments, joints, and tendons. Walking maintains flexibility in these structures, making the limbs less susceptible to injury. Bandages retain warmth and circulatory flow in the lower legs during the walking period. Leave splint boots or leg bandages on during the cool-down period to cool lower limbs slowly.

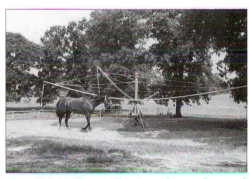

Fig. 6–27. A "hot-walker" can be used to cool muscles.

Drying the Hair Coat

Sweat scrapers are great for pulling extra moisture from the hair coat to regain loft and insulating capacities quickly. A brisk rubbing with a dry towel or brush also removes moisture from the coat, while exposing more hair surface to the air for faster drying. Toweling also "polishes" a dull coat. If necessary, an electric hair dryer *(set on low heat)* can be used to speed up drying of a soaked coat.

Body Clipping

To avoid prolonged cool-downs in the wintertime, many horses are body clipped to facilitate heat loss during exercise. Shaving hair away from the chest, abdomen, neck, and shoulders exposes a large area for evaporative cooling. Shaving also helps large surface blood vessels in these areas radiate heat away from the horse. However, if a horse has been body-clipped and the insulating fur layer removed, it is very important to cover the horse during resting hours.

Cover-Ups

Blanketing serves as a substitute for natural hair on clipped horses, protecting a horse from wind chill or wet weather. Blankets may also give additional protection against the elements for horses with a full hair coat. Many varieties of horse blankets are commercially available, each appropriate for different conditions.

Coolers

"Coolers" wick moisture away from the hair coat while keeping drafts

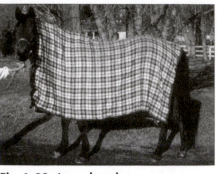

off the horse. A cooler is made of wool, acrylic, or a mixture of both. A wool cooler pulls moisture from the coat most effectively, while keeping a horse warm underneath. A cooler is poorly designed for trailer travel. It is too long and wide with no stabilizing straps. A horse can step on a cooler, and pull it off, risking it becoming entangled in the horse's legs.

Fig. 6–28. A wool cooler.

Anti-Sweat Sheets

An anti-sweat sheet works well to cool a hot horse. It is form-fitting and made of cotton or polypropylene. Holes or perforations in the sheet allow evaporation of moisture, while providing a protective covering similar to some brands of human thermal underwear.

Once a horse is cooled down fairly well, place another blanket on top of an anti-sweat sheet to produce a layering effect. The anti-sweat sheet

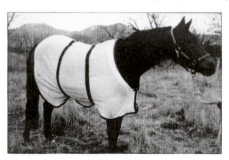

allows sweat to dry without holding in moisture that could become cold and clammy if kept close to the skin. Heat generated by the horse's muscles collects under the blanket layers, while moisture evaporates away, leaving a dry and warm horse underneath.

Fig. 6–29. An anti-sweat sheet.

Other Cover-Ups

A blanket with a wool liner helps to dry a wet horse while keeping it warm. The outer shell should be a "breathable" material so moisture can evaporate away from the horse's skin. Check with the manufacturer or tack shop if unsure about the properties of the outer shell.

Common materials used in horse blankets also include Gore-tex® or polypropylene. These materials create a water-resistant barrier. Yet, a wet horse cloaked in polypropylene or Gore-tex® dries quickly because of the unique "breathing" properties of these materials. The tight weave of these fabrics also creates a wind breaker effect.

Blanketing Wet Horses

Do not blanket a wet horse unless it is checked periodically for drying. A blanket soaked with sweat provides more surface area for evaporative cooling. More surface area increases the rate of body cooling, creating a "refrigerator effect," resulting in a chilled and miserable animal. Moisture evaporates from the skin faster than the body is able to warm the skin. Skin temperature decreases, and eventually chills the body as well. Certain fabrics such as cotton and Dacron enhance evaporative cooling, whereas wool can be wet and still retain some warmth.

Other Options

Enclosed Barn

Access to an enclosed barn provides greater cool-down options in inclement weather. A barn provides a draft-free environment with consistent temperatures. If a barn is well-insulated and warm, it is acceptable to wash the horse after a workout. If the hair is matted down by sweat, or caked with mud, vital body heat escapes. Washing sweat and dirt from the hair coat improves the insulating loft once it has dried. It is best to avoid bathing a horse during the winter months unless a warm barn is available to allow complete drying. *Repeated* bathing removes natural oils from a horse's hair and skin and reduces the water repellency of the hair coat. Bathing a horse in cold weather risks accidental chilling, even if using warm water. Use common sense: a dirty horse is better than a sick horse.

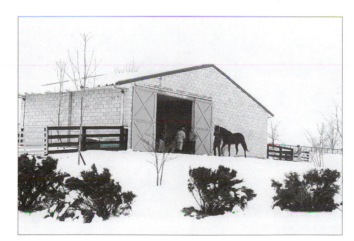

Fig. 6–30. An enclosed, well-insulated, warm barn is the best place to bathe horses in cold weather.

Management

Each horse tolerates climatic changes differently. Consider the horse's body weight, length and distribution of the hair coat, the stabling facilities, and blanketing options available. When cooling down a sweat-soaked horse, an educated approach coupled with instinct and common sense will prevent trouble. Keeping a horse current on respiratory vaccine boosters allows it to fend off chill-related respiratory viruses. Intelligent management can maintain a horse's conditioning program year-round.

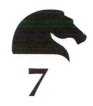

7

NUTRITION
FOR PERFORMANCE

With today's super-technology, hay samples can be submitted to a laboratory for identification of all available nutrients. With this detailed information and the assistance of an equine nutritionist and computer programs, owners and trainers can formulate a tailored diet for each horse. Although such ideal diets are within reach, they are not always practical for the average horse owner.

Consider each unique situation. A large operation may be able to put up its own hay. However, it is possible for repeated harvest of the same fields to deplete the soil of essential minerals. Hay grown in these fields is then deficient in mineral micronutrients and requires supplementation.

Fig. 7–1. Some farms may have access to good pasture for only a few months each spring.

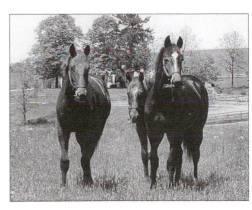

A small farm may only have access to a pasture turnout with ample grass for a few months each spring. As the pasture is overgrazed, other feeds are required to fulfill basic nutrition requirements. Paddock or stall-confined horses may need hay year-round. Hay is often bought monthly, as budget or storage space allows. It comes from different fields or different harvests, and varies in nutrient content with each truckload.

BASIC REQUIREMENTS

The equine intestinal tract is highly developed to extract nutrients from the digestion of plant matter. Roughage comes in the form of hay or pasture, and serves as the foundation upon which to build a feeding program. The high fiber content of roughage is essential to normal intestinal function and health.

Energy is one of the basic requirements in a daily diet, yet misconceptions persist about how horses obtain energy. Metabolism of roughage in the large intestine, and fermentation and breakdown of fiber generate large amounts of *volatile fatty acids* (VFA). These along with sugars (glucose) can be used immediately, or are stored as fat. Combining high quality roughage and high-power concentrates (grains and vegetable oil) in a sensible manner allows control of a horse's energy intake, and customizes a ration for each horse's special energy needs.

There are guidelines which can help create a safe diet that best meets a horse's nutritional requirements:

- A horse can only consume 2.5% of its body weight per day in feed. That quantity is simply all the intestines can hold. If the horse weighs 1,000 pounds, its daily feed limit—grain and roughage combined—is 25 pounds.
- At least half of the daily ration, by weight, should consist of roughage in the form of hay or grass, or a combination of the two. A 1,000-pound horse with a maximum daily ration of 25 pounds should consume at least 12.5 pounds of that in roughage. This amount does not provide the entire daily supply of essential nutrients, but it is a starting point on which to build.
- The higher the proportion of roughage, the safer the diet. The more high-power concentrate in a ration, the greater the risk of disease, including founder, colic, and various limb deformities that affect growing horses.
- Measure all feed by **weight** and not volume, as the weight of bales of hay or different grain products vary. Weighing the food provides consistency at each feeding.

Hay

Grass Hay

Alone, quality grass hay provides a nearly adequate diet for a mature, idle horse, meeting its needs for protein, energy, and fiber. However, grass hay is relatively low in calcium, and high in phosphorus. Therefore, this diet may need calcium supplementation in the form of ground limestone. This supplement satisfies an adult horse's requirement for a calcium-to-phosphorus (Ca:P) ratio of no less than one part calcium to one part phosphorus (1:1).

Cereal Grain Hay

Cereal grain hays, such as oat hay, are similar in nutritive value to grass hays in many respects. However, once the grain heads have fallen from this type of hay, all that remains is straw which is vastly reduced in energy value.

Legume Hay

Legume hays, such as alfalfa or clover, are grown throughout the country. Legume hays are 20% higher in energy, twice as high in protein, 3 times as high in calcium, and 5 times higher in vitamin A than good quality grass hays. Legume hay, therefore, gives greater nutrient value than grass hay. However, depending on the amount of legume hay fed, the high calcium content may need to be offset with a phosphorus supplement such as monosodium phosphate.

Nutritional Value

A lot of the nutritional value of hay depends on the stage of harvest and the state of preservation. Most of hay's nutrition (⅔ of the energy and ¾ of the protein value) is within the leaves. Because good quality hay is abundant in leaves, inspect the hay to be sure it is leafy and soft, rather than stemmy and coarse. If hay is stemmy because it was harvested late in the maturation process, or if the leaves have turned to powder and fallen off because it was poorly cured, its nutritional value must be discounted proportionately.

The moisture content should be less than 20% to prevent mold and spoilage. However, excessively dry leaves fall away and the hay loses nutrient value. Shake a flake of hay to see how many leaves fall out, or if they crumble to dust. Smell it for mold, and break it apart to look for discolored areas. If the hay is green, smells sweet, holds together well, and is not irritating to handle due to sticks, stems, or weeds, then it passes the test for freshness and palatability.

Pasture

The nutritional content of pasture forage varies not only according to plant characteristics, but also by season. Energy and mineral content depend on soil type, but certain rules-of-thumb help determine how to supplement pasture during different seasons. With rapid spring growth, grasses are high in protein, minerals, and vitamins, but lacking in energy due to the high water content of sprouting plants. A 1,000-pound horse has to eat 3 times as much fresh spring grass as hay to meet its energy requirements. Pasture loses water content as it matures, but it also loses protein and mineral value as its fiber content increases.

Concentrates

Energy is the most critical part of a horse's diet. A primary source of energy is carbohydrates, which are found in the fiber components of hay and grass, and are commonly found in a concentrated form as grain. Grains provide much more energy per pound than hay.

Carbohydrates are easily digested to glucose. Glucose is readily absorbed in the bloodstream and made available to muscles for work, or is stored as fat in adipose tissue or as glycogen in the skeletal muscles and liver.

The National Research Council stipulates that:

- Light horses at light work (English or Western Pleasure, hack, or equitation) require a 25% increase in energy consumption per day.
- Medium work efforts (ranch work, roping, cutting, barrel racing, jumping), require an energy consumption increase by 50% per day.
- Intense work (race training or polo) requires doubling of energy consumption per day.
- Draft horses require a 10% increase in energy consumption for each hour of field work.

When a horse is burning more energy than it is able or willing to eat in forage, grain is the most efficient way to increase energy intake. Grains offer a concentrated source of energy, but are relatively high in phosphorus and low in calcium. Processed grains (rolled, cracked, or crimped) are slightly more digestible than whole grains.

Oats and Corn

Oats and corn are the two most popular feed grains. Oats are higher in fiber content and lower in digestible energy than other grains due to a fibrous hull surrounding each oat kernel. Corn is twice as high in digestible energy as oats. Both oats and corn contain enough protein for mature horses, but oats have up to 12% versus 9% for corn.

Rye and Barley

Rye and barley fall between oats and corn on the energy scale. Barley must be processed to remove its indigestible outer hull. Rye, when fed alone, is unpalatable. These grains are usually fed in combination with other foodstuffs, in the form of a mixed grain or pelleted feed.

Fat

Fat is an excellent fuel source for working muscles if they are adequately supplied with oxygen during aerobic exercise. (Aerobic exercise generally occurs at speeds of less than 12 m.p.h., or at heart rates of less than 150 beats per minute.) By using fat as fuel and sparing glycogen reserves in the liver and skeletal muscle, a horse on a high-fat diet delays fatigue during aerobic performance. Glycogen remains available as an energy source for anaerobic activity of high speed or sprint efforts.

Fats are up to 3 times greater in energy density than an equal weight of grain. For example, 1 pound of fat (about 2 cups) provides the same amount of digestible energy as 3

Ration A:

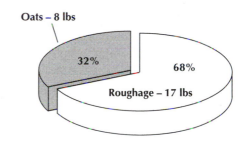

Oats – 8 lbs
32%
68%
Roughage – 17 lbs

Ration B:

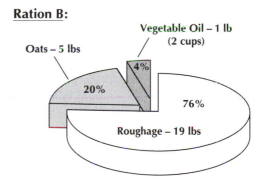

Vegetable Oil – 1 lb (2 cups)
Oats – 5 lbs
4%
20%
76%
Roughage – 19 lbs

Fig. 7–2. Ration B, with 3 pounds less oats, offers an equal amount of digestible energy as ration A.

pounds of oats, or 2 pounds of sweet feed. However, only a maximum of 12% – 15% of a ration can be fed in the form of fat. Other feeds such as roughage and grain must complement the use of fat as an energy source.

Vegetable oil as a form of fat is efficiently digested and metabolized. It is not as filling in the digestive tract as grain or hay, and less fat is required to supply a similar amount of calories and energy as found in grain. If the vegetable oil is stored properly so it will not spoil or become rancid, it is highly palatable when mixed with grain or bran.

Another source of fat comes in powdered form. Pace® for horses is powdered animal fat and sugars, which is well-digested and does not freeze in winter.

Protein

Because humans have a high demand for dietary protein, they often assume horses have a similar need. Protein is therefore commonly over-fed to horses. Horses use it as an energy source only if they lack carbohydrates (hay and grain) or fats. Protein is metabolically inefficient for the horse to process and excrete when fed in excess.

Every horse needs protein, but mature horses require only moderate amounts (8% – 10% of the ration). Growing horses, pregnant and lactating mares, and aged horses need up to 16%. Supplemental protein can be provided with legume hays, or with concentrated grain mixes of higher protein levels.

Corn and oats provide 8% – 12% protein. Grass hays or pastures are variable in protein content, and for exact values should be analyzed at a laboratory. Generally, good quality grass hay contains at least 8% protein. Alfalfa feed products generally provide at least 15% protein, and can be as high as 28%.

As a youngster grows, or as a horse exercises, its appetite normally increases to ingest more energy. With greater feed consumption, the additional protein needs of the growing or exercising horse are usually met.

Calcium/Phosphorous

A quality, well-balanced diet probably provides a horse with the vitamins and trace minerals it needs. However, calcium and phosphorus must be present in a horse's diet, not only in sufficient amounts, but also in the correct ratio, and they may require some adjustment. Grains and grasses tend to be high in phosphorus; legume hays provide excess calcium. Therefore, a judicious combination of grain or grass hay with legume hay often achieves an adequate balance of calcium to phosphorus. The ideal ratio of calcium to phosphorus for a mature horse is between 1.2:1 and 2:1. (The maximum Ca:P ratio tolerated by mature, idle horses is 5:1, while a growing horse has a critical need for a ratio of about 1.5:1.)

MEETING NUTRIENT REQUIREMENTS
The Pregnant Mare

A pregnant mare has specific dietary demands that affect the health of the growing athlete she carries. Some of the nutrients she receives will be stored by the foal before birth, and used after birth when the mare cannot provide them in her milk. Lack of these nutrients, especially in late gestation, can seriously impair the foal's athletic potential.

For the first two trimesters of a mare's pregnancy, she needs only a normal maintenance diet. Excess vitamin and mineral supplements fed in the beginning months of gestation have negative effects on the fetus, while excess energy causes a mare to become fat.

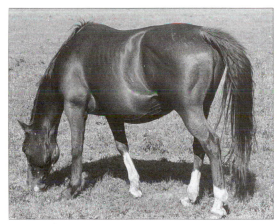

Fig. 7–3. Pregnant mares on pasture need mineral supplements.

The Last Trimester

By the ninth month of pregnancy, the fetus starts to grow rapidly; the mare now needs to eat for two. A mare on pasture in her last trimester needs additional supplements to provide adequate nutrition for her growing fetus.

During the last trimester of pregnancy, trace minerals are deposited within fetal liver tissues. Liver reserves of trace mineral micronutrients sustain a foal through a phase of rapid growth during its first 2 – 3 months. If a mare in late stages of pregnancy does not receive enough of specific micronutrients, the potential athlete *in utero* may not store enough reserves in its liver for healthy bone growth. A young athlete's predisposition for developmental orthopedic disease may begin during late gestation.

Most mares enter this last trimester in late winter or early spring. Rapidly growing spring pasture grass has such a high water content that a mare would have to eat 50 pounds daily to consume the 15 pounds of dry matter her late pregnancy requires. Not only are her intestines incapable of holding that much forage, but she would have to eat around the clock.

Grain

Mares can be supplemented with about 2½ pounds of corn, or 5 pounds of oats or sweet feed each day (½ – ¾ pound of oats or sweet feed for each 100 of her 1,000 pounds). Be careful with feeding corn—while it is excellent for the hard working athlete, it is easy to overfeed corn to a broodmare.

Sweet feed typically consists of oats, corn, and barley, mixed with 5% molasses to decrease dust and improve flavor. Molasses, with its high calcium content, assists in offsetting the relatively high phosphorus content of the grains. Sweet feed is available with protein levels ranging from 10% – 16%.

Weigh the grain rather than feeding it by volume, as oats and corn vary considerably in weight. Choose a sweet feed with a 14% or 16% protein level specifically formulated for broodmares.

Copper

In addition, pregnant mares experience an increased copper need in their last months of pregnancy because copper is transferred through the placenta and stored by the foal. Ideally, in her last trimester she should receive 30 ppm (parts per million) of copper daily, and it must be balanced with zinc and other minerals. Lack of minerals in the forage can be compensated for only by supplementing pregnant mares with a balanced mineral mix added to grain.

Calcium and Phosphorus

Some grain mixes come already prepared with added minerals. For a mare on grass pasture or hay, buy a specifically formulated mix to ensure she receives an adequate balance of calcium and phosphorus. She will also need a ground limestone supplement to supply ample calcium in her diet if she receives grain without added minerals.

During the last trimester, as the fetus grows and the mare gains weight, gradually increase her grain intake. By the time she foals, she can be eating as much as 6 – 8 pounds of grain each day. Another option is to supplement grass hay or pasture with up to 10 pounds of good quality alfalfa each day, omitting the grain. Alfalfa provides ample calcium and protein, while pasture furnishes the phosphorus alfalfa lacks. A mare on an alfalfa-rich diet will need phosphorus supplements.

The Lactating Mare

During the first 2 months of lactation, a mare's energy demands increase by 150% over maintenance. Milk *composition* is not influenced by diet, but its *quantity* depends on adequate energy and protein intake. In early lactation, a mare produces as much as 3% of her body weight in milk each day—approximately 30 pounds, or 7.5 gallons.

A pasture will mature in summer, losing nutritional value just when a mare needs it most. If her requirements were met with grain, that would be

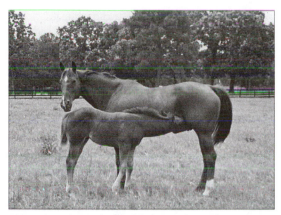

Fig. 7–4. From a foal's third month until weaning the mare's energy demands drop to 50% above maintenance.

1.75 pounds of grain per 100 pounds of her body weight. This would amount to 17 pounds of grain a day—a dangerous quantity for any horse. Instead, limit the quantity of grain to 8 pounds and provide an equal weight of alfalfa.

Concentrations of trace minerals such as copper, zinc, and manganese in the mare's milk are generally quite low, and cannot give a growing foal its dietary requirements. Despite supplementation of the mare with extra copper, zinc, or manganese, milk concentrations of these micronutrients do *not* increase. A foal depends on liver reservoirs formed in the last trimester of pregnancy, and on dietary supplementation once it begins eating solid food.

From a foal's third month until weaning, it will consume much of its diet as hay and creep feed, reducing its need for milk. Offer 1 pound of grain for each month of age, up to 6 pounds a day. As a result, the mare's energy demands drop to only 50% above maintenance. Reduce her ration of grain and alfalfa accordingly, or she is at risk for founder or colic.

The Growing Athlete

The young, growing horse has very specialized dietary demands to build a strong musculoskeletal system for future athletic stress. Normal development of bone, cartilage, joints, ligaments, and tendons requires more than just ample amounts of nutrients; the nutrients must also be balanced in respect to each other.

An example of an imbalanced diet would be feeding alfalfa only. Alfalfa has a high protein content (18%), high calcium-to-phosphorous ratio (more than 5:1), and high energy content. It is therefore a valuable feed source, but if fed alone, can trigger growth surges that cause *developmental orthopedic disease* (DOD).

Developmental Orthopedic Diseases

Long Bones

Under normal conditions, the cartilage of growing bone is gradually removed and replaced with bone cells, allowing long bones to elongate while still bearing weight. If this process goes awry, cartilage is retained in some areas where it should have mineralized into bone.

Thickening of cartilage layers in a defective area is accompanied by malnourishment and necrosis (death) of underlying layers of bone *(subchondral bone)*. Weakened bone develops microfractures, with subsequent pain. Or, subchondral bone and defective joint *(articular)* cartilage can separate, forming *osteochondrosis* lesions, which indicates DOD.

Growth Plates

Rapid bone growth due to excessive amounts of protein and energy in the diets of young foals has been implicated in DOD, as has an imbalance of calcium and phosphorus in the diet. An inherited predisposition

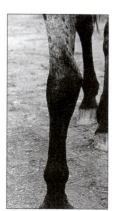 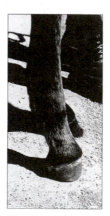

to rapid growth may also be a component of a DOD syndrome. In a fast-growing foal, nutrients which are essential for healthy bone development are depleted as cartilage matures too rapidly into bone at growth plates and joint surfaces.

Imperfect maturation of cartilage into bone within growth plates results in *physitis* (commonly known as *epiphysitis*), a form of DOD. *Angular limb deformities* are associated with unequal growth rates along a

Fig. 7–5.
Epiphysitis in knee.

Fig. 7–6. Contracted tendon.

growth plate, or with malformation or collapse of the multiple bones in the knee or hock joints.

Flexural deformities such as contracted tendons develop as a result of osteochondrosis or epiphysitis, causing pain in joints or growth plates. Upright pasterns, or *club feet* is another example of a flexural deformity.

Vertebrae

If the vertebrae in the neck develop abnormally, spinal cord compression and "wobbler" syndrome result as yet another manifestation of DOD.

Abnormally developing cartilage is susceptible to traumatic injury, because even normal activity can damage improperly developing cartilage. Many youngsters do not show evidence of defective cartilage in joints or growth plates until their maturing body weight excessively loads the malformed joint surfaces.

Preventing DOD

To prevent these crippling syndromes, an intelligent feeding program is essential for a young horse. Feed a ration combining grass hay, alfalfa hay, and grain concentrate. Alfalfa boosts the nutritional value of the grass hay, and grain provides phosphorus to balance alfalfa's high calcium content. Grain also provides nutrients without overloading the foal's intestines.

High Quality Diet

Offer the young horse all the hay it will eat, mixing grass to alfalfa in a 2:1 ratio. The alfalfa provides plenty of energy, calcium, and protein, including lysine, which is the only amino acid known to be essential for growing horses. Neither grain nor grass hay is a good source of lysine.

A young horse can be supplemented with as many pounds of grain as it will eat in hay, *up to 6 pounds*. If, for example, an 8-month-old horse will eat at least 4 pounds of grass hay and 2 pounds of alfalfa hay per day, it can also be fed a *maximum* of 6 pounds of grain. Vegetable oil or Pace® can be substituted for some of the grain to provide safer amounts of digestible energy. With alfalfa already providing considerable protein, the foal does not need more than a 10% protein sweet feed, or straight corn.

If quality alfalfa is unavailable, replace it with free choice grass hay. Still provide grain as above, but make sure it is 14% protein. Also feed a calcium supplement such as dicalcium phosphate (2 parts calcium to 1 part phosphorus) to replace the calcium alfalfa would have provided.

Trace Minerals

Insufficient dietary intake or a poor quality diet offered to a growing horse reduces the availability of specific micronutrients, such as trace minerals, that are important to healthy bone formation. Trace minerals such as copper are critical for normal musculoskeletal development of the young horse. Copper needs vary from region to region and must be balanced to the amount of available zinc. Trace

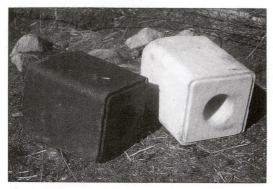

Fig. 7–7. Trace mineral and regular salt block.

mineral salt blocks do *not* supply the necessary quantities of minerals. Such blocks are 98% regular salt (sodium chloride) and have very minute amounts of trace minerals. These blocks were developed for *ruminants,* such as cattle, sheep, and goats. Free choice consumption by horses does not achieve desired levels of mineral intake each day.

To provide ample concentrations of trace minerals to a growing foal, the minerals must be supplemented in grain. Ask the veterinarian or equine nutritionist for specific recommendations on a trace mineral supplement.

A young horse's skeletal system continues to form until it is at least 3 years old. During this time, it should remain on a carefully balanced ration. Once near mature size and weight, it can tolerate a greater range of protein and mineral content in the diet without risking athletic potential.

The Idle and Lightly Worked Horse

An idle, mature horse that is not currently in training needs no special dietary considerations other than maintaining just the right weight. Idle, mature horses fulfill their energy needs effectively with good quality roughage, and need only be supplemented with free choice salt and a balanced mineral mix.

When running the hand along the horse's ribs, only the last two should be felt. Usually the idle horse thrives on a maintenance diet of 1.75 pounds quality grass hay per 100 pounds. (A 1,000-pound horse would receive about 18 pounds of hay per day.)

Light Training

When reintroducing a horse to a light training schedule of 3 or 4 days a week of trotting and cantering, feeding demands need only provide 15% more energy than maintenance. To provide the lightly exercised horse with the fuel it needs, feed up to 1.5 pounds of sweet feed for each hour of exercise, in addition to quality grass hay. Protein needs do not increase with light exercise, so for an adult horse a 10% protein mix is adequate.

Alternatives to Grain

Hay

Because horses evolved to graze at frequent intervals throughout the day and night, they would much prefer to graze over a long period than to eat only a small portion of grain that disappears quickly. If the horse cleans up its feed and looks for more, offer it extra grass hay while it stands idle in the stall or paddock, or turn it out to pasture.

Beet Pulp

Instead of extra hay, a horse's need for fiber can be satisfied with up to 2 pounds (10% of the ration by weight) of beet pulp. Beet pulp is a good roughage substitute because it is relatively low in nutrients and high in fiber (18%). Wet beet pulp swells to many times its original volume. To ensure it will not swell inside the horse and cause colic, soak it in large amounts of water for at least 5 hours before feeding.

Bran

Another low nutritive, but filling, grain product commonly used is wheat bran. Bran is high in fiber, low in energy, and about 15% protein. Not only is it extremely high in phosphorus, but it also binds calcium in a horse's body. This characteristic makes bran useful to balance high calcium diets of legume hays. Half a pound of bran a day is a nice treat and may increase a horse's water consumption, especially if fed as a mash. Although the presence of bran in a horse's diet may increase the volume of its manure, bran is not a laxative. In fact, if bran is overfed, a horse could become constipated.

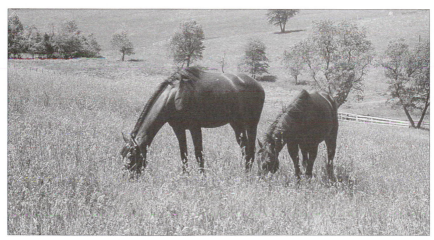

Fig. 7–8. Horses evolved to graze at frequent intervals.

If a horse is putting on a bit too much weight from an enhanced diet, then exercise it more, or reduce grain. Initially, some adjustments in the diet will be necessary to find just the right amounts of extra feed to keep a horse comfortable and happy while it builds muscle through exercise.

The Hard Working Athlete

The goal of a feeding and conditioning program is to improve muscular efficiency and provide fuel reserves for the working muscles. The mental and physical stress of hard exercise on an athletic horse radically increases its energy and trace mineral demands. An equine athlete must be supplied with a quality ration that can be consumed within its intestinal limits (2.5% of its body weight) while providing fuel for locomotion.

Horses involved in sports requiring intense bursts of speed (racing, polo, hunting, gymkhana, roping, and cutting) will use aerobic metabolism, but they will also rely on fuel supplied under anaerobic conditions in the muscles. Without ample fuel supplies, a horse will lose its competitive edge as it tires.

Horses in endurance sports (endurance racing, long distance competitive trail rides, and eventing) need large amounts of energy to sustain them through the rigors of prolonged athletic output, in both training and competition. At speeds less than 12 m.p.h. (a fast trot), horses work within aerobic limits, with ample oxygen supplied to working muscles. *(See Chapter 3 for more information.)*

Replenishing Energy

The diet of an equine athlete must not only fulfill normal metabolic function, but it must replenish energy supplies depleted in strenuous daily workouts. Hay does not offer enough energy to meet the fuel demands of the athletic horse, even if it eats its full intestinal limit of 2.5% body weight every day. The sheer bulk of hay limits a horse's necessary intake.

Although it is difficult to maintain body fat on the hard working horse, there are ways to maximize a horse's caloric and energy intake without jeopardizing its health or digestive function. To compensate for energy expenditures of rigorous athletics, it is necessary to supplement with concentrates. Up to half the daily intake (by weight) of feed can be supplied in a concentrated form.

Addition of Vegetable Oil

Vegetable oil, mixed into grain, is easily digestible by horses and contributes little to intestinal fill. It provides almost three times as much energy as a similar volume of grain, making it an excellent source of energy. In energy content, 2 cups of vegetable oil (16 ounces) is equivalent to 3 pounds of oats or 2 pounds of sweet feed. For example, feeding 5 pounds of corn and 2 cups of vegetable oil a day (divided into 2 – 3 equal feedings), achieves the same nutritional results as 7 pounds of corn. The reduced volume of concentrate allows the horse to eat more hay, and the ration is safer. As a bonus, the vegetable oil enhances the luster of the coat.

A powdered source of fat is available, called Pace®, and it also provides energy for the performance horse. It consists of animal fat and sugars. On a vegetable oil or Pace® supplemented diet, a horse needs to eat 15% less volume to fulfill daily energy needs.

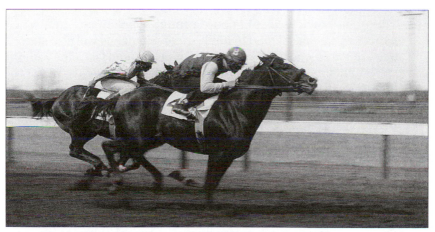

Fig. 7–9. Hard exercise increases an athlete's energy demands.

Free Choice Hay

The active performance horse should always have free choice hay so it can eat whenever it has the urge. A horse can consume more dry matter nutrients from hay than it could from pasture, because more than 80% of hay's water content evaporates during the curing process. Use a combination of grass (or oat) hay and alfalfa (up to half), making sure the alfalfa is leafy and of good quality to provide maximum nutrients.

Additionally, roughage in the intestines provides a continuous energy source for an exercising horse, and serves as a reservoir to hold water in the intestines, restoring sweat losses and avoiding dehydration.

Electrolyte Supplements

Although electrolytes are not technically considered "food," they are essential to a horse's well-being. During training and competition, an athlete may need electrolyte supplements besides the salt block. A good mixture is made with 3 parts Lite® salt (potassium chloride and sodium chloride) to 1 part ground limestone. Another useful mixture combines 2 parts table salt, to 1 part Lite® salt to 1 part limestone. Add about 2 ounces of either mixture per day to the grain, if necessary. Or, give 2 ounces mixed with water by syringe every 2 hours during strenuous exercise. (If limestone is unavailable from the feed store, obtain the calcium component of this mixture from Tums® or ground eggshells.)

Other Supplements

The equine athlete does not need protein supplements. In most cases, an increased intake of food to fulfill energy demands will also supply the added requirement for protein, trace minerals, and vitamins without excess supplementation. A particularly heavily stressed horse may benefit from vitamin B and C supplements.

The Aged Horse

As a horse ages, it is often difficult to maintain body weight. Flesh seems to vaporize from the body no matter how much hay is eaten. Harsh winter climates increase the metabolic demands on an old horse's system, making it doubly challenging to keep it in good flesh.

Many geriatric horses are retired campaigners who may live another decade or more when supported by preventative health care (deworming, dental attention) and high quality nutrition. An "old timer" may not have enough useful teeth to grind hay; it may be starving in the midst of plenty. To help out, replace hay with a soft gruel of pelleted feed that requires no chewing or grinding for digestion. Alfalfa pellets are an excellent source of fiber, protein, and energy. Pellets can be bought "straight" as compressed alfalfa, or in the form of a "complete feed" containing up to 25% ground grains in addition to compressed alfalfa. Alfalfa pellets contain at least 27% crude fiber. Ample fiber in the diet is necessary for normal digestive processes for old and young horses alike.

Feed the same amount of pellets *by weight* as hay—do not assume a 1-pound coffee can holds 1 pound of pellets. If a horse needs 25 pounds of hay per day, then give 25 pounds of pellets instead, divided into 2 – 4 daily feedings. When soaked in a feed tub for an hour with ample water, pellets swell and soften into a gruel which an old horse can gum and swallow easily.

Advantages of Pellets

Besides supplying highly digestible nutrients, pellets have other advantages. They are easy to transport and store, reduce manure quantity, and because of their compressed size, a horse can eat almost 20% more pellets than hay. Increased intake improves weight gain over the winter months.

Increased Requirements

An "old timer" reverts to the increased dietary needs similar to those of a growing foal. Protein requirements increase to 16%, Ca:P ratios need to be balanced at 1.5:1, and energy needs increase because of reduced intestinal effi-

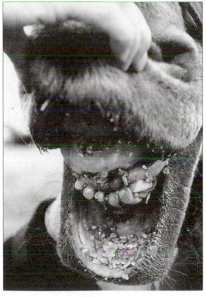

Fig. 7–10. An old horse may not have enough useful teeth to grind its feed.

ciency. The high calcium content of an alfalfa-based diet should be balanced with a phosphorus supplement, like monosodium phosphate. The geriatric horse may also need vitamin supplements, especially B and C. Normally a horse's body manufactures these vitamins in the intestine, but with old age, intestines do not function to full capacity.

Extra Energy

For extra energy, pour 1 cup of vegetable oil over the pellet mash twice a day. To satisfy a horse's psychological need to chew, also offer 5 pounds of grass hay. The horse may even get some nutrition from it, but the hay must be soft and leafy. Coarse, stemmy hay is irritating to the intestines if not properly ground by the teeth, and can lead to diarrhea or impaction colic.

Age and Obesity

Some older horses tend to become obese due to hormonal changes associated with age. Usually a diet of excellent quality grass hay avoids obesity and helps to prevent laminitis. These overweight individuals do not need supplementation with alfalfa, grain, Pace®, or vegetable oil, but their micronutrient needs must be met with vitamin and mineral additives that balance the ration.

HOT CLIMATE FEEDING

In the summer, many horses are exercised more than during winter months. Exercise burns calories and energy supplies, yet ironically, many horses reduce their feed intake by 15% – 20% during heat spells.

Water requirements vastly increase. Without ample water, a horse may stop eating when it actually needs to replenish its fuel resources.

A horse dissipates heat from actively working muscles through sweating, or evaporative cooling. As a horse sweats, loss of water and electrolytes leads to dehydration and diminished performance unless it can replenish those losses. To compensate for reduced feed intake and loss of electrolytes, it is important to increase digestibility of the diet, and to supply adequate nutrients to an exercising horse. A fit and properly nourished athlete with no excess body fat sweats efficiently. Conservation of body water and electrolytes delays the onset of fatigue or performance failure.

Heat Increment

Diet plays an important role in keeping a horse "cool" during exercise. Just as working muscle produces internal heat, so does digestion.

The body metabolizes every foodstuff at different levels of efficiency. Digestion and metabolic processes, and the muscular activity involved with eating and digesting each food type produces a different amount of heat. This amount of heat is a food's *heat increment* (HI). Understanding which foods have low heat increments allows dietary manipulation to improve a horse's cooling ability during hot summer days. The lower the heat increment, the less internal heat digestive processes generate, and the less heat a horse must dissipate in hot weather.

Heat Increments of Different Feeds	
HAYS	
• Grass Hay	30% – 33%
• Alfalfa Hay	15% – 18%
GRAINS	
• Corn	10% – 12%
• Oats	15% – 18%
• Barley	15% – 18%
FAT	
• Vegetable Oil	3%

Fig. 7–11.

Grains Versus Roughage

Grains are substantially lower in their heat increment than fibrous roughage feeds. Roughage, such as grass hay or pasture, has a heat increment value of 33%, while oats, barley, and alfalfa hay have HI values ranging from 15% – 18%. Corn has a HI of 10% – 12%. Compare these values to fat at a HI of 3%.

Because it is important to limit heat production in hot climates, and because high environmental temperatures reduce a horse's appetite, the grain portion of a ration may be increased to accommodate special needs. Concentrates are mostly digested and absorbed in the small intestine with little heat generated by metabolism, whereas bacterial fermentation of roughage in the cecum and large intestines generates heat. (This is one reason why extra hay should be fed to horses in wintertime, as large intestinal fermentation generates heat from within.)

Excess Grain

The proportion of grain should **never** exceed 50% of the ration. At least 1% of body weight must be consumed as roughage each day because fiber is essential to healthy equine digestive processes. If grain is fed at greater than 50% of the ration, the high starch content of grain overwhelms the ability of the small intestine to digest it. Excess fermentation of rich carbohydrates can lead to colic, gastrointestinal ulcers, laminitis, or tying-up. Grain concentrates give a horse calories to burn during exercise, but too much grain contributes to deposits of body fat. Insulating fat deposits slow heat dissipation to an extent greater than any value gained by over-feeding grains for their low heat increment.

Corn Versus Oats

Contrary to popular myths, corn is not a "heating feed." This mistaken impression may be earned from the fact that corn is about two times higher in digestible energy than oats. If corn is substituted for oats at the same *volume* as oats, a horse will receive twice as much energy. The result is a very "high" or "hot" horse that may become difficult to handle. An overly energized horse fusses and frets in efforts to vent its fire, and bad behavior patterns develop. References to such horses have dubbed corn with the misnomer of being a "hot" food. If corn is substituted for oats, cut the volume in half. However, it is best to *weigh* the feed so there is no question as to how much energy the horse receives.

The HI of corn is actually one-third less than the HI of oats. This difference is due, in part, to the indigestible fibrous hull of oat kernels. As the large intestine breaks down this non-nutritive fiber, internal heat is generated from its metabolism.

Feeding corn instead of oats increases energy supplies. The amount of roughage a horse must eat can then be reduced (within the 50% criteria), and only half the volume of corn needs to be fed as oats. A low HI and compact energy density make corn an excellent carbohydrate to feed in hot summer months.

Fat for Energy

Since the heat increment of fat is only 3%, it contrasts dramatically with other foodstuffs. Feeding 1 – 2 cups of vegetable oil each day provides a valuable source of digestible energy. Because vegetable oil is a fat, adding it to grain has multiple benefits. Vegetable oil is efficiently digested and metabolized, while minimizing heat production in the body.

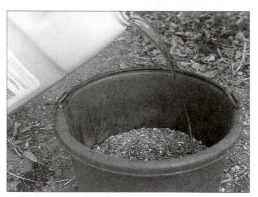

Fig. 7–12. Vegetable oil reduces the amount of concentrate needed and increases the digestible energy.

For horses that voluntarily limit feed intake during hot environmental temperatures, adding fat to the diet overcomes the difficulty of supplying ample energy. Fats are up to 3 times greater in energy density than an equal weight of grain. With fat supplementation, it is possible to reduce amounts of other foods and still meet daily energy needs. Feeding a cup of vegetable oil twice a day to a 1,000-pound horse reduces the amount of grain required to maintain body weight by as much as 25%. There is also a decreased risk of laminitis or tying-up by feeding fat because less grain needs to be fed.

Protein

Role in Sweating

Another mistaken belief of dietary folklore is that exercising horses need extra protein. Protein does *not* serve as a major fuel source during exercise efforts. An insignificant amount of protein is lost in sweat during exercise. Normally, proteins within sweat glands act as "detergents" to disperse sweat "water" evenly along the hair shaft, resulting in more effective evaporative cooling. In early stages of training, proteins contribute to the lather of sweat. As a horse is exercised daily in a conditioning program, proteins are not restored to the sweat glands between exercise periods. Therefore, as fitness improves, the sweat thins, and less protein is lost during exercise.

Protein Supplements

Normally, an adult horse thrives on a diet with 8% – 12% protein. Supplementing protein greater than 15% may be detrimental to an exercising horse. High protein foods also have a high heat increment, making them a poor dietary choice in hot climates. Despite the lower HI value of alfalfa hay (18%) as compared to grass hay (33%), it has a high protein content (as much as 28%). Therefore, feeding alfalfa exclusively has adverse effects.

Protein Requirements

Increased protein in the diet is unnecessary. Any slight increase in protein needs as a response to exercise is usually compensated for by an increase in appetite. During high environmental temperatures, horses that voluntarily limit their food intake need only *minimal* protein supplementation by adding small amounts of alfalfa pellets or alfalfa hay to the ration.

Results of Excess Protein in Hot Climates

Muscle Fatigue

Muscle fatigue during performance is directly related to a build-up of excessive lactic acid. The high protein in an alfalfa diet increases blood and muscle ammonia levels, which results in an increased production of lactic acid in the muscle tissue. Accumulation of lactic acid in the muscle tissue can lead to fatigue and tying-up.

Increased Water Requirements

Nitrogen is a component of ammonia by-products. Excess nitrogen in the body is toxic, and the body eliminates it through the urinary tract. The horse drinks more water to meet the needs of extra urine production. Increased water loss caused by urinary excretion of nitrogen compromises any horse in a hot climate, particularly an exercising athlete.

Respiratory Problems

Besides increased urine production, the nitrogen in urine produces ammonia. Ammonia accumulation in stalls injures the respiratory tract, compromising how well the respiratory system can oxygenate the tissues, and limiting performance. The respiratory tract also helps dissipate heat from the body. While evaporative cooling dissipates most of the heat, respiratory cooling contributes 20% to the cooling process. The healthier the respiratory system, the more a horse benefits in all ways.

Water Requirements

Horses on a hay diet drink almost twice as much water as horses on a grain supplemented diet. The more hay is provided in the diet, the more water the horse needs for digestion. Ample quantities of cool water must always be available to a horse to ensure efficient digestion and to replenish losses from sweat.

Pellets

Pelleted and extruded feed contains small particles which pull water into the large intestine during digestion. Feeding pellets results in softer manure, but pellets require more water for adequate digestion. Feeding a pelleted ration as a sole feed source may be unwise in a hot climate, because dehydration is a limiting factor of performance.

Roughage

Roughage (hay and pasture) is excellent for retaining water in the intestinal tract. Within reason, water lost in sweat is immediately replenished from a reservoir of water in the digestive tract. During prolonged competition of endurance sports, roughage also supplies energy to a horse long after the meal. It is best to feed 3 – 4 hours before an event, but not too generously, as excess bulk in the intestines limits performance. Balanced proportions of grain, fat, and roughage provide maximal energy.

Electrolyte Supplements

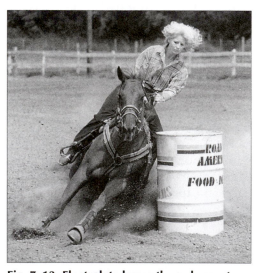

Fig. 7–13. Electrolyte losses through sweat are unavoidable and *cannot* be prevented by supplementation before exertion.

Electrolyte losses through sweat are unavoidable and *cannot* be prevented by supplementation before exertion. However, the long distance athlete may benefit from a dose of electrolytes the morning of the competition, in addition to continued replenishment throughout the event. It is unnecessary to supplement light working or idle horses with electrolytes even in hot weather. Such individuals replenish their own needs from a free choice salt block and good quality hay.

Improving Performance

Manipulating meal times and quantities can increase the opportunity for internal heat (generated by digestion and metabolism) to be dissipated throughout the day. Small meals at frequent intervals optimize body cooling mechanisms. During hot weather, feed the largest proportion of roughage at night. While a horse is resting during the cool hours of night, it metabolizes and ferments the fibrous portion of the diet. When there is less fiber in the intestines during exercise on hot days, heat produced from feed is not a limiting factor to performance.

In implementing a dietary program for a horse, there are no hard-and-fast rules. Each horse must be fed according to its individual needs. Not all horses need grain in their diet, while others require large amounts. Athletic pursuits and exercise regimens vary between horses, and from day to day for any individual. Genetics and age considerably influence the efficiency of nutrient use. By following some basic principles about which foods are "cooler" than others, and by discarding obsolete myths about feeding requirements, a horse's diet can be modified to improve mental and physical performance in hot climates.

OBESITY

The subject of a malnourished horse conjures images of an emaciated rack of bones. However, malnourishment has another extreme—obesity. An overweight horse is a statement of dietary imbalance, one that is overabundantly supplied with energy.

Eating Behavior

A horse accumulates fat for the same reasons people do. Either too many calories for its level of exercise are provided, and/or a bored or greedy horse eats more than it needs. Eating behavior in horses evolved in an environment where survival of the "fittest" implied a well-nourished and robust individual.

Free Choice Diet

Natural range forage is relatively low in energy, with variable nutritional content, depending on season and terrain. In the wild, horses consume moderate amounts of forage at frequent intervals, each meal being about 1 – 3 hours long. Unlike humans, the amount of food consumed is not governed by signals of stomach distention, or "feeling full," conveyed to the brain, unless the distention approaches pain. A horse with free choice food stops eating before the stomach is fully distended. Therefore, in the wild, stomach distention does not usually occur.

The amount of food a horse eats is governed by the rate of emptying food from the stomach, or the nutritive value of food in the stomach. Cues are sent to the brain from hormonal and nerve receptors that are integrated throughout the gastrointestinal tract and the body. They recognize satisfaction of nutritive needs, and accordingly regulate hunger or fullness by an appetite control center in the brain.

In a natural state, these integrated signals do not influence the amount or length of a particular meal. Instead, these cues affect the time until the next meal, and the amount ingested at the next meal. A horse in this environment eats only enough to maintain good body health.

In an artificial environment where humans dictate when and how much a horse eats, this natural control of eating no longer plays as significant a role. Knowing this fact, we can modify feeding practices to an advantage.

Meal Intervals

Horses with free choice food do not voluntarily fast longer than 2 – 3 hours at a time. A horse that receives only 2 meals a day is psychologically "starved" by the next meal because of imposed and lengthy fasting between meals. The horse then consumes large amounts rapidly at each feeding, rather than "grazing" throughout the day. If free choice food cannot be arranged, it is best to feed a *minimum* of three times per day.

Palatable Foods

The actual presence of food induces a horse to eat, but how much it eats is determined by the food's palatability and how easy it is to obtain and eat. A horse's perception of smell, taste, and texture decides palatability of the food.

In this modern era, plentiful amounts of tasty and easily consumed feed are available without a horse having to seek it. Many horses eat until all the food is gone. Access to appealing foods may override normal "regulatory cues" from the gastrointestinal tract and metabolic pathways. A horse continues to eat even though it is physiologically sated in energy and nutrients. Then the extra pounds stack up.

Seasonal Effects

An extensive layer of fat under the skin protects horses from the elements. This insulation diminishes the penetrating effects of wet and cold. Insulating fat deposits maintain a precise body temperature range, and they serve as a readily available source of energy when food is scarce.

Equine feeding behavior evolved in adaptation to an environment with ample nutrition in the summer, and sparse supplies in the winter. During mild months, horses stored sufficient body fat and energy to last through a winter of limited forage. Horses have not yet adapted to the constancy of modern feeding practices that carry them through winter without need of surplus fat depots.

Competition

Competition within a herd stimulates dominant horses to run others away from the food. Assertive individuals may then have access to more food than they need.

If we combine an evolutionary tendency to "plump" up with easy accessibility to highly palatable and energy dense food, the result is an overweight horse. If exercise is restricted and a horse remains relatively idle, instead of building muscle, it continues to put on fat.

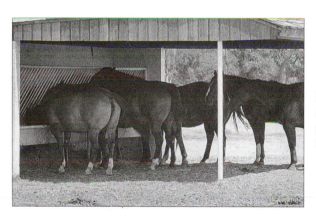

Fig. 7–14. An overly assertive horse often gets more food than it needs.

The Human Factor

It is much too simple to blame equine obesity on a tendency to overeat; the human factor is important. In some cases, the physiologically ideal body weight a horse carries may not correspond to ideal as viewed through an owner's eyes. Human desires sometime improperly plump up a horse to "show" condition.

It is our role to learn what constitutes a healthy body condition so we do not overindulge a greedy individual. It has been proven repeatedly that one of the greatest health hazards for horses is obesity.

Condition Scoring System

One report concluded that racehorses have an optimal racing weight within a range of plus or minus *16 pounds.* This range is a fine tuned balance, considering a horse can drink or urinate almost 16 pounds in a matter of moments. An average pleasure horse is considered overweight if it carries an excess of 100 – 300 pounds of body flesh.

We can fairly evaluate body condition to determine what is the correct weight for an individual, regardless of breed or conformation. Use of a *condition scoring system,* developed by Dr. Gary Potter and associates of Texas A&M, accurately estimates stored body fat more effectively than weight, height, or heartgirth measurements.

Thickness of fat over the rump and back correlates well with total body fat. Also evaluate rib fat; although it is not as reliable an indicator, it should be considered as part of the whole picture. By feeling the fat cover and visually appraising areas over the back, croup and tailhead, ribs, behind the shoulder, and the neck and withers, a horse is assigned a numerical condition value. This scale is from 1 – 9, from least body fat to most body fat.

Emaciated

An emaciated horse in poor condition has a score of 1. The spinous processes, ribs, tailhead, and hip bones project prominently. The bone structure of the neck, withers, and shoulders are pronounced, and no fatty tissue is felt.

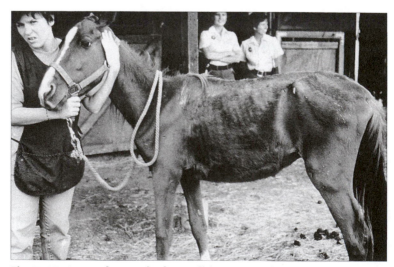

Fig. 7–15. A poor horse—body condition score of 1.

Thin

A thin horse has a score of 3. There is some fat covering the spine—about halfway up the spinous processes, but they are still easily seen. The ribs are visible but have a slight fat covering. The hip bones, tailhead, withers, shoulders, and neck are more full, but are discernible. Thin horses do not have enough body reserves to support long distance performance. They also chill easily in inclement weather. Many racing Thoroughbreds have a body condition score of 4.

Ideal Condition

A score of 5 corresponds to a "moderate" condition — the back is level, and the ribs are not visually distinguished but are easily felt when running a hand across them. Fat around the tailhead begins to feel spongy, the withers appear rounded over the spinous processes, with the neck and shoulders blending smoothly into the body. This condition is *ideal*.

Moderately Fleshy

In some cases, it is appropriate for the modern horse to build a "moderately fleshy" (score 6) body condition. On a horse with a score 6, the fat around the tailhead is soft, the fat over the ribs is spongy, and there is fat deposited along the withers, shoulders, and neck.

When a horse is continually exposed to inclement weather in harsh climates, with no access to shelter, a thin layer of fat "traps" heat within the body. Also, a lactating mare needs plenty of body reserves to manufacture and provide enough milk for her foal, and she should not be maintained too lean.

Overweight

Many overweight horses tend to be fleshy (score 7) or even fat (score 8). Although individual ribs are felt in a fleshy horse, there is noticeable fat between ribs, there is a crease down the back, and the withers, neck, and areas behind the shoulders are riddled with fat. It is difficult to feel the ribs at all in a fat (score 8) horse, and the neck is noticeably thickened and "cresty." Shoulders, croup, and buttocks ripple with fat.

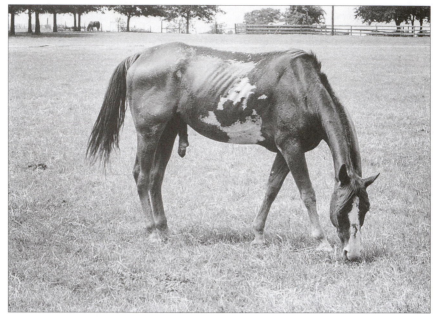

Fig. 7–16. A very thin horse—body condition score of 2.

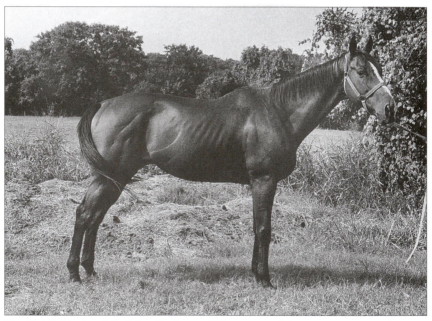

Fig. 7–17. Moderately thin—body condition score of 4.

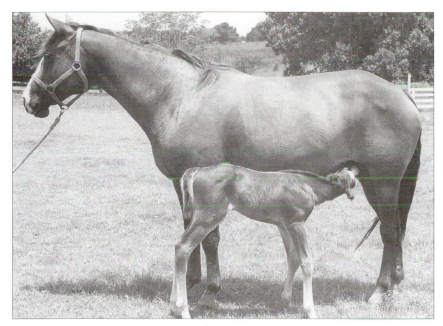

Fig. 7–18. A moderately fleshy broodmare—body condition score of 6.

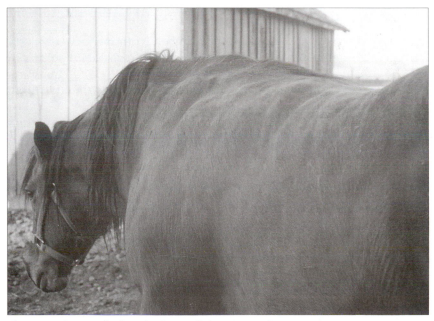

Fig. 7–19. Extremely fat—body condition score of 9.

Extremely Fat

An extremely fat horse tops the scale with a score of 9. Such a horse has a pronounced rain gutter-like crease along its back (which in fact will hold water), and patchy fat over the ribs. Fat also bulges around the tailhead, along the withers, behind the shoulders, and along the neck. The flank lacks definition and is filled in with flesh. Ample fat along the inner buttocks causes them to rub together. Serious metabolic problems threaten such a horse if a weight loss program is not begun immediately.

Combining a scoring system with conventional methods, such as weighing a horse or measuring heartgirth, achieves fine tuned control of body condition. Gradual weight gains are difficult to appreciate with daily observation. Weight tapes are not very accurate, but are useful to evaluate changes over time. Snapping a photograph of the horse at intervals permits an objective, visual comparison of body condition.

Obesity-Related Diseases

Obesity is a systemic disease that can lead to serious consequences and metabolic problems in the horse. A list of these problems includes:

- laminitis
- exercise intolerance
- heat exhaustion
- intestinal lipomas
- colic
- tying-up
- musculoskeletal injuries

Obesity also contributes to developmental orthopedic diseases such as malformation of joint cartilage (osteochondrosis) or inflammation of the growth plate (epiphysitis) in a growing horse. Pregnant mares may have difficulty foaling due to reduced muscle tone attributable to lack of exercise associated with obesity.

Although they are listed above as a group, each individual syndrome is a separate debilitating condition, potentially resulting in permanent lameness or death. At the very least, an overweight horse cannot perform to potential.

Musculoskeletal Injuries

Another problem arises when a "weekend warrior" is over-fed daily to compensate for its athletic output which only occurs on Saturday and Sunday. Instead of removing supplemental energy sources from the diet on weekdays when the horse stands idle, an owner continues to provide appetizing food, full of calories. The rider wonders where the horse's exuberance has gone, and why it is now so sluggish and dull. "Maybe it needs more grain" is a common response to the malady. Insult is heaped onto injury. Feet, tendons, ligaments, joints, and bone must withstand excessive concussion and strain. Musculoskeletal injuries develop as the legs are loaded with excessive weight.

Laminitis

Perhaps one day an owner notices the horse is tender on its front feet. The liver can no longer detoxify the continual carbohydrate overload of grain, rich alfalfa, or lush pasture. The resulting systemic metabolic crisis causes severe problems with the blood supply in the feet. The diagnosis: laminitis.

Lipomas

What is seen as deposits of bulging fat on the outside of a horse is a reflection of what is being deposited internally around organs and within the *mesentery*, which is the fan shaped tissue encircling the small intestine.

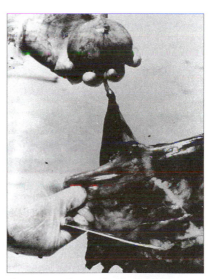

A horse develops intense abdominal pain, a sudden onset colic crisis that is not responsive to medical therapy. On the operating table, it is discovered that fat stores have been generously deposited within the mesentery. Fat globules have formed a fatty tumor *(lipoma)*. The lipoma hangs from a long stalk that has wrapped around a part of intestine, strangulating it.

Fig. 7–20. Lipoma in the intestine.

Obesity and the Growing Horse

Excessive body fat in a young, growing horse can overload an immature, undeveloped skeleton, contributing to bone and joint abnormalities. Obesity also amplifies concussive forces on maturing cartilage, resulting in orthopedic disease.

Cartilage was removed from the knees of growing Thoroughbreds and analyzed after 3 months of a high energy, push-fed diet where the horses were encouraged to eat too much too often. Abnormal cellular development of cartilage was evident. After 9 months on a push-fed diet, clinical signs were obvious. Lameness, limb deformities, growth plate abnormalities (epiphysitis), and retarded formation of the cartilage (osteochondrosis) developed from the unbalanced diet.

Hormonal and Mineral Imbalance

Hormones influence cellular processes of maturation, differentiation, and synthesis of cartilage and growth plates. The amount of carbohydrate energy a foal ingests regulates the growth of bone and cartilage by affecting hormonal control. Overnutrition interferes with normal circulating levels of hormones such as *somatomedin* (a growth regulator), *insulin, thyroxine,* and *cortisol.* With accelerated growth rates, mineral demands for adequate bone development also increase. Relative excesses or deficiencies of specific minerals result in developmental orthopedic disease.

Musculoskeletal Failure

An increase in energy and protein consumption of up to 30% greater than the values recommended by the National Research Council does not enhance the biomechanical strength of growing bones of yearlings. Additional body fat loads bones with additional body weight without a proportional increase in structural stability. Under these circumstances, failure of bone, ligament, tendon, or joint structures is inevitable. These syndromes are commonly seen, particularly in overweight individuals.

Preventing Obesity

These medical maladies are easily preventable. Reduce high energy diets of rich alfalfa hay, lush pasture, or supplements of grain or pellets. Substitute instead a diet including grass hay—providing it free choice if possible. Some individuals, however, thrive on a limited amount of grass hay fed daily, so free choice feeding may not be practical.

Within 2 – 3 days of a free choice grass hay diet, appetites usually stabilize. A horse consumes only what is physiologically necessary to maintain a healthy weight. Grass hay is palatable, but not overly appealing as are alfalfa or concentrates. Neurohormonal cues from the gut can once again naturally regulate hunger and satiety.

A common dilemma is in following feeding guidelines. They are just that—guidelines. Each horse has a unique metabolic constitution that dictates how easy or difficult it is to maintain its weight. How much energy a horse burns on a daily basis is determined by:

- age
- temperament

- rider's weight and expertise
- environmental temperature and humidity
- intensity and duration of work
- terrain
- level of conditioning

Losing Weight

It is dangerous to "starve" an obese horse for rapid weight loss, as starvation leads to high levels of circulating fatty acids *(hyperlipemia)*. These fatty acids are deposited in the liver, resulting in liver damage. Weight loss should be gradual. Ample roughage will ensure healthy gastrointestinal function, and mental peace of mind. Feeding at least 1 pound of hay per 100 pounds of body weight each day maintains intestinal movement and health.

Place an obese horse on a strict diet by restricting high energy foods, or substituting with less energy-rich foodstuffs. Switch from alfalfa hay to grass hay, pull the horse off rich pasture or limit its access to only a few hours a day, and eliminate grain and vegetable oil.

A weight-loss diet for a horse is no different from a human attempt to defeat an overweight problem. Reduce the amount and the quality of food ingested, and provide regular exercise. Not only will a horse look better, but it will feel better, and be able to perform to potential.

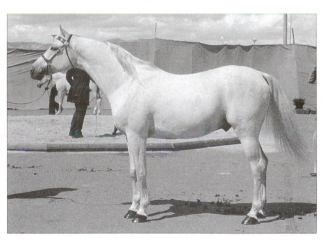

Fig. 7–21. An overweight horse benefits from exercise and a lower energy ration.

Training the Overweight Horse

Along with a sensible diet, exercise is the best way to reduce fat deposits. Walking is an excellent way to slowly increase heart rates and warm muscles. Start the first week with 15 – 20 minutes, every other day or three days that week. Work two-thirds of the time at a walk, and one-third at the trot. The second week, work for 30 minutes, 3 – 4 days. Slowly increase distance in the third week, but keep the speed the same until the horse is working for 30 – 60 minutes. Finally, add longer trot intervals and 1 – 2 minute canter intervals (changing leads) in the fourth week. At the end of one month, the horse should be fit enough to further increase mileage, and then speed.

Inability to Control Heat

Working muscles expend energy at 20 – 50 times the resting metabolic rate, and one natural by-product is heat. As internal body temperatures initially rise, most of the blood from cardiac output is diverted to the skin, away from the working muscles. Blood vessels of the skin dilate, transferring excess heat from the muscles to the body surface. This increased blood flow elevates skin temperature, and activates sweat glands to begin evaporative cooling.

As environmental temperatures rise, or as humidity increases, evaporative cooling becomes less efficient. For heat loss to result, the outside air must be cooler than the inside of the horse. Also, sweat must evaporate to transfer heat from the skin to the air. High humidity limits complete evaporation, and therefore reduces the effects of evaporative cooling.

An athletic horse should have enough fat reserves to burn going into the training season, but there can be too much of a good thing. For the athletic horse, fat can dramatically hamper performance.

An obese horse is in extreme danger of being unable to regulate its own temperature even under the best conditions. Extremes in environmental temperature and humidity increase this danger. In the summer, follow a careful exercise approach for the overweight horse.

Reduced Heat Dissipation

A fat horse carries an added insulating layer under the skin. A fat and unconditioned horse must work harder at a given effort, generating more body heat than a fit horse. It is difficult for a fat horse to dissipate heat away from working muscles because fat slows the conduction of heat to the skin periphery. The same fatty tissue that conserves body heat in cold weather interferes with evaporative cooling on hot days.

Because they cannot efficiently conduct or sweat the heat away from the body, fat horses are prone to exercise intolerance, fatigue, and heat stress. As a horse sweats in large quantities, it loses vital body fluids and salts, contributing to dehydration and electrolyte imbalance. At first, performance may suffer, but with continued fatigue there is a rapid decline toward heat exhaustion and metabolic failure.

Tying-Up

Once surface evaporation can no longer keep up with the heat build-up, internal temperature continues to rise. This heat impairs muscle contraction, adding to fatigue and exhaustion. Loss of electrolytes through the sweat, and an increased muscle temperature spark a chain of abnormal biochemical events in the muscles, resulting in the paralyzing cramps of tying-up.

Inversion

If a horse cannot rid itself of enough heat, it may start panting to remove heat through the respiratory tract. This problem is seen as an *inverted* pulse rate to respiratory rate ratio, with the breathing rate above the heart rate.

Slow Cardiac Recovery

Cardiac recovery is difficult as the body struggles to eliminate internal heat. The circulatory system cannot keep up with the competing demands of the working muscles, the increased metabolic rate, or the need to increase blood flow to the skin.

Elevated Temperature

Continued inadequate dissipation of heat leads to rising and persistently elevated body temperature. Rectal temperature over 105.8° F results in heat-induced injury of nerves, with irreversible systemic collapse, shock, and death.

These events may also occur in a horse that is not overweight, but is underconditioned for the work effort, or in any horse exercised in excessively hot and humid climates.

Increased Energy Needs

Body condition has a more pronounced effect on performance than environmental temperature. Not only does additional body fat impair performance, but the effort required to move additional body mass also increases a horse's energy expenditures. After exercise, faster pulse and respiration recoveries are noted in moderate body condition (score 5) horses than in fleshy (score 7) individuals. Unconditioned horses do not metabolize fat as efficiently as fit horses because their enzyme systems have not been "trained" to effectively use fat as fuel.

Heat dissipation requires additional calories. A fat horse tends to consume more energy-dense feed after a work effort than does a fit, sleek horse. A fleshy horse requires an increase in total energy intake for both maintenance and performance simply to remain in an overweight condition. The average obese horse consumes about 5 pounds more feed per day than a moderately conditioned horse. Such an appetite compounds the problems of obesity.

(Editor's Note: For a detailed look at all areas of equine nutrition and related subjects read **Feeding To Win II** *published by Equine Research, Inc.)*

8

FITNESS EVALUATION

The goal of the rider or trainer in any equine sport is for the horse to compete in top form with minimal stress. At the end of the performance, the horse should have enough zest to continue if asked. This is the ultimate test of stamina, strength, speed, and *heart*.

Each horse is a unique individual. The best way to keep a horse out of metabolic danger is to know the horse. Know its normalcies, abilities, and most of all its limits. Metabolic problems often begin subtly. The rider or trainer should be able to recognize warning signs of impending fatigue, or metabolic disaster. An aware and sensitive rider can stop the spiral leading to exhaustion and crisis before it begins.

FITNESS INDICATORS

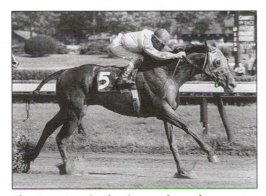

Fig. 8–1. Terrain, footing, and weather must be considered when evaluating a horse's fitness for an event.

Competition places critical physiological demands on a horse at every moment. A horse's level of fitness is not the only influence on its ability to perform well. Also consider the horse's metabolic condition and body weight, the age, the weight of the rider relative to the horse's size, the terrain or footing, and the weather.

Specific criteria determine how a horse is holding up to stress, and its ability to continue a performance. One general fitness indicator is the horse's attitude. The look in the eyes, the degree of alertness, the impulsion of stride, and the way the horse holds the body and ears indicate its overall well-being.

Heart Rate Recovery

One objective criterion is the horse's *heart rate recovery* after a performance. During exercise, the heart rate can increase to eight times the resting rate, increasing blood flow and oxygen to working muscles. For example, if a horse's resting rate is 30 bpm, its heart rate at maximal exertion could be 240. In a normal recovery the heart rate falls rapidly in the first minute after exercise, then decreases more slowly over the next several minutes.

The recovery rate depends on fitness, environmental temperature, and the type of athletic exertion. For an endurance horse, the heart rate should drop below 60 – 70 beats per minute (bpm) within 10 minutes after exercise has stopped. For a sprint horse, the heart rate should drop to 150 – 180 bpm after 30 seconds, and 100 – 140 bpm after 1 minute. Within 30 minutes, the heart rate should be below 60 bpm after any kind of exertion.

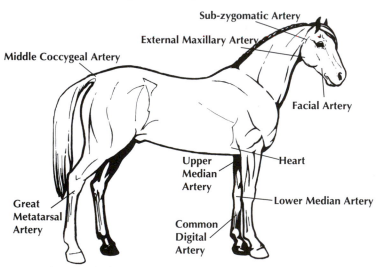

Fig. 8–2. Points on the horse to count the heart rate.

Cardiac Recovery Index

Once the horse's heart rate is less than 60 – 70 bpm, a *cardiac recovery index* (CRI) is enormously helpful in discovering subtle problems before they become serious. Determine the resting level by counting the heart rate for 15 seconds. Trot the horse out 125 feet and back the same 125 feet. This distance usually takes about 25 seconds to complete. Start the stopwatch as the horse begins the trot, and stop it at 1 minute *(about 35 seconds after the horse returns)*. At this point, count the heart rate for 15 seconds. The heart rate of a normal horse that is not suffering from metabolic or musculoskeletal problems returns to the resting rate, plus or minus a beat, at the minute check.

A CRI heart rate that is two or more beats above the resting rate may indicate exhaustion or pain. An example of its use is in endurance events. The CRI is one of the parameters used to determine if a horse should be held at the check for a longer rest period, or should be taken out of the competition.

Capillary Refill Time

Gums should be a healthy pink color, and if blanched (pressed) with a fingertip, they should become pink again in approximately 2 seconds. This method shows that the circulatory system is in good shape, pumping blood to all parts of the body. The time required for this response is called the *capillary refill time*.

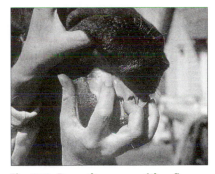

Fig. 8–3. Press the gums with a fingertip to check capillary refill time.

Jugular Refill

Another method of evaluating circulatory efficiency and hydration is achieved by pressing a finger into the jugular furrow (groove) and watching how long the jugular vein takes to fill with blood. Every horse's exact jugular refill time will be different, however, the jugular vein should fill to the size of a pencil within 2 seconds. Checking the jugular refill time at the beginning of the event helps the rider monitor dehydration during the event. If the refill time is longer than it was at the beginning of the event, then the horse is dehydrated because the circulating blood volume is lower.

Gut Sounds and Intestinal Activity

Intestinal activity and the associated gut sounds heard on both sides of the flank are important indicators of normal physiological function. An exercising horse may have fewer gut sounds because a large percentage of blood goes to the muscles. Less blood reaching the intestines slows intestinal activity. However, the intestinal tract should not be silent. Also, a horse's appetite should be active, preferably greedy, at rest stops or after a performance.

If a horse is operating anaerobically, it can be watered and fed hay after it is cool to the touch on the chest—after about 20 – 30 minutes. After 30 minutes to 1 hour, the horse can safely be fed grain.

If a horse is operating aerobically, and it continues to exercise after a rest period (1 hour maximum), it is safe, indeed necessary, to allow the horse to drink water and eat hay or grass. If desired, a small amount of grain may be given to a horse that is still operating aerobically. After exercise, cool the horse out as above before watering or feeding, to allow time for the blood to flow back to the intestines.

Veterinary Evaluation

When available at equine sports events, a veterinarian can play a crucial role in achieving safe and successful competitions. Rely on this resource. Communicate with the veterinarian, and ask questions. Point out inconsistencies in the horse's performance.

In addition to evaluating a horse's metabolic condition at rest stops during endurance events, veterinarians also recognize swelling in the limbs, or an obvious lameness that might prevent a horse from competing. They may also point out nicks, scrapes, minor injuries, and sores from improperly fitted tack that the rider may overlook.

STRESS INDICATORS
Persistent Heart Rate Elevation

Persistent elevation of heart rate may indicate an impending metabolic collapse. The heart rate remains high if a horse is near exhaustion. Pain also elevates the heart rate. If other metabolic signs such as attitude, gut sounds, level of fatigue, level of dehydration, and body temperature seem normal, seek out a source of pain, particularly in the limbs or muscles.

Respiratory Rate

The respiratory rate should decrease with the heart rate recovery. Preferably, the respiratory rate will drop below the heart rate after about 10 minutes. However, environmental conditions, hair coat, obesity, and level of fitness influence this drop. For example, in hot and humid climates, horses may pant in rapid, shallow respirations. A high respiratory rate is also associated with high body temperatures.

Inversion

Whenever the respiratory rate remains faster than the heart rate, it is called an *inversion*. Even an inexperienced eye will observe that an "inverted" horse appears to pant. Respiration is shallow and rapid, and the horse's flank moves in and out with each breath.

If the heart rate recovers within 10 minutes, but the respiratory rate remains high, the horse is not necessarily in trouble. It may need help in ridding its body of the extra heat. After extended exercise, spend a few minutes walking the horse so the circulation continues to flush heat and lactic acid from the muscles. Soak the head and neck with water to speed cooling.

Dehydration

There are many levels of dehydration, and there are variable indications of it. A rough estimate of dehydration is made by pinching a fold of skin on the point of the shoulder or the eyelid, and noting how quickly it snaps back into position. If a horse is not dehydrated, blood flow to the skin is normal so the skin snaps back immediately. Pinched skin that remains "tented" and does not return to normal indicates a dangerous level of dehydration.

A horse with mild dehydration of 2% – 3% may have a prolonged capillary refill time, a dry mouth, or dry mucous membranes. Other signs of dehydration include depressed intestinal activity, and slow heart rate recovery. However, even low levels of dehydration can adversely affect the performance horse. At about 5% dehydration:

- the eye sockets appear sunken
- skin elasticity is markedly reduced
- the horse is weak, and appears dull

Mild dehydration with a slight decrease in circulating blood causes the sodium, chloride, and potassium (electrolytes, or body salts) in the bloodstream to stimulate thirst. With progressive dehydration and an excessive loss of sodium, chloride, and potassium, the stimulus to trigger thirst is eliminated. By not drinking, a horse worsens the dehydration problem. Just because a horse will not drink does not mean it does not need fluids. It may be on the edge of a serious electrolyte imbalance, and in need of immediate intravenous fluid and electrolyte therapy.

On a hot day, it is possible for a 1,000-pound long distance horse to

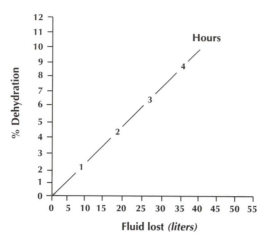

Fig. 8–4. Liters of fluid lost, and the increase of dehydration during a long distance activity on a hot day.

lose 2 – 3 gallons (7.6 – 11.4 liters) of fluid each hour of exercise, or 6 – 12 gallons (22.7 – 45.5 liters) during the entire activity. This amount of fluid loss can lead to **severe** dehydration of 7% – 10% and circulatory collapse.

A racehorse can lose up to a half gallon (0.4 liters) of fluids during a mile race. On a hot, humid day, even mild dehydration can affect race performance.

If an overheated horse abruptly stops work, blood pools in the muscles. This accumulation reduces the amount of circulating blood, contributing to the horse's relative dehydration. If an exhausted horse refuses to move, massaging the major muscle groups in a rhythm with the heartbeat can help circulate blood through the muscles.

Preventing Dehydration

Conditioning helps prevent dehydration. The more fit a horse is, the less demand exercise has on the body, and the less heat is produced by exercise. Therefore, conditioning reduces fluid loss from sweat. By sweating less, the body conserves vital electrolytes and body fluid.

Allow the horse to drink at every opportunity. A hot horse can be allowed to drink as long as it continues to move afterwards. Otherwise, cool out slowly and offer small amounts of water at frequent intervals.

Doctoring Drinking Water

Some horses simply do not like the taste of strange water and will refuse to drink. If a horse is finicky about water, begin to "doctor" the drinking water at home with a small amount of cider vinegar or sugar about a month before competitions. The vinegar or sugar disguises the strange water source and encourages a horse to drink. As an alternative, carry water from home to a competition.

Body Temperature

Working muscles expend at least 20 times the energy of their resting metabolic rate, with the natural by-product being heat. A *thermoregulatory center* in the horse's brain sets the normal temperature and maintains it within a very narrow range. To control body temperature within this limit, the body needs to dissipate the heat produced by working muscles. A high body temperature often corresponds with a high respiratory rate, and both these factors are monitors for thermoregulatory control within the horse.

The rectal temperature is a good indicator of internal temperature. It is normally 98° – 101° F. After prolonged exercise, it is normal for the rectal temperature to reach 103° – 104° F, but the temperature should return to normal within 15 – 30 minutes after exercise.

A rectal temperature persisting above 105° F reveals metabolic problems, and may result in weakness and incoordination. Loss of muscle control and strength can lead to serious accidents. An exhausted horse may stumble and fall, or it may not safely clear an obstacle—placing both horse and rider in jeopardy.

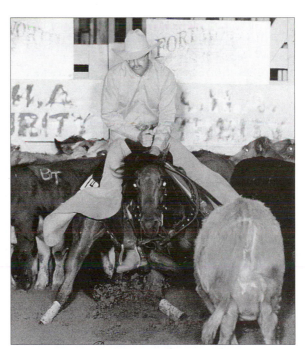

Fig. 8-5. Sweating is the primary method of heat dissipation.

Natural Cooling Methods

The body dissipates a vast amount of heat produced by muscle metabolism through evaporation. A smaller amount of heat is lost through respiration.

Evaporative Cooling

To remove most of this heat, a horse sweats. As body temperature initially rises, most of the blood is diverted to the skin for heat dissipation, and away from the working muscles. Water vapor on the skin, produced from the sweat glands, pulls heat from the blood vessels and the outside air evaporates the warm water. This process is called *evaporative cooling.* Along with heat loss, evaporative cooling also releases large quantities of fluid and electrolytes.

Respiratory Cooling

As body temperature rises, another far less effective mechanism helps dissipate heat. Just as a panting dog moves air across its hanging tongue, a horse breathes rapidly to cool the body. Warm blood, flowing from heated muscles, circulates to the lungs. Warm air in the lungs is exhaled. With each incoming breath, cool air (including oxygen) is exchanged for warm air. Respiratory cooling does not release fluids or electrolytes, but it contributes only a small amount to the cooling process.

Other Cooling Methods

Cool Water Application

Soaking the neck, chest, and legs with water creates the same effect as sweating. Cool water applied over the large, superficial blood vessels of the

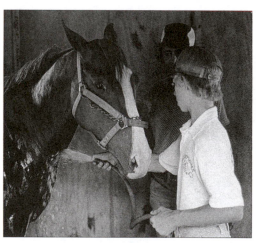

head, jugular region of the neck, armpit, and forelegs dissipates internal heat. The water temperature is not critical provided the large blood vessels in these areas are repeatedly soaked. A single bathing is not enough. Continuously apply water until the respiratory rate lowers, or drape wet towels over the head and neck while the horse walks.

Fig. 8–6. Soaking the neck cools the horse.

Cooling down a horse too rapidly leads to chilling and shock. The body temperature of a severely overheated horse should lower 1° F every 15 – 30 minutes when bathing the head and neck with water.

Never apply water to the large muscles in the back or hindquarters of an overheated horse! Walking and natural cooling best dissipates heat from these muscles. If these muscles cool too rapidly, muscle reflexes will cause the blood vessels to constrict away from the skin. Less blood flow to the skin surface allows heat to persist within the muscles.

Also, the muscle tissues still retain lactic acid that needs to be carried away by the bloodstream. Muscle cramping associated with vessel constriction also reduces oxygen to the muscles. After a hard workout, it may take a couple of hours until it is safe to give the horse a full body bath. After a pleasure ride that stimulates only a light sweat, the horse may be bathed after 20 – 30 minutes of cool-out.

Dangers of Cold Water

Applying cold water to the heavy muscles of the back and hindquarters can cause tying-up *(myositis)*. A tied-up horse has these symptoms:

- refuses to move or appears very stiff if it tries to move
- exhibits signs of "colic" due to pain from muscle cramping
- sweats, paws, or attempts to roll
- heart and respiratory rates climb in response to pain

A trainer or veterinarian can evaluate muscle suppleness, as well as tenderness to hand pressure along the large muscle groups of the back or hindquarters. A normal horse has a fluid stride in contrast to one that is beginning to tie up. Tight or excessively firm muscles, or obviously cramping muscles indicate fatigue and electrolyte abnormalities.

As muscle fibers spasm and contract, more heat is produced in already overheated muscles. Retention of body heat increases both heart and respiratory rates to cool the body. The result is a very slow recovery time, and metabolic problems. Avoid such a scenario by resisting the urge to fully sponge down a horse until it completely cools out. *(See Chapter 4 for more information.)*

Heat Stress

Heat stress occurs when the body temperature climbs above 105° F, and the body cannot efficiently cool itself. Internal temperature continues to rise. Usually, heat stress develops from overexertion leading to overheating, rather than external heating by the sun's rays. However, exhaustion or heat stress can develop if weather conditions have overtaxed a horse's ability to dissipate heat, or have interfered with proper fluid and electrolyte levels of the body.

Hot Weather

Hot weather limits a horse's ability to shed heat from the body. The horse sweats, but sweating is not always enough to stay ahead of the heat build-up. As either environmental temperature or humidity increase, the evaporative cooling of sweating becomes less efficient. In a horse experiencing heat stress, internal heat continues to rise once evaporation from the skin can no longer keep up to rid the body of heat.

Level of Conditioning

Hot weather is not the only factor contributing to heat stress. A horse that is ridden *too fast for its level of condition* produces excess body heat. A horse with many fat layers under the skin cannot dissipate heat effectively. Not only does excess fat impair normal cooling processes, but it directly relates to a horse's level of fitness.

Preventing Heat Stress

Conditioning builds muscle in place of fat. Conditioning also develops capillary beds, improving the circulation of oxygen in the tissues and flushing heat to the skin surface.

Training during hot and humid weather, especially interval training or multiple workouts can cause heat stress. The horse should be monitored closely for signs of heat stress on hot, humid days. Workouts should be less intense or shorter to prevent heat build-up in the working muscles. Also, wetting the neck, chest, and forelegs of the horse before and during exercise can delay heat build-up on a hot day.

Determining the Danger of Heat Stress

A simple formula adds the environmental temperature to the percent humidity, determining the danger of heat stress on any given day. If, for example, the temperature is 90° F and the humidity is 75%, the sum is 165. At this level, evaporative cooling may not be enough to cool the horse.

Levels of Heat Stress (Temperature + Humidity)
If the sum of temperature and humidity is less than 120, normal cooling mechanisms are sufficient unless a horse is obese or has a long hair coat.
If the sum is greater than 140, a horse relies mostly on sweating to dissipate body heat.
If the sum is greater than 150, and especially if humidity contributes to more than half of this amount, evaporative cooling is severely compromised.
If the sum is greater than 180, there are no natural means for the body to cool itself; internal temperature will continue to rise, resulting in heat stress.

Fig. 8–7.

As the horse loses vital fluids through sweating, it will steadily dehydrate if they are not replenished. Dehydration reduces blood flow to the skin. The body responds by limiting sweating to conserve body fluids. Heat continues to build within the horse with no outlet, stimulating a decline towards exhaustion.

Anhydrosis

In hot, humid climates, a horse may experience a syndrome called *anhydrosis.* This syndrome is a loss of the ability to sweat. A horse that does not sweat cannot cool itself. Body temperature rises, the horse pants, and performance suffers. A horse that has ceased to sweat needs medical attention and should be kept still and quiet.

Tissue Hypoxia

At higher temperatures, muscles (and all body tissue) have a greater demand for oxygen. If these metabolic demands cannot be met, muscle contraction is impaired, contributing to fatigue. If a horse's body temperature exceeds 106° F, the body demands more oxygen than can be supplied by the respiratory system. Tissue *hypoxia* (lack of oxygen) results, leading to kidney, liver, and brain damage. At temperatures greater than 107° F, a horse may go into convulsions or a coma, and die.

Warning Signs of Fatigue

The body has developed obvious alarm systems to alert the astute observer to beginning failure, preventing serious metabolic problems like dehydration, exhaustion, and heat stress. A knowledgeable rider or trainer will notice many of these signs of fatigue:

- slow heart rate recovery
- elevated heart rate for over an hour
- high respiratory rate, often shallow and inefficient
- deep, gulping breaths that persist for over 1 minute
- high rectal temperature for longer than 30 minutes
- dehydration with dry or pale mucous membranes, prolonged capillary refill time, jugular refill time, lack of intestinal sounds, and/or lack of skin elasticity
- depression
- disinterest in surroundings
- lack of appetite or thirst
- muscle tremors or twitching
- muscle cramping

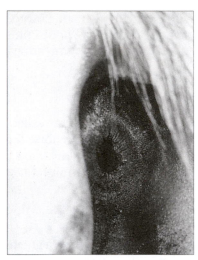

Fig. 8–8. Flaccid anal tone indicates exhaustion.

• thumps *(synchronous diaphragmatic flutter)*

An exhausted horse with these symptoms is in need of medical attention. Without therapy, it can progressively decline and go into shock.

Other Stress Indicators

Diarrhea is an indicator of stress, and contributes to loss of fluid and electrolytes through the feces. Dry and scant feces warn of marked dehydration. Anal sphincter tone should be strong; a flaccid anus is a sign of exhaustion.

ELECTROLYTES

For racing and other short-term events, a primary problem is heat dissipation from working muscles. For horses in longer events, the problem of *electrolyte* loss also must be addressed. Electrolytes are the body salts that contribute to all biochemical functions. A delicate balance in the amounts of these salts is essential for normal biochemical functions, such as muscle contraction, and normal intestinal function. Not only does extreme and prolonged sweating lead to dehydration, but horse sweat consists of more than just water. Sweat releases important electrolytes and minerals, including:

• sodium	• chloride	• magnesium
• calcium	• potassium	

Supplementing Electrolytes

Electrolyte losses through sweat are unavoidable and *cannot* be prevented by supplementation before exercise. Most long distance horses will need electrolyte supplements during an event. Lite® salt in an oral supplement contains potassium, sodium, and chloride.

If it is necessary to supplement electrolytes due to weather conditions or extreme athletic exertion, prepare the mixture by using three parts table salt (sodium chloride) to one part Lite® salt to one part limestone.

If limestone is unavailable from a feed store, obtain the calcium for this mixture from Tums® or ground eggshells. A commercial product, Enduralytes®, is an excellent electrolyte replacer for the long distance athlete, with an easily metabolized source of calcium.

Mix 2 oz. of the supplement with enough water to dissolve it and give the mixture by oral syringe during a rest stop. (Note that NATRC competitions do not allow administration of electrolytes by syringe; they must be top-dressed on the food, or added to the drinking water.)

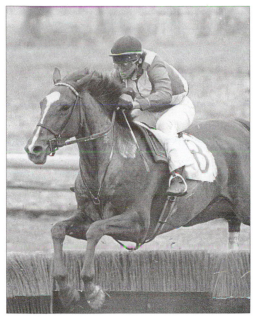

Fig. 8–9. Loss of electrolytes contributes to white, foamy sweat.

Lack of Electrolytes

Loss of abundant electrolytes contributes to a foamy, white, and thick consistency of the sweat when they are released from the skin. The better conditioned a horse is, the "thinner" the sweat becomes.

After a performance, small amounts of electrolytes are replenished by making a salt block available to the horse or by adding them to the feed. If losses are extreme, a veterinarian can give fluids and electrolytes by stomach tube or intravenously.

If essential amounts of electrolytes are lost in a horse's sweat and not replenished, a cascade of events contributes to a horse's decline. Correct balances of sodium, potassium, calcium, and magnesium control *neuromuscular irritability*, which is the ability of a muscle to respond to nerve impulses.

Neuromuscular Depression

A lack of certain electrolytes leads to neuromuscular depression, which means that the muscles respond slowly or not at all to nerve signals. Sodium, chloride, and potassium, three of these electrolytes, are major components of sweat. Working muscle releases these electrolytes through the sweat.

Loss of Sodium

A loss of sodium in the bloodstream depresses neuromuscular activity, impairing muscle contraction. A horse with a sodium deficiency is prone to fatigue and performance falters. Not only is sodium crucial to neuromuscular function, but it also helps retain body fluids so a horse does not become dehydrated. Sodium is not available to the horse in feed, so it must be offered as a supplement on the grain or by syringe.

Loss of Chloride

With exercise of a short duration chloride loss is not usually a concern, but extended endurance exercise stimulates the kidneys to compensate for a loss of chloride by retaining bicarbonate (similar to the bicarbonate of baking soda) from the blood. Bicarbonate retention by the kidneys results in a mild *alkalosis,* or high pH of the bloodstream.

The competitive endurance horse operates aerobically until it fatigues or must sprint or climb. During these difficult efforts, working muscles generate lactic acid by anaerobic metabolism. Yet, not enough lactic acid is produced to lower the pH level of the blood and counteract the bicarbonate. A long distance horse is therefore more likely to have a metabolic alkalosis than a racehorse, for example. In view of this alkalosis, it is **dangerous** to feed sodium bicarbonate or inject a sodium bicarbonate solution into an endurance athlete.

Loss of Potassium

Potassium is an important electrolyte controlling the force of contraction in the muscles, both skeletal and heart. It is also responsible for dilating small arteries to improve oxygen supply to the tissue. If oxygen and blood supply to the muscles are compromised with potassium depletion, tying-up develops. Potassium loss also results in fatigue.

Hay is rich in potassium so this mineral is normally replenished when a horse stops working and eats. If exhaustion or metabolic problems depress the appetite, potassium must be replenished by supplements.

Neuromuscular Hyperirritability

Neuromuscular *hyperirritability* means that the muscles respond too much, or cannot stop contracting. Calcium relates to hyperirritability in two ways. First, too much calcium in the muscle cell and a lack of energy molecules contributes to hyperirritability. Second, if a horse loses excess calcium or magnesium in sweat, the neuromuscular system becomes hyperirritable, seen as muscle twitching and nervousness.

Hard work increases the demand of calcium and magnesium for muscle contraction, and therefore accelerates their depletion. A horse with excessive losses of calcium and magnesium from the bloodstream may develop multiple syndromes, including:

- intestinal shutdown
- colic
- heart arrhythmias
- tying-up
- thumps (synchronous diaphragmatic flutter)

Electrolyte supplements may be necessary during a long distance event to prevent these syndromes.

Excess Calcium in Muscle Cells

Normal contraction of muscle fibers depends on a calcium balance in the muscle cells. Each muscle fiber has a "pump," fueled by energy molecules, that removes calcium from the cell. Without energy, the pump cannot remove calcium from the cells. Excess calcium in muscle cells creates persistent contraction, or spasms of muscle fibers.

Lactic acid accumulated in muscles changes the pH to an acid environment, which also interferes with the activity of the calcium pump and energy use. Imbalances of sodium, chloride, potassium, and magnesium also impair muscle function and pump activity. Fatigue and tying-up result. *(See Chapter 3 for more information on tying-up.)*

Lack of Calcium in the Bloodstream

Calcium or magnesium loss from the bloodstream through the sweat can lead to *stress tetany*, which is a visible form of hyperirritability. Muscles and nerves become hyperirritable; a horse becomes nervous and jumpy, the muscles twitch or spasm, or the limbs stiffen.

Thumps

Thumps, or synchronous diaphragmatic flutter, is not a disease in itself, but it is a distress flag indicating electrolyte imbalances. The *phrenic nerve* passes directly across the heart muscle as it runs to the diaphragm, and provides nerve impulses for contraction of the diaphragm muscle. Excess loss of calcium and magnesium through the sweat, and rising levels of lactic acid in the body sensitize the phrenic nerve. It begins to respond to the electrical discharges of the heartbeat. Then the diaphragm contracts at the same time as the heartbeat. This contraction is seen as a twitching in the flank, or felt as a thumping if the

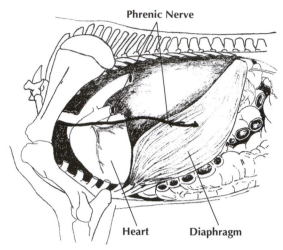

Fig. 8–10. The phrenic nerve and the interaction with chest anatomy.

hand is placed against the flank. The twitching is not related to respiratory movements.

Dietary Cause of Thumps

Hard work and hot, humid weather promote loss of calcium and magnesium through sweat. As a horse sweats, hormones from the parathyroid gland must remove calcium from the bones to the bloodstream, and the kidneys must retain the calcium to prevent its loss through urine. This system maintains calcium levels in the bloodstream.

Alfalfa hay is rich in calcium. A horse that is fed a diet primarily of alfalfa hay is predisposed to thumps and tying-up. A consistently high dietary intake of calcium "turns off" the parathyroid gland. It is unable to mobilize calcium from bone stores during periods of excess calcium loss in the sweat. A horse can be fed alfalfa hay during and after a competitive event to replenish these losses, but should not be fed excess alfalfa between events.

Electrolyte Imbalance: A Dehydration Cycle

Once changes in the electrolyte balance begin, deterioration proceeds in a domino-like cascade, preventing a return to normal. Continuing dehydration diverts the blood away from the muscle, liver, and kidney tissues, to the skin for heat dissipation through sweating. Additional electrolytes are lost through the urine and sweat, and dehydration continues.

Sweating may not be enough to cool the horse, and initially the body sweats more profusely, losing more fluids in an attempt to dissipate heat. As the horse's internal temperature rises, it succumbs to heat stress.

With less body fluid, blood volume lowers, and blood circulation to all tissues diminishes further, which reduces oxygen availability. Then lactic acid collects in oxygen-starved tissues, biochemical reactions falter, and cell death occurs. Ultimately all body parts fail together. Without medical intervention, the result of this process is shock and death. The key to a horse's safety and performance stamina is to prevent it from nearing a state of heat stress or exhaustion.

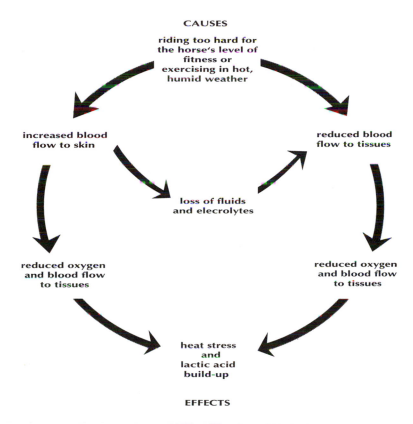

Fig. 8–11. Dehydration cycle leading to heat stress and lactic acid build-up.

PREVENTING METABOLIC PROBLEMS
Good Nutrition

Good nutrition, both during training and performance, can diminish stress and fatigue. Feed is the substance on which a horse refuels. The type of hay consumed (alfalfa or grass), the amount, and the quality are all important factors. At rest periods or after a long distance event, provide hay and salt to replenish the body's stores. Grain can be offered after the horse cools.

Energy reserves in the body fuel the muscles. Conditioning encourages the use of fatty acids as an energy source, saving glycogen for last. Fatigue is directly linked to the depletion of these energy stores.

Fiber

There are two ways to achieve abundant glycogen stores: conditioning muscles to use fat resources first, and a high intake of fiber. In studying diets of top level endurance horses, Dr. Sarah Ralston (Colorado State University, 1987) discovered that high roughage diets supply the fiber necessary to support prolonged aerobic exercise. Low fiber diets correlate with an increased risk of failure in performance.

Fat

When added to grain, vegetable oil is a valuable energy source. It provides almost three times as much energy as an equal amount of grain. Up to 2 cups of oil can be added to the daily diet of a 1,000-pound horse without adverse effects. Corn and soybean oils are the most palatable. However, any vegetable oil is useful.

There is a powdered animal fat product for horses called Pace® which is easily digested. Unlike vegetable oil, it will not freeze in winter.

Excess Protein

Protein-rich alfalfa hay tends to generate heat by metabolism, and indirectly affects a horse's performance by interfering with its cooling ability. Many horses easily tolerate this metabolic heat, while others do not.

Only 10% protein in the diet is necessary for most mature horses. No advantage is gained from protein supplements. Dr. Harold Hintz (Cornell University) observed that too much protein fed to horses results in the need for more water, placing a performance horse at a disadvantage in hot climates. Feeding mineral supplements on a regular basis also promotes urination, resulting in the loss of more body fluids.

Conditioning

To prevent metabolic problems, condition the horse properly before any event or race, and ride logically without overstressing it.

Properly warm up a horse for 15 minutes before a competition so that muscles, tendons, and ligaments receive adequate blood flow and flexibility before speed begins. An adequate cool-down is important after a stressful exertion to remove toxic by-products from muscle, and to dissipate heat from the horse's internal core.

Acclimatization

With training, a horse becomes accustomed to environmental influences. However, the athletic horse often performs away from home in a different environment. Ideally, if a horse is going to perform in a location that has dramatically different environmental conditions than it is used to, it should be moved to the location about 3 – 4 weeks beforehand. This will help to acclimate it to the different stresses. If the horse is not moved soon enough, performance may suffer.

Hot, Humid Climate

A competitor unaccustomed to a high heat index (combination of the temperature and humidity) can lose excessive fluids and electrolytes in the sweat. To properly prepare the horse for exertion in hot and humid climates, the horse must learn to sweat. The only way to achieve the desired training effect is to move the horse to that type of climate. Over 3 – 4 weeks of steady training, the skin and the sweat glands respond to the increased demand to lose body heat. The horse's muscles also learn to work more efficiently in hot, humid weather, minimizing internal heat build-up. Even so, a heat index of greater than 150 may overtax any horse's ability to cool by sweating.

High Altitude

Below 7,000 feet, the atmosphere usually supplies adequate oxygen to fuel the body. At 10,000 feet, a horse consumes 10% more oxygen for the same task performed at sea level. Working muscles operate less efficiently if oxygen supplies are not sustained. Rapid fatigue and excess body heat result.

The enormous storage capacity of oxygen-carrying red blood cells in the spleen allows a horse to respond immediately to a higher elevation. As a survival response to a lack of oxygen, the spleen dumps extra red blood cells into the circulation, providing more oxygen to the demanding tissues.

Low oxygen in the blood turns on a special hormone *(erythropoietin)* that stimulates the bone marrow to make hemoglobin, and more red blood cells to hold the hemoglobin. The blood thickens, but unlike the thickening associated with dehydration, the new red cells are more laden with hemoglobin and oxygen. This adaptive process takes several weeks. After this time, the body is supplied with ample oxygen. Within a month, a horse should be well-acclimated to the added demands of a high altitude environment.

Another temporary, but immediate response to altitude within the first week or two is an increased heart rate and cardiac output, pushing more blood and oxygen to the tissues. The horse breathes deeper, and the respiratory rate rises, gathering more oxygen to be absorbed into the bloodstream. The competitor that has not been properly acclimated may have slower heart rate recovery times than usual.

Initially after relocating to a higher altitude, a horse will urinate more frequently. Increased urination is a normal response to lower oxygen levels. However, it can lead to greater body fluid loss and relative dehydration. In addition, the reduced efficiency of working muscles produces more internal body heat. Then the horse sweats to rid the body of heat, losing body fluids and electrolytes. If the horse does not drink enough to compensate for fluid losses in the urine and sweat, the body slowly dehydrates.

Some individuals may also go off their feed in the first week after relocation. Then the horse will lose weight, and will not get valuable nutrients—energy, protein, and electrolytes.

Immune System

A horse that is moved to a new environment is exposed to strange bacteria and viruses. The psychological stress of transport and new surroundings depresses a horse's immune system, making it more vulnerable to viral and bacterial attack. The immune system can respond to these foreign bodies by making antibodies against them. At least 2 weeks is required to activate the immune system to provide disease protection. This protection is particularly important to prevent respiratory disease that can severely impair performance.

Observation

For endurance and other long distance events, allow the horse access to water and food to restore fluids and energy. Provide electrolyte supplements to restore those losses from sweat. Cool the horse down at rest stops by sponging the head, neck, and legs.

It is essential to take careful note of the horse throughout a performance. The horse cannot speak; its only defense against trouble is to communicate by body posture, or lack of interest or energy. Pay complete attention to the horse, and "listen" to it. In this way, an owner or trainer ensures the horse's durability and excellence in its competitive athletic endeavors.

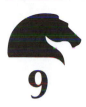

9

LEG SWELLING: CAUSES & CURES

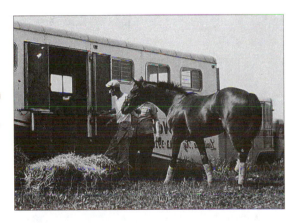

Fig. 9–1. Careful attention to a horse's safety is important in avoiding leg injuries.

DETERMINING THE CAUSE

After discovering a mysterious leg swelling on a horse, begin a systematic analysis of the situation. Leg swelling can result from a traumatic injury, or from a systemic illness which affects the entire body. Tissues of the leg do not have a great ability to expand. Limb swelling causes discomfort as the skin stretches to accommodate the enlarged size. The first step is to gather information.

Determine if the horse is lame on the affected limb. Observe it at the walk, and then if it appears to be moving well, observe it at the trot. Then examine the limb to identify the exact source of the problem, whether it be skin or soft tissue swelling, tendon swelling, or joint swelling. Look closely for nicks, scrapes, or puncture wounds. If the pastern area is

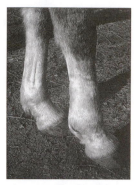

Fig. 9–2. Swelling in the left front cannon bone area.

swollen, pick up the foot and look for a nail or other sharp object. Take the horse's rectal temperature, which is normally less than 101° F. Check to see if more than one leg is swollen.

Reconstruct the workouts from the last few days. Was the footing good? Could the horse have slipped? Was it ridden on hard ground too long, or too fast? Was it turned out to pasture—alone or with others?

These questions may provide data to identify the cause of the swelling. An inflammatory response can be controlled in many different ways, and it is wise to consult the advice of a veterinarian before beginning any therapy.

TENDON AND LIGAMENT INJURIES

Any trauma, stress, or strain to tendons or ligaments in the leg may begin as a slight filling along the back of the cannon or in the pastern area. In any inflammatory condition, proteins *(polypeptides)* are released into surrounding tissues. They summon white blood cells (WBCs) to "clean up" the problem. Cellular "water" enters with them, and the limb swells more. As the WBCs finish their job and die, they release enzymes that are toxic to surrounding cells. More WBCs, and water, invade the area. The inflammatory cycle continues, and the swelling remains.

Edema

Normally, fluid that diffuses from the capillaries into tissues brings WBCs, nutrients, and oxygen to the cells. The function of the *lymphatic system* is to retrieve this fluid and return it to the circulatory system.

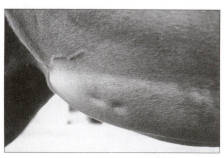

Fig. 9–3. Pitting edema on the belly.

With an inflammation, the lymph system cannot remove the fluid, and then the cells and intercellular spaces swell with the excess fluid. This swelling results in *edema*. If one pushes on the swollen tissues, the fluid may be displaced, especially in regions where the skin is able to stretch more, leaving an indented impression of the fingertip. This characteristic is aptly termed *pitting edema.*

Edema of the limb is self-perpetuating. When the tissue expands, it increases the distance over which nutrients must cross to reach the cells. Swollen tissue compresses blood vessels and further limits fluid movement out of the cells.

JOINT INJURIES

Joint swelling can be serious, and should receive veterinary attention. Trauma to a joint, such as a fall or a kick, or bone fracture responds well to immediate application of ice until the veterinarian arrives.

Windpuffs

Windpuffs, or inflammation, of the fetlock joint occur as a result of heavy work, nutritional deficiencies, or trauma. Windpuffs may also occur when a horse that has been heavily worked suddenly stops work for a few days. In this situation, the windpuffs may abate with exercise.

In most cases, there is no pain, heat, or lameness associated with windpuffs. Once a windpuff has begun, it may remain for life. A long-standing windpuff may also harden. However, unless lameness develops, treatment other than light exercise or improvement in the diet is usually unnecessary.

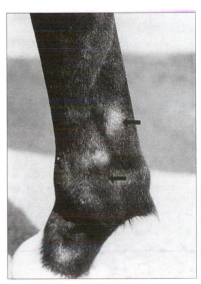

Fig. 9–4. Two windpuffs.

Dislocation or Punctures

Dislocation or punctures within a joint show pronounced swelling and lameness. Successful management of these injuries with return to soundness is dependent on rapid and aggressive professional treatment.

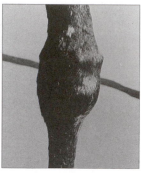

Fig. 9–5. A swollen knee on a foal.

Joint Inflammation in Foals

A foal with one or more swollen joints may be suffering from *navel ill*, an infection within the joints that entered at the umbilicus and spread through the bloodstream. In the very young foal, rupture of the *common digital extensor tendon* at the front of the cannon bone results in a full swelling on the outside of the knee or hock. A weanling or yearling may suffer from *epiphysitis* (inflammation of the growth plate) that appears as an hour-glass-shaped fetlock, or an overly knobby, swollen, and painful knee.

THERAPY FOR LEG SWELLING
Cold Therapy

By understanding the physiology of swelling, certain principles can be applied to control it. Examples of injuries that benefit from cold therapy are:

- strained tendons or ligaments
- splints
- muscle injury
- joint injury
- kick injury
- interference trauma (striking one leg with another)

Ideally, apply cold for the first 48 – 72 hours after an injury occurs, beginning immediately. Water immersion (in buckets, boots, or a running stream) or ice massages are the best forms of cold therapy. Wrap ice in towels to prevent freezing the superficial skin layers.

Effects of Cold Therapy
Decreasing Inflammation

Cold therapy stops the inflammatory process by decreasing blood flow to the area as capillaries constrict from the cold. By slowing microscopic bleeding and hematoma formation, fluid leakage into the injury site is controlled. Hemorrhage and edema disrupt tendon or ligament fibers. With healing, excessive fibrous scar tissue to grow and thicken the tendon. This scarring is minimized with the initial use of cold treatment and a compression bandage.

Pain Relief

Cold also provides pain relief *(analgesia)* because nerve signals are limited at temperatures of 50° – 59° F. Analgesia lessens the muscle and tendon spasms which occur because of pain.

By "cooling" a tendon, pain and lameness subside and give a false impression of a "cure." But cold therapy also increases the stiffness of the collagen in tendon or ligament fibers, reducing the elasticity of these structures. Although the horse may not be visibly lame, premature or strenuous exercise is extremely detrimental to the limb and may result in additional injury. **Rest** is the time-honored therapy for treatment of most tendon strains.

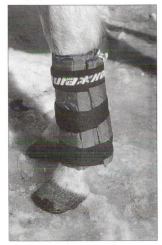

Fig. 9–6. A cold pack.

Length of Application

Muscle tissues require cold application for about 25 minutes to achieve the desired effect. Initially, muscle temperature rises due to a reflex which increases the circulation. Then the temperature begins to decline in the deeper muscle layers, and continues to drop up to 10 minutes after cold application has been discontinued. If no activity follows therapy, the muscle tissue will not warm up to normal temperature for 4 hours. Therefore, confining the horse ensures prolonged cold therapy effects. Deep muscle massage will also loosen spasms in the fibers.

Joints cool more slowly than muscle, and remain "cooled" for up to 2 hours. If a joint can be safely moved, intermittent flexion during cold therapy hastens the cooling process.

In deeper structures such as muscles and joints, cold deters swelling, but at temperatures less than 59° F, subcutaneous edema (beneath the skin) is increased. A light pressure bandage controls this swelling caused by cold therapy. However, the benefit derived from the cold therapy far outweighs this mild superficial edema.

Bandaging

After cooling down a strained tendon, a splint, or injured muscle or joint, carefully bandage the limb when possible. The benefits of bandaging include:

- reducing swelling
- encouraging the tissues to heal with limited scar tissue

• supporting damaged structures
• preventing the spread of swelling to other areas of the leg

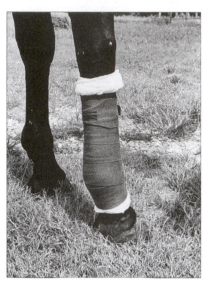

Fig. 9–7. A light bandage controls swelling and discourages scar tissue from forming.

Gravity encourages swelling of the structures below the injury site. Therefore, if the injury is above the fetlock it is best to bandage from knee to hoof, or hock to hoof. Also, a bandage is less likely to slip into a position where it hinders blood flow if the entire lower limb is bandaged.

If swelling appears above the bandage, or if a horse chews at the bandage or stamps its foot, check for excess tightness of the bandage. Cotton padding prevents inadvertent tightening of the bandage materials that could hinder circulation or compress tendons. Apply bandages uniformly, with no bumps or wrinkles.

Heat Therapy

Begin heat therapy **after** 2 – 3 days of cold therapy. Heat therapy works by warming the tissues around an injury site. This warming actually stimulates the body to "cool" the area by dilating vessels and increasing blood flow. The oxygen supply is improved, and blood components such as WBCs, antibodies, and nutrients are delivered to the tissues. The lymphatic vessels can once again remove waste products and excess edema fluid. Pain decreases, and wound healing is enhanced. Increased circulation to the area leads to mild edema in the subcutaneous tissues. Therefore, light bandaging after heat therapy is advantageous.

Hair and the thick layer of horse hide serve as an insulating barrier to heat, and more time is required to warm deeper structures than surface structures. Applying heat to a limb for 20 minutes is usually adequate. Problems that benefit from heat therapy include:

• contusions (bruising)   • mild sprains   • strains
• muscle or nerve inflammation   • joint arthritis

Water immersion or hot water bottles are more effective than dry heat, such as an electric heating pad. Place a towel between the skin and the hot pack to prevent burning and to insulate the pack. Never apply anything too hot to a horse's skin. A temperature about 125° F is sufficient.

If circulation and tissue metabolism were increased by erroneously applying heat immediately after the injury, further damage and swelling would occur. But now, 3 days later, microscopic bleeding has ceased, and the healing process has begun. At this time, heat therapy decreases spasms in the area to provide pain relief, and promotes cleanup of the injury.

Sweating

"Sweating" is another one-step method of heat therapy. An effective leg sweat is prepared by combining DMSO (dimethyl sulfoxide) and a nitrofurazone preparation. "Sweat" bandages work by increasing heat and circulation to an area to remove swelling. A plastic wrap placed under a standing wrap traps sweat produced by the leg, creating a fluid barrier and retaining heat by preventing evaporative cooling. To prevent skin rash, do not leave a sweat bandage on for more than 48 hours.

Epsom Salts

Adding Epsom salts (magnesium sulfate) to wet heat therapy helps draw swelling from the tissue. Dissolve 2 cups Epsom salts per gallon of warm water, and soak the injured site for 20 minutes.

Poultices

A commercial poultice preparation "pulls" swelling from an inflamed area in the same way Epsom salts do. Apply a poultice compound under a layer of absorbent material, such as roll cotton. A poultice pulls swelling away from the tissues, and creates a warm, moist, environment. Place a light pressure wrap over the cotton to hold the preparation in place, and to support soft

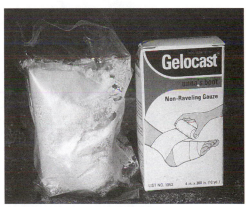

Fig. 9–8. Poultice-impregnated gauze.

tissue. Gelocasts®, zinc oxide-impregnated bandages, and Animalintex® pads serve as excellent, ready-made poulticing materials, and need only be covered with an elastic, adhesive bandage, such as Elastikon®.

Liniments and Balms

Many old-time horse liniments and leg balms also create heat and increase circulation by chemical action and by mild irritation of the skin. Human and equine athletes use these balms to advantage, but most should not be applied under a bandage as there is a real possibility of "burning" the skin. Always read the labels and follow the instructions of the manufacturer.

Other Beneficial Therapies

DMSO

When applied in the same manner as a poultice, dimethyl sulfoxide (DMSO) is a very effective anti-inflammatory agent. It occasionally irritates the skin, and may result in mild hair loss. Do not apply it to any raw or deep wound surfaces. Wear protective gloves when applying DMSO as it easily penetrates human skin.

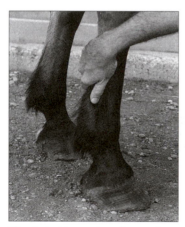

Fig. 9–9. Massaging the tendon.

Massage and Hydrotherapy

Deep massage is beneficial to an injured muscle or tendon along with cold ad heat therapy. It increases circulation and breaks down adhesions formed by scar tissue. Massage by hand manipulation, or by hosing the limb with a forceful spray of water (hydrotherapy). Whirlpool boots are also commercially available. A whirlpool can be made by reversing a vacuum cleaner to convert the sucking air into blowing air. The hose inserted in the water achieves a turbulator effect, but exercise extreme caution when using electrical cords and water in close proximity.

Exercise

Hand walking, or self-exercise in turnout, also enhances circulation to a limb, and reduces the build-up of fibrous scar tissue adhesions in tendon or ligament injuries. Light exercise can begin after the acute inflammatory stage has subsided, which may be from 2 days to 2 weeks after the injury. *"Stocking up"* from confinement, or swelling created by pregnancy responds quickly to light exercise.

Drug Therapy

Drug therapy is used in conjunction with hydrotherapy and rest of an injured leg. Commonly used drugs are the non-steroidal anti-inflammatory drugs (NSAIDs), such as phenylbutazone, Banamine®, or aspirin. NSAIDs limit the inflammatory process before it begins, and limit edema, swelling, and pain. However, NSAIDs can mask a severe problem. They may hide an injury that requires professional attention. They also enable a horse to inflict further injury by lessening a protective pain response.

SYSTEMIC ILLNESS

During the analysis of the injury, note if more than one limb is swollen. If so, it is advisable to contact a veterinarian immediately.

Do not overlook the obvious — simple stocking up from sluggish circulation caused by standing in a stall or small pen. Advanced pregnancy often slows circulation in the tissues, resulting in swollen, stocked up legs. However, complete swelling of more than one leg may signal a systemic problem which affects the entire body. These diseases include:

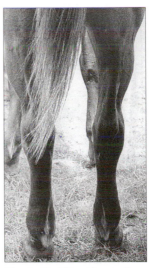

- heart disease
- a tumor or abscess that blocks the lymph system
- a dietary protein deficiency
- protein loss due to intestinal parasitism, or liver, kidney, or intestinal disease

Fig. 9-10. "Stocking up" caused by poor circulation.

- viral infections, such as equine influenza or *equine viral arteritis*
- vaccination reactions
- an allergic form of strangles *(Streptococcus equi)* called *purpura hemorrhagica* which causes blood vessels to leak *(vasculitis)*

Horse owners have treated sore legs with cold and then hot packs for centuries. Modern science has only explained the treatment in medical terms, and defined the limits of this method of therapy. Done properly, the system still works. *(Editor's Note: For information on diagnosing and treating all types of equine injuries, read **The Illustrated Veterinary Encyclopedia for Horsemen,** and **Veterinary Treatments & Medications for Horsemen,** both published by Equine Research, Inc.)*

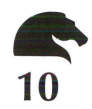

10

TENDON INJURIES: PREVENTING & MANAGING

As the horse evolved to flee predators, the bones in the lower legs telescoped in length. Longer bone provides a lever arm which increases the contraction of the muscles to propel a horse across the ground. When the strap-like tendons that connect muscle to bone cross over a joint surface, the bending motion of the joint amplifies muscle contraction. Elastic energy transmitted within a ten-

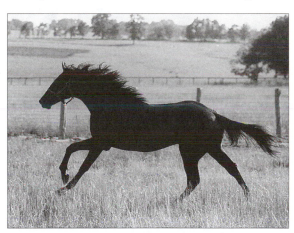

Fig. 10–1. Elastic energy transmitted within a tendon produces locomotion.

don produces locomotion. The athletic horse is at risk of tendon injury because every step stresses these elastic structures.

Tendinitis is an inflammation which involves only the tendon, while *tenosynovitis* is inflammation of the tendon and its sheath. An owner or trainer may see a tendon injury as a *bowed tendon*. A bowed tendon results from an inflammatory condition in the tendon that causes it to thicken with scar tissue.

There are several kinds of bowed tendons, each classified according to their position on the limb. A low bow is in the lower cannon area near the fetlock joint. A middle bow is in the middle of the cannon area. A high bow is in the upper cannon area. A full bow involves all three areas. If a horse suffers from tendinitis or a bowed tendon, its athletic career is not necessarily over. Proper management and healing of the original injury greatly influence how well a tendon regains function and resists repeated trauma.

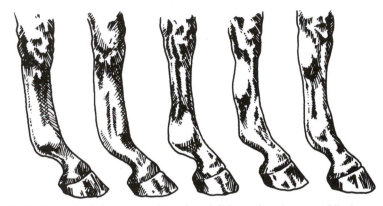

Fig. 10–2. From the left, a normal tendon, full bow, low bow, middle bow, and high bow.

A study by Dr. Roy Pool (University of California at Davis) found that 25% of clinically "normal," symptomless horses have some microscopic abnormality in the tendon, suggesting a degenerating area of tendon. If this unhealthy spot increases, and a tendon is continually or abruptly overstretched, clinical tendinitis results.

STRESS HANDLING OF TENDONS
Tendon Structure

Tendons are made of bundles of longitudinally oriented collagen fibers. Most tendons are surrounded by sheaths. The tendon sheath allows the tendon to glide smoothly over the structures of a limb. As the limb bears weight, a tendon normally extends within a narrow range of elasticity. When reasonably stretched (as with weight-bearing), the collagen fibers maintain their linear and parallel order. Then once the load is removed they snap back to the original position.

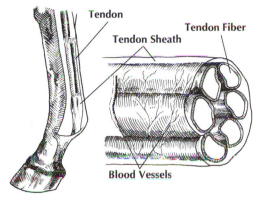

Fig. 10–3. Tendon structure and sheath.

Tendon Injury

Tendon and Muscle Interaction

One of the normal functions of the flexor tendons along the back of the cannon bone is to stabilize the fetlock. These tendons prevent the fetlock from collapsing onto the ground when the limb is supporting weight. Normally, the muscle decreases the stress on the tendon, which attaches the muscle to the bone. When the muscle fatigues, vibration in the muscle and tendon *(musculotendinous unit)* increases strain on the collagen fibers of the tendon. As groups of muscles fatigue, the limb sinks into unnatural configurations. An example is *dorsiflexion* of the fetlock, when the fetlock sinks toward the ground, overstretching the flexor tendons.

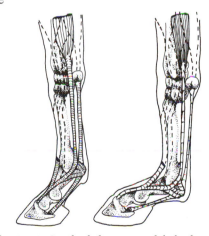

Fig. 10–4. On the left, a normal fetlock. On the right, dorsiflexion of the fetlock.

Overloading Tendons

Initially, a tendon adapts to the stretch, but increased loading of a limb may extend a tendon beyond its elastic limit. If a tendon is stretched beyond 5% – 6% of its length, the fibers stiffen, and irre-

249

versible structural damage results. Like a rubber band that has been overstretched, once the excessive weight-bearing strain is removed an overstretched tendon does not regain its original pattern. If a tendon is stretched beyond 8% of its length, it can rupture.

Conditioning Tendons

Overstretching a tendon through overloading results from excessive athletic demands for which the horse is not conditioned. Conditioning is one way to prevent and manage tendinitis, or a bowed tendon. Light and repeated loading of tendons through conditioning and training stimulates the tendons to respond to mechanical strain. They become more elastic and resist being overstretched.

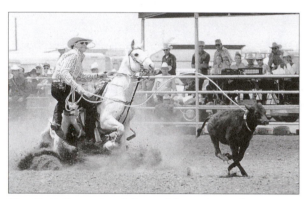

Fig. 10–5. Sports involving sudden twists and turns can cause tendon injury.

If a horse is fatigued, or if a training program incorporates too much speed, jumping, uneven terrain, or sudden twists and turns, tendons lose stability when the corresponding muscles become exhausted or are overloaded. It is therefore important to properly condition a horse for the intended sport. Other mechanical factors, such as poor footing, unbalanced feet, poor conformation, and high risk activities also contribute to tendon injury and should be avoided.

Mechanical Factors Leading to Tendon Injury
Poor Footing

If a foot is not picked up quickly enough as the body advances across the ground, the *superficial digital flexor tendon* is overstretched. The *superficial flexor muscle* contracts as a horse propels forward. The complementary tendon should be shortening, but if the pastern is not picked up and moved forward quickly enough, the fetlock sinks to the ground (dorsiflexes) while the body continues forward. The tendon will then overstretch.

Situations that can cause poor footing and tendon injury include:

- Slippery ground that encourages a hoof to slide backwards, simulating a situation where the leg is too far under the body where it cannot advance or be lifted quickly
- Deep footing, such as mud, sand, or snow which causes a foot to sink—it may not elevate in time to avoid tendon injury

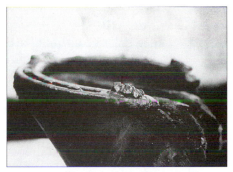

- Shoe caulks, trailers, or studs on the shoes which make the foot "stick," delaying lift and advancement of the foot as the body moves forward
- Uneven footing which excessively loads the tendons beyond normal stress limits

Fig. 10–6. Shoe caulks can make a foot stick, thereby delaying lift and advancement of the foot.

Unbalanced Feet

Unbalanced feet simulate uneven footing, causing a leg to twist unnaturally because it is unevenly loaded. Once it was thought that raising the heels on a tendon-injured horse would decrease the stress on the tendon. This idea is incorrect: raising the heel lengthens the distance the tendon drops with weight-bearing and increases tension on an already-injured tendon. A serious bow may benefit from slightly lowering the heels, but it is best to trim the feet at a proper and reasonable angle.

A broken hoof-pastern axis angle also interferes with a smooth breakover of the limb. For example, a long-toe – low-heel (LTLH) configuration slows lift and delays advancement of the foot as it travels.

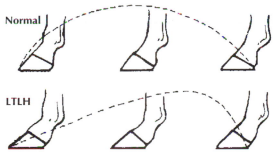

Fig. 10–7. A long-toe – low-heel configuration delays lift and advancement.

Poor Conformation

A calf knee conformation functionally mimics a LTLH hoof, delaying breakover and stressing the flexor tendons. A long, upright pastern conformation predisposes to tendon injury by increasing the fetlock drop experienced with weight-bearing.

High Risk Activities

Certain activities contribute to dorsiflexion of the fetlock, increasing the risk of overstretching a tendon. Jumping not only abnormally loads the forelegs upon landing, but often involves sudden and tight turns, or uneven terrain. Roping, barrel racing, cutting, and polo are other examples of activities that abruptly load the forelegs as a horse is turning or moving at speed. Long distance riding, negotiating downhill terrain, or the speed work of racing place excessive demands on the entire musculotendinous unit.

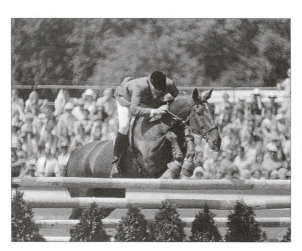

Fig. 10–8. Jumping is a high risk activity which can injure a tendon.

In some cases, it is necessary to change the athletic pursuit of an injured horse to ensure a successful career. For example, a jumping horse can be converted to a pleasure or equitation candidate. A cutting, barrel racing, or reining horse can become a western pleasure or trail horse. A racehorse can become a hunter/jumper, dressage, or driving horse.

INJURY PRONE AREAS

Cannon Bone Area

There are several areas on equine legs where injuries most often occur. The *superficial digital flexor tendon* along the back of the cannon bone is predisposed to injury because it is under the greatest amount of tension. It is also farthest from the center of rotation of the fetlock joint. Many injuries occur at the point where the superficial digital flexor has the smallest cross-sectional area, which is in

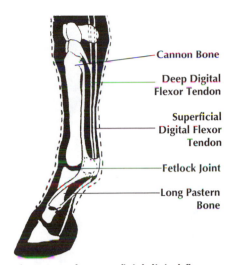

Fig. 10–9. The superficial digital flexor tendon is especially prone to injury.

the middle of the cannon bone area. As the tendon's cross-sectional area decreases, it becomes stiffer and less elastic. In addition, there is an increased force per unit area on this narrower segment of the tendon.

Fetlock Area

Another area highly susceptible to injury is the fetlock area. If the *deep digital flexor tendon* is injured, a low bow results. Tendon injuries in the fetlock area or below have a poorer prognosis than injuries higher on the limb. Because of the digital sheath over the tendon in this area, more connective tissue develops beneath the skin (subcutaneous) in the healing process. This tissue restricts gliding of the tendon through the sheath.

The *volar anular ligament*, a non-elastic band of dense connective tissue, runs horizontally across the back of the fetlock, and may be involved in a low bow. The volar anular ligament does not stretch as the deep digital flexor tendon swells, therefore the ligament binds down the inflamed tendon. This unrelenting pressure reduces blood flow to the tendon over time. Fiber death, reduction in gliding motion,

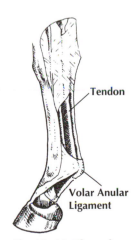

Fig. 10–10. The volar anular ligament will bind down an inflamed tendon.

253

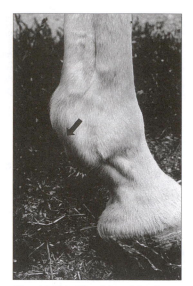

Fig. 10–11. The "dent" in the swelling is due to volar anular ligament constriction.

and development of adhesions which bind the two structures together result from a reduced blood flow. The ligament constricts, resulting in a visible depression over the back of the fetlock, with a pronounced bulge above and/or below, near the digital tendon sheath.

With immediate surgical intervention to release the constricting ligament, there is a more favorable prognosis for a horse to return to function. If adhesions are allowed to progress too long before surgery, they "glue" the structures together, permanently restricting the tendon and causing pain.

TENDON REPAIR

What begins as small microscopic tears in the orderly tendon fibers may expand to a large tear. Accompanying inflammation produces clinical symptoms of pain, heat, or swelling. Capillary bleeding within the tendon triggers an inflammatory response. Edema and bleeding interrupt the normal tendon fibers' pattern of tight, longitudinally-oriented, and parallel bundles. The tendon is weakest at 5 – 7 days after injury, with the acute inflammatory stage lasting up to 14 days.

Tendons are excellent at repairing themselves if given the time and help they need. To better understand how to aid healing, and speed a return to function, it is helpful to study the healing process within an injured tendon.

Fibrin and Granulation Tissue Repair Process

Fibrin is a blood component which binds together torn tendon collagen. In the first 3 weeks after injury, this fibrin forms a *fibrovascular callus* around the injured tendon. The fibrovascular callus connects the wounded structures, in effect, hardening the fibrin cells into a scaffold, in preparation for repair. Then, like a skin wound, the body repairs the tendon injury with *granulation tissue* and more fibrous connective tissue.

The blood supply within the tendon only nourishes about 25% of the tendon volume. But because inflammation limits internal blood flow, healing components must come from the tissue around the tendon (peritendinous). The more the peritendinous cells contribute to healing, the greater the development of adhesions and scar tissue. Adhesions restrict the normal gliding ability of the tendon through the sheath, and scar tissue limits its elasticity.

During this repair period, granulation tissue forms and then organizes into fibrous tissue. The inflammatory process permanently thickens a tendon with scar tissue, giving the visual impression of a bow where there had been a straight structure.

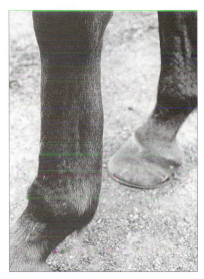

Fig. 10–12. A bowed tendon is thickened with scar tissue.

During the next few months, a tendon repair "matures." Collagen fibers redevelop to a normal, longitudinal orientation. Usually, by 6 weeks after injury, collagen formation exceeds collagen breakdown within the tendon. By 3 months, collagen fibers begin to form discrete bundles. The bundles are similar to normal tendon by 4 months.

Exercises That Promote Healing

During the repair process, controlled passive motion exercises realign collagen fibers longitudinally by placing mild tension on the tendon. These slow, range-of-motion exercises include manual flexion and extension of the limb for 10 – 15 minutes, 2 or 3 times a day. After the acute inflammatory stage, begin light hand walking.

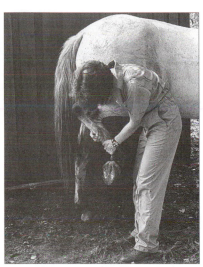

Fig. 10–13. Manual flexion of the injured limb realigns collagen fibrils.

Progressively increase these exercises over the months. It is not known how much passive physical therapy is appropriate, therefore it is wise not to overdo this practice.

Aggressive physical activity interferes with repair, and reinjury can occur. Attempts to forcibly break down adhesions are counterproductive, whereas gentle lengthening and stretching of scar tissue gives better results.

Healing Time

The time required for healing varies, depending on the extent of the injury. A minimum recovery period for slight tendon tearing may require only a month. More severe injuries require *at least 10 months* for a tendon fiber to completely heal. It may be necessary for a horse to recover for 1 – 1½ years to achieve optimal repair. It is essential that veterinary recommendations be followed, so that a performance horse is given a long enough recuperative period to prevent a relapse.

Indications of "healing" can be misleading. Many horses at 10 weeks after injury may not respond to finger pressure over the tendon. They may also have no heat or swelling in the area. However, there are still areas of tendon damage that are in the earlier healing stages and require a longer rest period than other areas of the same tendon.

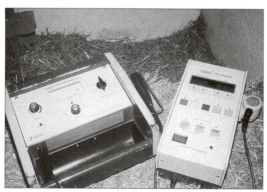

Fig. 10–14. Two types of ultrasound machines.

Ultrasound Evaluation of Injuries

Ultrasound is a useful tool to evaluate tendon injuries and to monitor healing. Before the introduction of ultrasound, only certain clinical signs could be used to evaluate tendon healing. A study by Dr. Virginia Reef (University of Pennsylvania) revealed that specific, outward, clinical appearances have little relationship to the severity of a tendon injury as evidenced by ultrasound.

In her study, heat was felt in only 17% of injured tendons. Heat diminishes long before healing is completed, therefore it is not a reliable indi-

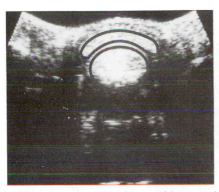 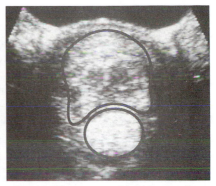

Fig. 10–15. Ultrasound is used by veterinarians to diagnose and monitor an injury. For example, on the left is a normal deep digital flexor tendon and superficial digital flexor tendon. On the right, the deep digital flexor is still intact, but the superficial digital flexor tendon is disrupted and severely injured.

cator of readiness to return to work. Similarly, only 19% of the horses in the study were sensitive to finger pressure over the afflicted tendon. Only 40% had an associated lameness, while swelling or filling of the leg was apparent in 85% of the horses. These numbers illustrate that the degree of lameness or swelling is *not* a reliable indicator of the severity of an injury. Accurate assessments of the extent of tendon damage and the progress of healing require the use of diagnostic ultrasound technology.

How it Works

With diagnostic ultrasound, high frequency sound waves are transmitted to a tendon. The denser the tissue, the more resistant it is to sound waves, and the sound waves bounce back off the tissue surface as an "echo." The denser the tissue, the grayer the projection seen on the screen *(echogenicity)*. If the sound waves pass freely through blood, fluid, or edema, the image appears black on the screen because the sound waves do not produce an echo.

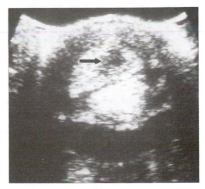

In this way, a tendon is "imaged" to measure the extent of an injury in both width and length. The monitor shows areas of fiber disruption, or swelling of a tendon.

Fig. 10–16. The black dot in the middle is a central core lesion.

For example, a common tendon injury is a *central core lesion* associated with severe fiber disruption and hemorrhage. On the screen, the lesion appears as a black hole in the center of the tendon. The size of the hole determines the severity of the injury and prognosis for return to athletic soundness.

Both mild and severe injuries initially give similar outward appearances of pain, swelling, and heat. However, the prognosis for healing is radically different between a severe central core lesion and a tendon that is merely swollen. Ultrasound discerns these differences at the onset.

Monitoring Healing

Ultrasound is useful to monitor the healing process over time. The increasing grayness on the screen reflects the stage of healing. This information helps to plan a strategy for returning a horse to performance. After an appropriate lay-up period, and as the echogenicity of the lesion increases, longer and faster workouts can be used to restore tendon strength. Exercise reorients the fibers along the plane of tension. Ultrasound diagnostics are repeated at 2–3 month intervals to monitor progress for as long as 1–3 years after an injury has occurred.

RECURRENCE OF TENDON INJURY

A recurrence of a tendon injury is possible if the tendon is prematurely stressed while an injury is visible on ultrasound as a "discrete healing lesion." Also, not all fully healed tendon injuries are immune to further damage. A prior tendinitis does not result in loss of strength in the tendon, but it does result in reduced elasticity. A previously injured tendon, bowed or not, may be unable to withstand normal stresses placed on it by exercise.

Transition Zone

Subsequent tendon damage does not necessarily occur at the site of the original injury. It often occurs just above or below the point where tendon structure least resembles normal structure. These areas are called *transition zones* because they are between the normal areas and previously injured areas of the tendon. Adhesions in the transition zones may prevent the fibers from orienting longitudinally as they heal. Instead, they orient abnormally and may prematurely tear before they reorganize in a longitudinal pattern. Fibers with a loosely structured and random pattern are a weak link in the collagen chain.

Adhesions are unyielding, causing the inelastic tendon tissue above or below the original injury to "super stretch." Continued microtrauma in this area enlarges the traumatized area, and causes lameness due to chronic inflammation.

TENDON THERAPY

There are many approaches to therapy for tendinitis or a bowed tendon. The ultimate goal is to restore elasticity and gliding function to the tendon. As indicated, lameness, heat, sensitivity, and filling of the tendons are unreliable indicators of actual injury in the area, yet these may be the only indicators if ultrasound is not available. Once these symptoms appear, take emergency measures to minimize damage.

Controlling Swelling

Local swelling and hemorrhage further damage tendon fibers. Therefore, controlling swelling is essential if the tendon is to heal well and with limited adhesions. If a horse shows lameness in a previously bowed limb, or if it is sensitive to pressure over an affected tendon, ice the leg immediately or hose it with cold water to limit swelling. A light pressure bandage controls swelling beneath the skin, which is associated with cold therapy, until a veterinarian arrives. Non-steroidal anti-inflammatory drugs control swelling. DMSO applied to the tendon area under a light bandage also exerts strong anti-inflammatory effects. After acute inflammation has stopped, warm soaks improve circulation and elasticity of the tendon and assist the healing process. Depending on the extent of the injury, the acute inflammatory stage may last from 2 days to 2 weeks.

Surgery

For superficial digital flexor injuries, Dr. Larry Bramlage (Rood and Riddle Equine Hospital, Lexington, Kentucky) has suggested cutting the superior check ligament just above the knee to release tension on the scarred tendon. Performing this surgery during the initial repair stage significantly reduces scarring in the tendon. The superior check ligament becomes longer as it heals, reducing tension on the injured tendon. Its transitional zone is not subjected to much stress because both the muscle and tendon above the knee actively assume some of the load of weight-bearing.

Bandaging

After a layoff for a tendon injury, support wraps are useful during reintroduction to work by delaying the onset of fatigue in an injured leg. It is speculated that a bandage also limits dorsiflexion of the fetlock when the limb is fatigued. A leg bandaged with the Equisport® (3-M) bandage can absorb up to 39% more energy, for example, dorsiflexion of the fetlock, than an unbandaged leg. With its elastic properties, the bandage assumes the elastic function of the tendons as the fetlock sinks with weight-bearing, reducing strain on the tendons.

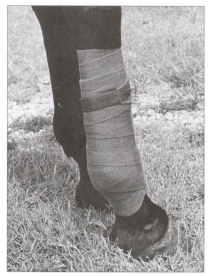

Fig. 10–17. Bandages support injured tendons and are sometimes used to protect sound legs from tendon injury.

The supportive capabilities of a bandage depend on the tension with which it is applied, and the bandage configuration. The tighter the bandage is applied, the greater is its energy-absorption capacity. Be sure not to apply the bandage so tightly as to cut off the circulation. If in doubt, consult a veterinarian.

The most versatile method of applying the Equisport® bandage is at half-stretch tension in a low figure eight, starting just below the knee and spiraling down with a two to three layer figure eight over the fetlock, and the bandage spiraled up again to the knee. Applied in this manner, the bandage does not inhibit fetlock mobility, and at half-stretch tension it should not impair local circulation or constrict the tendons.

Materials that absorb the most energy also tend to wear out fastest. Bandage support of a limb declines rapidly with an increasing number of fetlock dorsiflexions. Studies with the Equisport® bandage focus mainly on racetrack application where the bandage only needs to aid limb support for about 2 – 5 minutes. This limitation must be considered when bandaging a long distance trail horse, dressage, or jumping horse. Bandages may be more of a hindrance than a help if they are too tight and impair local circulation, or if they partially restrict the range of motion of the fetlock joint.

MANAGEMENT

After a tendon injury, the horse should be stalled for at least 2 – 3 weeks to restrict movement of the limb. This enforced rest prevents further damage to the tendon.

To promote proper realignment of the fibers by passive motion therapy, the ankle can be alternately flexed and extended for short periods several times daily after the acute inflammatory stage has subsided.

Ultrasound documents the initial injury, and monitors its progress to recovery. Follow a conservative approach based on recommendations by a veterinarian and ultrasound information before returning a horse to active work.

There is no substitute for appropriate conditioning or proper choice of athletic function. In managing an old injury, the importance of a warm-up and cool-down for a horse (and tendons) cannot be overstated. Good circulation in the limbs improves the elasticity of the musculotendinous unit and helps to avoid tendon injury. *(Editor's Note: For information on diagnosing and treating many types of equine injuries, read **The Illustrated Veterinary Encyclopedia for Horsemen,** and **Veterinary Treatments & Medications for Horsemen**, both published by Equine Research, Inc.)*

11

HIGH-TECH THERAPY FOR INJURIES

For any athlete, pain can be the difference between a poor performance and one that is brilliant. Equine athletes may only be able to communicate subtle pain by a decline in their athletic output. High-tech therapies, used along with conventional medicine, can relieve pain and heal injuries.

HIGH-TECH THERAPY APPLICATIONS

Diagnosis

An honest evaluation of a technique's effectiveness requires accurate diagnosis of the injury. Adding technological advances, such as heart rate monitors, to a training program lends insight into the level of discomfort a horse experiences while at work. Previously "inexplicable" impairments in performance can now be documented. A sustained, higher than normal heart rate at a given work level reflects pain induced by exercise stress.

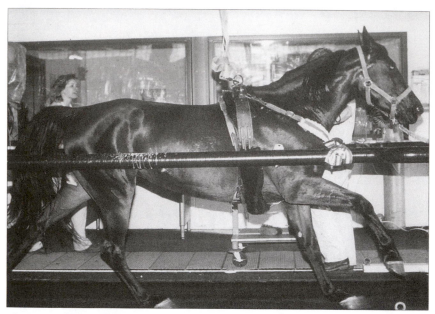

Fig. 11–1. Gait analysis using a treadmill and video camaras can help detect subtle problems before they become serious.

A gait analysis monitor is an imaging device that shows how well a limb is moving on a treadmill. In addition, video cameras can record and exactly measure the length and cadence of strides to detect subtle problems before they become serious. Infrared thermography is a diagnostic tool which images heat gradients. It detects inflammatory conditions, particularly of the lower limbs, spine, face, and superficial muscles. Such devices often foretell impending failure.

Injury Management

Not only is sophisticated technology used to define a problem, but these tools are also applied to manage a healing process, and to facilitate the horse's rapid return to soundness. Recently, researchers have dedicated their efforts to evaluating high-tech therapies—such as lasers and ultrasound—for injury management. In many cases conventional medicine is insufficient to "cure" a lameness. Therefore it is understandable that a frustrated owner or trainer may seek high-tech alternatives to alleviate a chronic problem that has not responded to standard treatment.

Relieving Pain

No single approach is infallible, especially when it comes to the healing process. The medical profession can only assist nature and manipulate biological processes to proceed along a desired course. Many high-tech options such as *Transcutaneous Electrical Nerve Stimulation* (TENS) provide pain relief without actually "curing" the injury.

When an injury occurs, the body's guarding response increases muscle tension with a subsequent decrease in blood flow. This decrease causes waste products to accumulate in the injured area. In addition, the body's natural inflammatory response to the injury includes continued production of prostaglandins and other chemicals that reinforce inflammation, heat, swelling, and pain. Pain relief limits the inflammatory response, enabling the body to heal quickly. Although the problem remains, it does not interfere with performance to the same degree. TENS, electroanalgesia, lasers, and ultrasound provide pain relief. Laser radiation and ultrasound, however, also promote healing.

Promoting Healing

Using scientific evidence about biological factors that promote healing, high-tech options such as lasers and ultrasound attempt to stimulate circulation to the tissues. Electrical Muscle Stimulation (EMS) also promotes healing. Healing requires adequate circulation of oxygen and nutrients to the tissues, and removal of waste products from the tissues. Lasers, ultrasound, and EMS accomplish these goals similar to how conventional procedures use pharmacological drugs, hot and cold therapy, or poultices.

When a horse is in obvious need of conventional surgical or medical treatment, alternative therapies do little to repair the injury. However, the use of high-tech alternatives along with conventional surgery, pharmacological drugs, and physical therapy enhances the probability for successful treatment.

ANCIENT ARTS, NEW TECHNOLOGY

Several new technologies capitalize on "modern" knowledge of the healing process, while instituting the ancient principles of the arts of *acupuncture* and *acupressure* to manage an injury. These high-tech therapies are a blending of Eastern and Western medical philosophies.

Acupressure and acupuncture operate by stimulating specific nerve tracts and meridians that directly interact with the injured body part. These "points" can now be stimulated by high-tech tools in a variety of ways.

Acupuncture

The ancient art of acupuncture stimulates specific nerve fibers with needle penetration. There are many good books on the market today regarding the pure forms of acupuncture and acupressure. This chapter deals only with the modern applications of those arts, using high-tech equipment. High-tech ways of stimulating acupuncture points are:

- heat application to the points
- acu-injection of drugs or saline at the points to prolong stimulation of the nerve
- electrical stimulation of the points

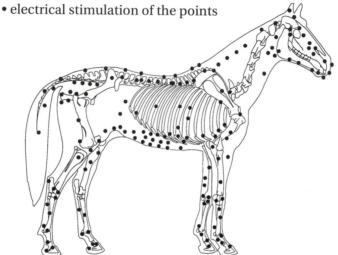

Fig. 11–2. An overview of the numerous acupuncture points of the horse.

Acupressure

Acupressure is an off-shoot of acupuncture. It seeks to stimulate the same points as acupuncture, but without penetrating the skin. Because it requires no technical knowledge, there are many ways to use acupressure. One way to use acupressure on the horse is massage therapy. Another common acupressure tool is the twitch.

The Twitch and Endorphin Release

A nose twitch "sedates" and relaxes the horse while a mildly painful procedure is performed. Heart rates decrease up to 8% while using a twitch, just the opposite response expected from a painful or frightening experience.

It is hypothesized that the twitch stimulates specialized sensory fibers in the skin, resulting in a release of chemicals from the central nervous system. These chemicals, similar to morphine, are called *endorphins* and *enkephalins.* They reduce and suppress perception of pain. Scientists at the University of Utrecht, Netherlands, analyzed levels of these substances in the blood and discovered that endorphin levels increased by 81% during twitching, and returned to normal within 30 minutes after the twitch was removed.

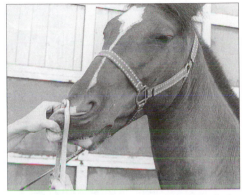

Fig. 11–3. Pressure from the use of a twitch releases endorphins and enkephalins.

ELECTRICAL THERAPIES
Transcutaneous Electrical Nerve Stimulation
Relieving Pain

One method of electrically stimulating acupuncture points is Transcutaneous Electrical Nerve Stimulation, known as TENS. This point stimulation provides relief from pain symptoms.

Conventional TENS therapy provides a voltage of electrical pulses high enough to stimulate the acupuncture points, but low enough to avoid sustained muscle contractions. Impulses are passed to the nervous system using a padded electrode placed over the skin. The electrodes send impulses to nerve receptors in the skin and in the superficial tissues. Sensory information is relayed to the central nervous system by specific pain receptors *(nociceptors).*

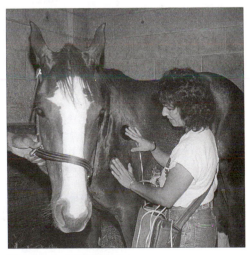

Fig. 11–4. A TENS set-up.

267

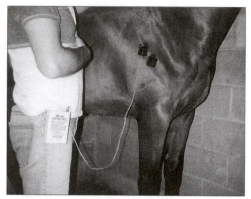

Fig. 11–5. Another TENS set-up.

These nociceptors are located in areas of motor and trigger acupuncture points. A motor point excites muscle tissue and causes it to contract. Trigger points define hypersensitive areas afflicted with inflammation and tenderness.

Many acupuncture points are located in the superficial skin layers, where nerves and nociceptors transmit impulses from both the internal and external environments to the central nervous system. Stimulation of these nerve fibers and pain receptors by TENS results in the production and release of endorphins and enkephalins from the brain. Although the half-life of enkephalins is as brief as 1 minute, endorphins have a half-life of 2 – 3 hours, providing opiate-like pain relief.

The Gate Theory

TENS provides pain relief by a "gate theory." Repeated, *non-painful* stimulation of the sensory nerve fibers causes the nerve endings to fatigue. Then they are unable to transmit pain sensation to the brain. This overload of stimulation also causes a release of *serotonin*, a chemical which blocks pain impulses and reception by the brain, and, in effect, "closes a gate." Then the brain "ignores" the less intense stimulus of the injury.

Diagnosis

TENS is also a valuable diagnostic tool, particularly if used in conjunction with infrared thermography. Infrared thermography shows heat gradients, detecting inflammatory conditions. An inflamed area is already stimulated by pain reflexes because it hurts. Therefore, less voltage is required from TENS to "fire" a trigger point nerve. TENS finds the more sensitive nerve tracts, which are in an inflamed area. This method confirms an infrared thermograph which shows acute inflammatory heat patterns. Conversely, in structurally sound areas with no inflammation, infrared thermography shows "cold" patterns. Appropriate therapy can then be directed at the specific injury site.

Electroanalgesia

Another type of electrical stimulation, electroanalgesia, is very similar to TENS therapy, but uses different frequencies than TENS. Unlike conventional TENS, electroanalgesia mildly amplifies electrical output to produce visible muscle twitches.

Low-Frequency Electroanalgesia

Low-frequency electroanalgesia (LFEA) may provide pain relief for 1 – 3 days. LFEA is especially helpful for the chronic pain of degenerative joint disease because it stimulates large nerve fibers in the joint to elicit a central pain suppressing effect.

High-Frequency Electroanalgesia

At a higher frequency than used for TENS, electroanalgesia also provides pain relief by the gate theory (ignoring the less intense stimulus of the injury), and by releasing endorphins. *High-frequency electroanalgesia* (HFEA) relieves pain more quickly than LFEA, but pain relief is sustained for shorter periods than LFEA.

Electrical Muscle Stimulation

High voltage *Electrical Muscle Stimulation* (EMS) has been reported to exercise atrophied muscles by passively producing muscle contractions. Muscles are strengthened through this process because it "retrains" the biochemical and enzymatic reactions vital to adequate muscle contraction. A limb that needs rest for bone, joint, ligament, or tendon repair can be "exercised" without weight-bearing and is not unduly stressed while healing. Also, the pumping action of these electrically-produced muscle contractions indirectly improves circulation to the area. Therefore, improved blood flow enhances the healing process while removing waste products, and edema formed by a stagnant circulation is reduced. EMS may also improve cases of laminitis by improving circulation to the foot.

Pulsing Electromagnetic Fields

Still another high-tech method allegedly improves oxygen supply and increases temperature within the tissues (particularly bone) by improving dilation of blood vessels and circulation. This in turn promotes healing. This technique uses *Pulsing Electromagnetic Fields* (PEMF). It is sometimes used for bone injuries, especially long

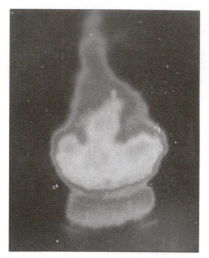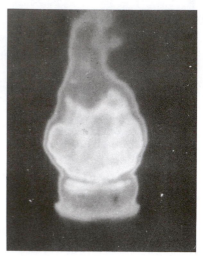

Fig. 11–6. Thermograph showing increased blood flow into the foot after EMS. On the left, before treatment. On the right, after treatment the light area, signifying blood flow, is lighter and larger than before.

bones, such as bucked shins or splints.

Usually two electromagnetic coils are placed on opposite sides of the injured area, with each coil "capturing" the electromagnetic field of the other to align it into a uniform field. This uniform field supposedly produces a uniform electric current within the tissues.

Normally, bone has an electrical polarity. The pulsing field generated on the coils mimics the long bone's normal electrical potentials, stimulating faster healing.

Theoretically, varying wave patterns and pulse rates determine the biological response. There is still no evidence as to which specific pulses and waves affect what or how. It is speculated that magnetic fields increase oxygen levels in tissue and improve energy production to fuel healing processes. Improving circulation and oxygen to the tissues may also limit the pain created by lack of oxygen.

A similar principle attempts to use biomagnetic, flexible, rubber or plastic pads surrounding a foil. The foil contains a magnetized iron compound, producing alternating magnetic fields. Foil pads are bandaged in place to increase circulation when applied over blood vessels.

The principle of PEMF is good in theory, but controlled research projects comparing different electromagnetic devices show no improvement in the healing rates of bone or tendon.

LASERS

A recent method of wound healing and pain relief is using *Laser* radiation as a "light-needle" to stimulate acupuncture points. The word "laser" is an acronym for *Light Amplification by Stimulated Emission of Radiation.*

Laser radiation is generated by electromagnetic waves of the same wavelength that are aligned in both time and space, and travel in nearly parallel directions. These characteristics allow the waves to be focused as a thin beam onto a very small spot. The intensity of this beam can be

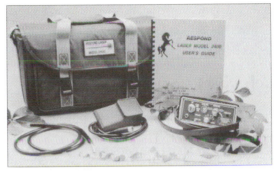

Fig. 11–7. Portable laser unit and components.

magnified to cut directly through living flesh. Laser radiation is used as a surgical tool for intricate procedures such as eye or urogenital surgery. A less intense beam can coagulate tissues to control bleeding during surgery.

The most common commercial laser uses 85% helium and 15% neon to produce a beam of radiation at the far end of the visible light spectrum. Because a red beam is visible to the human eye, it can be accurately applied.

Benefits of Soft Laser Treatment

The intensity of the laser is lowered by deliberately broadening, or de-focusing the beam to be used on a larger area of the horse. The result is called "cold" heat, or soft laser treatment (SLT). SLT may stimulate wound healing reportedly by modifying biochemical responses, particularly collagen (connective tissue) repair, and increasing energy production. It may also alleviate pain by releasing endorphins.

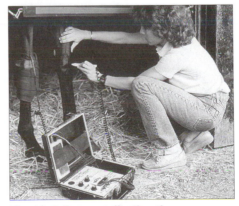

Fig. 11–8. Laser application therapy.

A threshold of laser energy must be delivered to affect the tissues, but not enough energy to be destructive. In some situations, a pulsing wave is more beneficial than a continuous beam. With a continuous beam, damage to the tissues due to overheating is possible. As yet, the threshold level has not been exactly defined, and depends on the type of tissue, whether bone, muscle, tendon, or ligament.

More important, the tissues must receive the laser energy at a wavelength that can be absorbed and not reflected. Commercially available lasers differ in the amount of energy they deliver to the tissue, and these products are not standardized.

Relieving Pain

The most profound effect of laser therapy may be pain suppression by stimulating acupuncture points. Cells absorb laser energy readily due to the laser's interaction with normal cell processes. For example, lasers favorably affect the sodium-potassium pump that is the essence of intracellular communication and biochemical reactions, which causes cellular functions to speed up.

Because absorption is so great, laser energy usually penetrates 3.6 – 15 millimeters, which although only skin deep may activate acupuncture points to release endorphins. Endorphin and enkephalin levels increase in the blood and in the cerebrospinal fluid to provide pain relief. SLT also suppresses pain transmission by nerves, reducing nerve tissue excitability.

Promoting Healing

At present, researchers are still speculating how SLT accelerates healing. The laser energy itself may affect the tissues as a whole by "vibrating" the cells at a specific wavelength. Or, a particular frequency of applied energy may effect specific cellular functions of the "lasered" tissue.

Biochemical functions may be stimulated to rapidly respond to an injury. The "cold" heat generated by soft laser energy excites protein synthesis, cell replication, and communication between the cells. The biochemical signals tell the injured body part to heal faster, which intensifies the immune response.

Developing blood vessels within the tissue improves circulation, reducing swelling and edema. Fibroblasts, the precursors of connective tissue, are stimulated to produce collagen faster and correctly.

Wounds

Because it excites the natural immune response, soft laser therapy can be used to heal open wounds. The wound is stimulated to heal more quickly than with conventional medicine alone.

Day 1   **Day 15**   **Day 35**

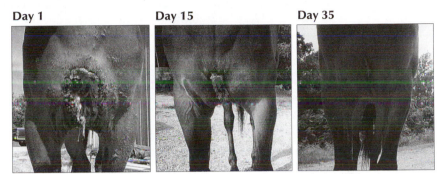

Fig. 11–9. The accelerated healing process of a wound treated with soft laser therapy and penicillin.

Laser is particularly applicable to horses with retarded healing processes such as old wounds with necrotic, or dead and dying tissue. Collagen deposit is enhanced in such cases, reawakening and accelerating healing without risking excessive scar formation.

Internal Injuries

Use of cold laser is not limited to open wounds. It helps heal bowed tendons, curtails ligament injuries, and curbs sore throats from an over-reacting lymph system. Used correctly, it is a safe tool for non-invasive therapy, where cellular membranes remain intact, and no detectable changes occur in the cells.

This non-invasive characteristic is the magic of laser therapy. Initially, therapy is applied once or twice a day. Then the intervals between applications are progressively lengthened.

The arts of acupuncture and acupressure have been used successfully for thousands of years by Eastern approaches to medicine. Through our unfailing worship of high technology, the West may have inadvertently stumbled onto the healing applications of these ancient arts.

ULTRASOUND

Ultrasound has been a major benefit to medical diagnostics. It identifies illness or injury of internal body organs or musculoskeletal structures. *(See Chapter 10 for more information.)*

Ultrasound is also a therapeutic tool because it "heats" musculoskeletal components that may be too deep, too large, or too dense to benefit from hot soaking. We are all familiar with the healing effects of deep heat. For human athletes, heating pads, hot whirlpool baths, hot tubs, and saunas relax aching muscles and improve circulation in the body. Since it is impractical to immerse a horse in a steaming water bath for 20–30 minutes, we must resort to other measures.

The penetrating warmth of ultrasound therapy reduces spasms in muscles or tendons, particularly in the large muscles over the back, buttocks, and shoulders. It is especially difficult to use conventional heat therapy in these areas because only superficial warming would result. (Ultrasound should **not** be used over open and contaminated wounds, because it can drive bacteria further into the tissues, spreading infection.)

Mechanics of Ultrasound

Ultrasound's therapeutic advantage comes from its mechanical effects. As sound waves enter the tissues, the tissue molecules "vibrate." Energy created by the friction of sound waves entering the tissue generates heat. Ultrasound energy is barely absorbed by skin, but is well-absorbed in tissues with a high protein and low fluid content, such as muscles, tendons, and ligaments. Muscle absorbs 2½ times as much of this energy as fat, and bone absorbs 10 times as much energy as muscle.

Types of Ultrasound
Continuous Waves

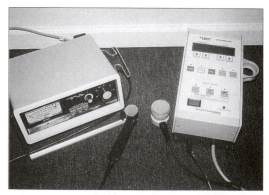

Ultrasound is used as either a continuous wave, or a pulse at regular intervals. Continuous wave ultrasound provides deep heat, improving elasticity and pliability of tight, thickened, and scarred tissues. Horses involved in sports that require collection, pushing from behind, or stretching the back can form scar tissue

Fig. 11–10. Ultrasound machines with different sized heads for different areas of the horse.

in their backs. These sports include endurance racing, eventing, jumping, and dressage. Or, scar tissue can form as *fibrotic myopathy* within the thigh muscles. The deep heat of ultrasound therapy benefits these injuries.

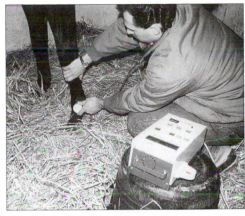

Fig. 11–11. Ultrasound application.

Problems With Continuous Wave

If ultrasonic waves are generated continuously, excessive heat builds in the shallow tissues. Ultrasound can raise tissue temperature by 7° – 8° F at 2 inches below the skin surface if applied continuously over one spot or for too long. This method is counterproductive because too much heat injures the tissues, resulting in permanent damage to bone and surrounding tissue. The appropriate amount of time depends on the type of tissue and the injury involved, and as yet have not been defined.

Bones are very dense, and the sound waves cannot pass all the way through them. The energy reflects back to the source, overheating the bone and surrounding tissue.

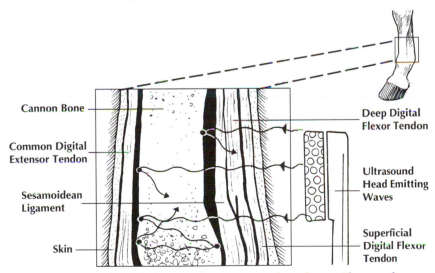

Fig. 11–12. The effects of ultrasound waves on various tissues. The sound waves bounce off of and inside the bone, causing heating.

Ultrasound treatment of fractured, inflamed, or growing bone results in excessive blood circulation to the bone, with resultant demineralization and thinning of the affected area. Excessively heating bone and surrounding tissues destroys the blood supply, causing part of the bone to die and separate from the healthy bone.

Pulsing Waves

Pulsated waves can be compared to waves crashing on a beach. Unlike the ocean, however, medical pulsing waves can be adjusted to penetrate the exact distance desired into the tissues, limiting overheating. For example, a greater intensity of ultrasonic waves increases the tissue absorption of the waves. Not only can the ultrasonic waves be adjusted to limit penetration, but the interval between pulses allows heat dissipation from the tissues.

Applications of Ultrasound
Reducing Swelling

Ultrasound therapy is useful for tendon, ligament, or joint injuries to the limbs. A useful application of ultrasound is to combine it with cold therapy. Apply an ice pack or cold water for 20 minutes, then pulse at 25% frequency (every fourth wave) for 20 minutes. A massaging effect known as "micro-streaming" or "acoustical streaming" encourages moving molecules to go from areas of high concentration to areas of low concentration. Applying ultrasound in this way improves circulation, limits the onset of edema and pulses the swelling out of the limb.

Place a "sweat" bandage on the limb for 24 hours after using a combination of cold and ultrasound therapy. The second day, use ultrasound over topical medication *(phonophoresis)*. Ultrasound encourages small, molecular-weight molecules, such as topical corticosteroids, to penetrate up to 2 inches. For this reason, ultrasound is **not** used over open and contaminated wounds, because it can drive bacteria deep into the tissues, spreading infection.

Relieving Pain and Promoting Healing

The deep heating of ultrasound relieves pain by changing the rate at which the nerves react and by limiting tissue spasms. Warmth restores the pliability of collagen fibers and relieves joint stiffness. Deep heat enhances circulation and production of energy which accelerates the healing process.

Ultrasound and Physical Therapy

When combined with range-of-motion exercises, optimal results are achieved from ultrasound. These exercises include physical therapy in the form of flexing and extending the limb immediately after ultrasound treatment.

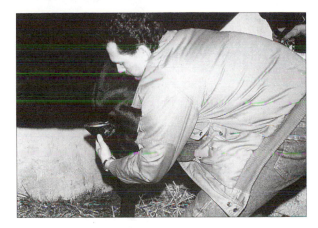

Fig. 11–13. Ultrasound therapy should be followed by physical therapy.

Many injuries can be avoided with adequate conditioning and training. However, chronic injuries such as arthritis or constrictive scar tissue deposits benefit from the enhanced range-of-motion and pliability afforded by ultrasound.

BENEFITS OF HIGH-TECH THERAPY

To return an equine athlete to soundness, the owner or trainer must achieve specific goals. It is paramount to reduce pain, to regain full use and movement of an injured area, and to restore or enhance strength to the injured area.

High-tech alternatives can provide pain relief, and in cases of reparable injuries, may help speed the healing process. Physical therapy by flexing and extending the limb, along with controlled exercise and balanced shoeing, can also help return a horse to performance.

Ours is a highly technological society, and some people have invested an enduring faith in promoting the "magic" of such wonders. To date, few specific *scientific* studies have been conducted that support the results of any of the high-tech equipment in use. Currently, most results are based on trial-and-error experimentation, along with individual, anecdotal testimonials to the success of these devices. Many products claim successful results where other, conventional modes of treatment, including prolonged rest, have failed.

Expectations must remain realistic—these devices will not cure the incurable. Instead, a horse may regain enough strength, elasticity, and pain relief to be serviceable in instances where pharmacological alternatives provide little comfort.

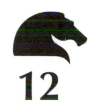

12

MANAGING CHRONIC LAMENESS

For the performance horse, one occupational risk is the development of a lasting lameness. Not all chronic pain can be corrected or cured, but some solutions offer the horse relief from continual discomfort. A complete list of potential debilitating lameness conditions would be exhaustive, but the most common situations include:

- chronically bruised feet
- navicular syndrome
- chronic back pain
- conditions of *degenerative joint disease* (DJD)

Bruised feet result from improper trimming or shoeing. For example, a flat-footed horse is prone to sole bruises. Bruises may also be caused by riding on rough terrain.

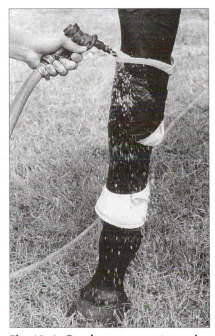

Fig. 12–1. Good management can give a horse relief from chronic lameness.

Improper shoeing may also be a cause of navicular disease, especially in horses that engage in rigorous, concussive activities such as jumping, racing, or polo. Inflammation of the feet causes damage to the deep digital flexor tendon and its associated navicular bone, resulting in chronic lameness.

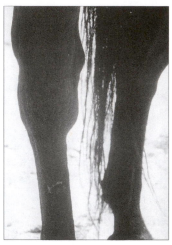

Fig. 12–2. Bone spavin.

Chronic back pain may develop as a consequence to pain in one or both hind legs, or by a poorly fitted saddle or poor riding technique.

Examples of degenerative joint diseases include:

• bone spavin (arthritis of the hock)
• high ringbone (arthritis of the pastern joint)
• low ringbone (arthritis of the coffin joint)
• stifle arthritis
• arthritis in any other joint

A veterinary lameness workup will identify the cause, allowing the problem to be appropriately addressed.

CAREER OPTIONS
Changing Disciplines

Every horse has a different pain tolerance. Some sports are too demanding for a horse with chronic pain, and a solution is to change disciplines. Jumping, hard stops, speed work, and collection aggravate many chronic pain conditions. A horse that cannot perform to a minimum standard in a sport should be converted to another career. Changing disciplines is better than causing excessive pain while trying to achieve the impossible. Suitable alternatives include using the horse as a school horse for beginning riders, or as a trail horse or equitation horse for light pleasure riding.

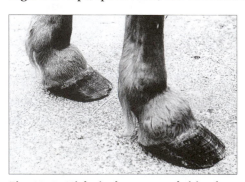

Fig. 12–3. High ringbone, or arthritis of the pastern joint.

Lowering Expectations

A horse that can withstand a rigorous athletic task to some degree may be able to continue competing in that sport, yet the owner should lower his or her expectations of the horse. Accept a lower level of performance in the chosen discipline. Entering fewer events each season, and spacing them apart can also help the chronically lame horse. Also, be prepared to scratch from a competition at the last moment if the horse is moving poorly that day.

If the horse cannot perform to a level of expectation, retire it, or put it in an environment with lower athletic demands. Lowering our expectations is more humane than asking a horse to suffer pain.

TRAINING AND FITNESS LEVELS

The greatest problem with managing the chronically sore athlete is maintaining a competent level of training and fitness. The work required to keep such a horse fit may make it impossible to participate in demanding sports like racing, cutting, reining, polo, or jumping.

The better the horse is trained when a chronic lameness problem surfaces, the less effort is required to retain its level of training. Moving a novice horse with chronic pain to higher levels demands far more effort than maintaining a lame but highly skilled horse at current levels. A novice horse may be unable to progress through the transition phases of training. Set realistic expectations and goals, and modify both as the horse's condition allows.

Not only is the horse's level of training important, but conditioning the whole body is critical to success. Maintaining the horse in as good a condition as possible for its intended athletics helps the body compensate for the lameness. Strengthening

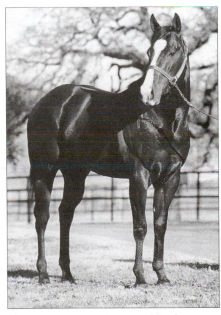

Fig. 12–4. Maintaining good body condition minimizes stress on the musculoskeletal system.

muscles, ligaments, and tendons compensates for the load on a sore joint, muscle, or tendon. A tired horse is likely to take a misstep or over-tax the musculoskeletal system. Fitness minimizes the development of fatigue.

Another example of maintaining condition is body weight. It is impor-tant to maintain the horse's body weight at a reasonable level. Obesity compounds the stresses on joints and support structures in the limbs. A horse that carries excess weight, either its own or too heavy a rider, over-loads the injured area.

Record Keeping

A log of the horse's performance can track its responses to athletic demands, without guessing about what is and is not working. Including these items in the log helps avoid guesswork:

- training schedule
- productive output
- mental and physical attitude
- types and frequency of medication and therapy
- daily performance results

Rushing Training

Do not rush a horse to compete by a predetermined date. Allow the horse to progress at its own pace of learning and conditioning. Rushing the training overtaxes both its physical and mental states, and inevitably leads to a debilitating lameness.

BALANCED SHOEING

One of the most critical steps in managing the chronically lame horse is a regular schedule of balanced shoeing. A balanced foot is better able to dissipate concussion stresses evenly up a limb. Unlike in foals, con-formational defects are not correctable in a mature horse. Stresses and strains continue on twisted joints and ligaments despite the best shoe-ing techniques. Yet, without the stable foundation of a balanced foot, conformational defects are magnified to seriously crippling levels.

Of utmost importance is correcting a broken hoof-pastern axis angle to reduce stress on the navicular bone, deep digital flexor tendon, and support structures of the coffin joint. *(See Chapter 4 for more informa-tion.)* For example, eliminating a long-toe–low-heel foot configuration reduces stress on these structures, improving navicular disease, low ringbone (coffin joint arthritis), and high ringbone (pastern joint arthritis). In addition, each foot should be balanced so that it impacts the ground equally on both sides.

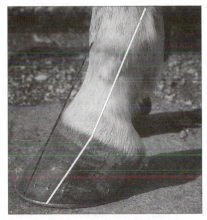

Fig. 12–5. A broken hoof-pastern axis angle, shown by white line. The black line shows the proper angle.

Special Shoes and Pads

Horses with lower limb problems like hoof cracks, high ringbone, low ringbone, or navicular disease benefit from an *egg-bar shoe*. Egg-bar shoes enlarge the foot's base of support for loading forces down the limb. Bone spavin (arthritis of the hock) also benefits from egg-bar shoes because the shoe limits the twist on the painful joint, and provides stability and support throughout the limb.

Conditions like bruised feet or inflammation of the coffin bone (pedal osteitis) improve with protection from stout hoof pads. A wedge pad is often used to treat navicular disease by raising the heel to decrease the pull on the deep digital flexor tendon as it passes behind the navicular bone and bursa.

TREATMENTS
Medications

Many horses with a chronic lameness condition can continue to train and perform if appropriate medications are given. However, different associations and state racing commisions have variable rules concerning anti-inflammatory drugs. Always check with the show steward or racetrack officials about the types and amounts of anti-inflammatory drugs legal for competition. Find out what forms must be filed and when. If a drug must be

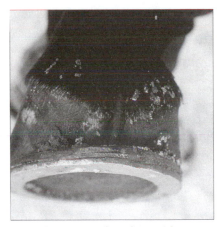

Fig. 12–6. An egg-bar shoe with a wedge pad.

withdrawn before competition, find out how long is required for withdrawal. If a veterinary certificate is required, contact the veterinarian soon enough to obtain the necessary document.

NSAIDs

Anti-inflammatory medications are an essential part of chronic pain management. The most common pain relievers are the non-steroidal anti-inflammatory drugs (NSAIDs) like Banamine®, Ketofen®,

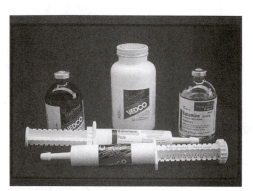

phenylbutazone, and naproxen. It is sometimes helpful to use low doses of NSAIDs the day before, the day of, and the day after a demanding exercise period. However, maintaining the horse on daily doses could create intestinal or gastric ulcers.

For endurance or competitive trail, NSAIDs must be withdrawn 3 – 4 days before the event. The American

Fig. 12–7. Common NSAIDs.

Quarter Horse Association also forbids NSAIDs. The American Horse Shows Association limits the amount of NSAIDs that can be given, and they must be withdrawn 12 hours before competition. Each State Racing Commission has its own rules and/or restrictions concerning NSAIDs and other drugs. *(For more information on NSAIDs, see Chapter 18.)*

Adequan® Therapy

For joint pain, additional options are available. Intramuscular injections with Adequan® provide horses in both the acute and chronic

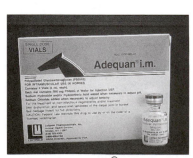

stages of DJD with considerable relief. Adequan® improves the lubricating properties of joint fluid and exerts some anti-prostaglandin effects, reducing the destruction of joint cartilage by inflammatory enzymes.

An oral supplement containing mussel shells (Synoflex®, Flex-Free®) allegedly increases the chondroitin sulfate component of joint fluid to achieve similar effects to the

Fig. 12–8. Adequan® therapy.

Adequan® therapy. There is no current scientific proof of these compounds' true value, but anecdotal reports tell of favorable results, particularly if the horse starts these oral supplements after Adequan® therapy.

Hyaluronic Acid Injection

Multiple injections of *hyaluronic acid* (HA) at 2–3 week intervals into a singly affected joint is an effective deterrent to the progression of arthritis. HA improves joint lubrication and has anti-inflammatory effects, but its usefulness is limited to inflammatory conditions in joints that have not yet developed cartilage damage.

Corticosteroids

Injecting a corticosteroid, a potent anti-inflammatory drug, gives immediate but short-term relief. Long-term use can lead to irreversible cartilage degeneration, therefore corticosteroid injections should be restricted to joints that are not responding to other methods of therapy. Moreover, the potent anti-inflammatory effects of a corticosteroid injection may mask enough pain that the horse will overuse the joint and further damage the cartilage. Usually a couple of weeks' rest following a steroid injection minimizes the potential of overuse damage of the joint.

Topical Anti-inflammatory Medications

DMSO (dimethyl sulfoxide) is a powerful anti-inflammatory agent that will reduce inflammation in the soft tissues around a joint, and is particularly beneficial for ligament or tendon injuries. However, topical anti-inflammatory medications cannot penetrate to joint depth when applied to the skin, and are not considered useful for joint therapy. For this reason, topical liniments or blistering agents also have limited value for joint pain.

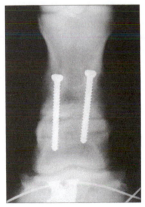

Surgery

Joint Fusion

Some lameness conditions respond favorably to surgery. It is possible to surgically fuse *(arthrodese)* specific low-range joints in the horse, such as the lower joints of the hock or the pastern joints. Rehabilitation takes up to a

Fig. 12–9. Surgical fusion of the pastern joint.

year to return a horse to athletics. Success rates range from 60% – 80% depending on the original problem. Conditions that also involve soft tissue injury, like a rupture of the collateral ligament, may not heal as quickly or as successfully as those with strictly joint problems.

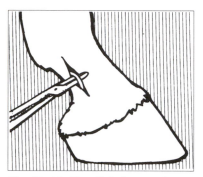

Fig. 12–10. The digital nerve is cut in a neurectomy.

Neurectomy

A common surgical option to treat navicular disease is neurectomy, which is a complete cutting of the nerve supply to the back third of the foot. This surgery can keep a horse working comfortably for a year or more. A neurectomy provides pain relief for up to 3 years for about 60% of navicular horses. This procedure is not a cure; it simply buys time. *(See Chapter 4 for more information on navicular disease.)*

WORKOUTS FOR THE LAME HORSE

Daily physical therapy encourages limberness in a chronically sore horse. These horses are often tense and rigid in many parts of their bodies from attempting to guard against anticipated pain. Relaxed muscles are less prone to injury.

Warm-Up

The chronically lame horse needs to be especially coddled in warm-up and cool-down periods. Warm it up with slow, low-stress work, incorporating stretching exercises into the routine. Start with at least 10 minutes of brisk walking followed by 10 minutes of light trotting before asking for more demanding work. A proper warm-up increases circulation to the muscles and improves suppleness while gently stretching tendons and ligaments before applying extreme stress to the limbs. Walking is an excellent way to limber a horse and improve blood circulation throughout the body with a minimum of stress impact.

Massaging and Stretching

Massaging the heavy muscle groups of the hips, thighs, and back improves relaxation. Also, manually stretching each leg several times before exercise helps the suppling process.

Mounted stretching exercises are particularly valuable for treating a horse with back pain. Encouraging a horse to work in a long and low frame stretches the topline and relaxes back muscles. The reins should be loose so the rider's hands create no restriction to a full stretch. *(See Chapter 6 for more information.)*

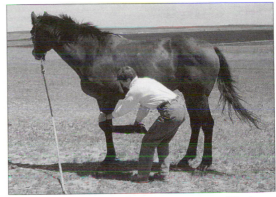

Fig. 12–11. Manual stretching relaxes and limbers up tense muscles.

Strengthening Muscles

Strengthening the support structures of muscles, ligaments, and tendons allows them to assume some of the load, placing less stress on the stifle joint. Resting a horse with stifle lameness can be counterproductive. A horse with stifle arthritis particularly benefits from conditioning and development of the muscles in the hind legs. Easy trail riding can benefit a horse with hock problems by strengthening the gluteal and quadriceps muscles. Circle work, however, places increased torque (twisting) stresses on the limbs. Therefore, minimize its use as a training technique for the chronically lame horse.

Each day of exercise, allow the horse to dictate how much it can tolerate in the workout. Be sensitive to behavioral clues that signal increasing soreness. A horse in pain develops bad habits, and its attention is distracted from the training and the task at hand. If the horse hurts, it is better to quit for the day than to persist at the athlete's expense.

Soft Footing

A horse with navicular problems works best on soft footing. For the foot sore horse, minimize downhill riding to reduce the concussion impact on the horse's feet. Jumping, uneven terrain, and hard stops are activities that worsen foot soreness, and they should be avoided.

At a competition, remember that the footing in the barn or training area may be better than the footing at a competition or in the warm-up arena. Seek another area for a warm-up if the footing is unsatisfactory.

Cool-Down

Walking after exercise relaxes the chronically lame horse. A 15-minute walking cool-down removes toxic by-products and heat from the tissues, and safely restores stretch to muscles and tendons.

Hydrotherapy

Hydrotherapy is an ideal means of managing arthritic joints or sensitive tendons. Hosing a limb with cold water or icing a limb immediately after a workout session minimizes the inflammatory response to exercise. Joints may need 30 – 60 minutes under an ice wrap to cool down enough to elicit an anti-inflammatory response. After icing, apply a standing bandage to limit rebound swelling.

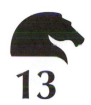

13

AVOIDING
DIGESTIVE DISORDERS

For the performance horse to reach maximum potential, it must be in the best of health. Good feeding management and good health care maintenance play key roles in maintaining a strong metabolic constitution and avoiding digestive disorders.

THE DIGESTIVE PROCESS
Eating Habits

The horse evolved as a grazing animal, serenely munching on sweet grasses of the plains, moving with the herd in search of available forage. The intestinal system was accustomed to small and frequent meals. Horses ate plants moist with dew and containing natural water. It cropped grasses as they grew, slowly adapting the microflora in the intestinal tract to changes in the nutrient value of plants as they responded to season and climate. As available food sources dwindled, the horse moved on, not stopping long enough to contaminate its feed with droppings that might reinfest it with parasite eggs. In this idyllic state, the horse moved about, maintaining muscle tone and good circulation.

Today, horses live quite differently. Urban development and time constraints compel us to confine horses for convenience. Horses in a natural state graze continually—by providing meals designed by humans we drastically alter how the intestinal tract handles food. People are now faced with management of an animal not naturally equipped to deal with imposed diets, feed schedules, and exercise routines.

The Teeth

Once food is in a horse's mouth, the teeth begin the digestive process by grinding the food, making it easier to digest. Horses chew their food in a rotary grinding motion, and the teeth of the upper jaw are wider than those in the lower jaw. These factors cause an uneven wear pattern. The outer edges of the upper teeth and the inner edges of the lower teeth develop sharp points, creating ulcers and sores in the cheek or tongue.

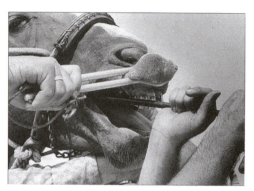

Fig. 13–1. Floating smooths sharp points.

The teeth should be checked annually by a veterinarian so the sharp edges can be smoothed by rasping them down with a file, a process known as *floating*. If the teeth are not regularly floated, large hooks often develop on the front premolars and the rearmost molars. These hooks pose problems for chewing and bridling.

Wolf Teeth

Examine a young horse for *wolf teeth*, which are vestigial premolars located at the front of the molars in the upper jaw. A wolf tooth should not be confused with canine teeth. Most male horses grow canine teeth which sit in front of the bit, about halfway between the incisors and the molars. Some mares also grow canines, but not as commonly as male horses.

A wolf tooth is very small, but its location coincides with the place a bit rests in the horse's mouth. To avoid bad habits, wolf teeth should be removed before training begins. Horses with tooth problems from either large hooks or wolf teeth resist the bridle, and many throw their heads to avoid the painful bumping of the bit on the offending tooth.

Wave Mouth

Older horses often lose teeth, which causes no immediately apparent problems. But the absence of a tooth allows the corresponding tooth on the opposite jaw to overgrow. The horse's teeth eventually develop a *wave mouth*. Then the teeth cannot efficiently grind the food for digestion. These horses are prone to diarrhea, impactions, colic, or choke.

The Digestive System

Changes in a daily routine can result in digestive disorders. A detailed look at the equine digestive system shows how sensitive it can be to management situations.

The Stomach

The stomach of a 1,000-pound horse is equivalent in size to the stomach of a large man. The relatively small equine stomach capacity is approximately 4 gallons.

Eating stimulates regular stomach contractions to move feed into the small intestine. Normally, the stomach empties its contents, called *ingesta*, into the small intestine within 2 – 3 hours. When the stomach contracts, the intestines contract as well. Progressive propulsion of ingesta towards the large intestine is essential for digestion, nutrient absorption, and gas elimination. Roughage moves out of the stomach rapidly, while grain concentrates remain longer.

A horse is unable to vomit due to muscular limitations of the esophagus, even if the stomach overdistends with fluids or gas. Excess fermentation and overfilling of the stomach can cause pain, and can lead to rupture and death.

The Small Intestine

The small intestine regulates passage of the ingesta into the cecum and prevents backflow of gas from the cecum. Feed moves rapidly (compared to the rest of the digestive process) through 70 feet of small intestine taking only 3 – 4 hours to be admitted into the cecum's fermentation chamber.

The Large Intestine

Fermentation

A horse's intestinal tract is like a fermentation vat, capable of processing fiber and cellulose due to the bacteria and protozoans within it. In the horse, fermentation occurs after the small intestine in the cecum and large colon. Here, proteins, carbohydrates, and cellulose are broken down by bacteria into nutrients, which are absorbed along with fluids. Cellulose breakdown by bacteria produces large volumes of gas that have no escape through the esophagus, and must travel hundreds of feet through the intestinal loops to the rectum.

Within the large intestine near the *pelvic flexure*, is a regulator that coordinates muscle movement of the intestines and the progression of ingesta through the various loops of bowel. Large particles may be delayed for up to 72 hours to allow bacterial digestion to degrade fiber into fuels. At the same time, more easily digested foodstuffs and gases are propelled towards the rectum for elimination.

The Large and Small Colon

The large colon has five segments. At several junction points where the segments anatomically blend into one another, the diameter of the bowel abruptly decreases. It is at these points of stricture that ingesta or foreign bodies can cause an obstruction, and prevent normal outflow of gas and materials. The small colon has a similar function as the large colon, but it is smaller. The ingesta therefore becomes smaller as the feces are prepared to be passed from the body.

All segments of the intestine are interrelated by allowing normal function of the other parts to continue. Consistent waves of contractions *(peristalsis)* and a healthy blood supply to and from the intestines are vital to a horse's overall well-being. Interruptions in either of these features can set off a series of events that result in digestive disorders.

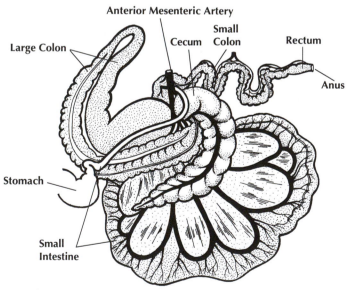

Fig. 13–2. The digestive system, with the fan-like mesentery supporting the small intestines.

DIGESTIVE DISORDERS IN FOALS

Foals are notoriously bad about tasting and eating everything in sight. Foreign body obstructions often cause colic in young horses. Fibers from rubber tire feeders, baling twine, wood pieces, and rubber balls have all been incriminating items. Twigs, rubber tires, and plastic have been implicated in some esophageal obstructions. Foals are also susceptible to sand colic as early as the first few months of life.

Foals will often consume their mother's manure *(coprophagy)*. This makes them subject to heavy parasitism, which can also cause impaction colic. Their environment should be routinely cleaned and the mare and foal dewormed every 6 – 8 weeks.

Foals have a markedly smaller diameter and volume digestive tract than an adult horse, which hastens the onset of signs. A very young foal may show signs of a colic by rolling onto its back with legs in the air, neck outstretched in obvious pain.

Manage the foaling environment appropriately. A newborn foal is susceptible to *meconium impaction* if the first fecal balls are not passed soon after birth.

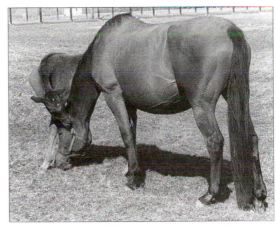

Fig. 13–3. Foals will taste everything in sight.

Meconium is a dark, pelleted feces which consist of accumulated cellular debris and waste materials during fetal development.

Up to a year of age, foals are prone to *gastric ulcers* if medicated with non-steroidal anti-inflammatory drugs. *(See Chapter 18 for more information on NSAIDs.)*

COLIC

Colic is not a disease in itself, but rather it is the word used to describe abdominal pain. It is a symptom indicating a digestive disorder. Colic is a word that conjures up visions of a horse in distress—nostrils flared, pawing at the ground, kicking or biting at the belly, rolling on the ground, and sweating. The horse may stretch out as if to urinate, but it is

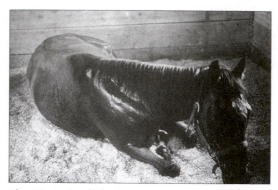

Fig. 13–4. A colicky horse may sweat and lie un-comfortably.

too uncomfortable to apply an abdominal press to empty the bladder. It may stand depressed and dull, not wanting to eat. It may lie down, then get up, only to lie down again to relieve the discomfort coming from within the belly.

Colic must be differentiated from other problems not directly related to the gastrointestinal tract. Examples are pain from:

- ovulation
- foaling
- founder
- tying-up
- bladder stones
- laminitis
- fever
- etc.

The horse has a unique intestinal system. The distinctive anatomy of the intestines predisposes to a variety of syndromes that cause pain. Pain of colic is a result of excess tension or stretching of the bowel lining (*mesentery*), that serves as a supportive sling of the intestines within the abdomen. Spasms of the bowel lining, due to irritation or a decrease in blood supply, also result in pain.

Horses require up to 2.5% of their body weight in feed intake per day, equivalent to 25 pounds for a 1,000-pound horse. At least 50% of that feed should be in the form of roughage. This fiber component stimulates intestinal movement. Also, a horse that is fed complete pelleted rations, condensed hay cubes, or limited quantities of hay suffers from boredom. Its natural urge to chew finds it devouring fence boards, eating dirt and sand off the ground, or consuming its own manure.

Spasmodic Colic

Spasmodic colic is due to a gut that moves too much. Nervousness and excitability, sometimes induced by sudden weather or barometric pressure changes, may result in this colic. Stress from transport or athletic competition can upset normal nerve impulses to the intestine and change intestinal movement. Toxic plants, or blister beetles in alfalfa hay are exceedingly irritating to the intestines and can be fatal. Certain drugs and organophosphate dewormers also overstimulate intestinal movement.

Severe changes in intestinal movement may cause a segment of bowel to telescope into an adjacent segment. This *intussusception* effectively acts as an obstruction, yet the condition of the horse rapidly deteriorates as gangrene and bowel death *(necrosis)* develop. It is an exceedingly painful and potentially lethal syndrome, requiring rapid surgical intervention.

Impaction Colic

An obstruction, or *impaction* in the large colon takes many hours to days to fully form and cause outward signs of pain or discomfort. Once an impaction becomes extensive enough, it places pressure on the bowel, or alters normal movement of the intestines. Abnormal intestinal contractions or gas distention causes pain. This mild or intermittent pain may be accompanied by depression and lack of appetite.

Intestinal tumors or abscesses can mimic an impaction. The tumor or abscess pushes on the bowel lining, causing discomfort, or it reduces blood flow and alters normal movement. Although the horse did not have an impaction before, changes in the normal intestinal function can cause an impaction, called a *secondary impaction*.

Causes of Impaction Colic

Obstructions of the bowel are commonly caused by decreased muscular movements of the gastrointestinal tract. As foodstuffs accumulate and sit in the bowel, water is removed. Once an impaction begins, the smooth muscle of the intestinal walls contracts in an attempt to move it along. This contraction may not only generate pain, but it also squeezes out more fluid, worsening the problem. Now the ingesta is no longer pliable and movable, and forms an obstruction. Impaction colic can be caused by:

- limited exercise
- coarse food
- enteroliths
- consumption of foreign materials
- decreased water intake
- consumption of bedding
- heavy parasite load

Limited Exercise

Limited exercise reduces blood circulation to all muscles, including the intestinal muscle. A sluggish circulation changes normal intestinal movement, which may cause an impaction. During cold or wet weather, horses used to being outdoors may be brought into a stall. Then even low-level exercise is restricted.

Decreased Water Intake

Digestion of the great amounts of fiber a horse eats each day requires large volumes of water to fuel normal metabolic processes and maintain body fluid levels. A horse consumes 5 – 15 gallons of water each day in cool weather. Excessively hot weather, sweating, and dehydration may remove water from the gut and dry out the ingesta. Obstructions also occur due to limited access to clean or ice-free water. Frozen water or even excessively cold water discourage drinking.

As horse owners, we have been told that feeding extra hay during cold weather generates internal heat as a by-product of fiber breakdown in the large colon. So, obediently, we add hay to the pile, which under normal circumstances is the correct thing to do. However, if a horse is not drinking enough, this practice compounds the problem by increasing intestinal bulk without adequate water to process it. Moreover, coarse feed materials or concentrated food requires more water to properly digest.

Coarse Feed

Excessively dry or coarse feed can create an obstruction within the bowel. In addition, any dental problems can add to the problem by decreasing the ability to adequately grind coarse feed. Coarse feed irritates the bowel lining, causing diarrhea or constipation.

Consumption of Bedding

Shavings or straw bedding may seem unnaturally palatable to a bored horse. A horse may overconsume bedding to satisfy a fiber deficiency. These materials commonly form an impaction. Or, a pregnant mare may eat her bedding when suddenly confined in a new environment for observation and foaling.

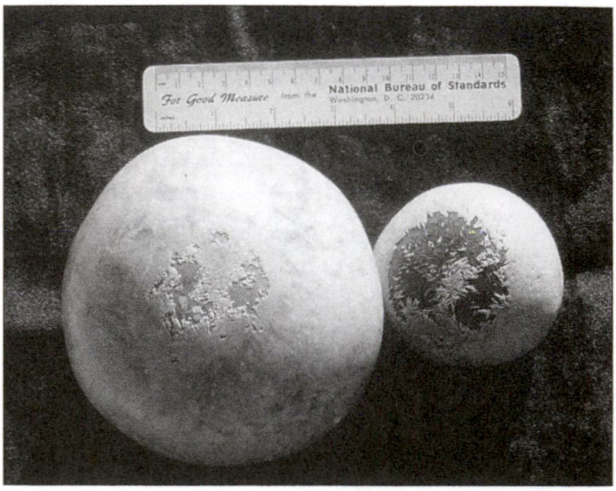

Fig. 13–5. Enteroliths can vary greatly in size depending on their age.

Enteroliths

In certain areas of the United States, particularly the West and Southwest, water and soil conditions contribute to an *enterolith* obstruction. Enteroliths are mineralized salts surrounding a pebble or small object. Over long periods, progressive layers of mineral deposits build around the central core. Once an enterolith enlarges enough to obstruct flow of ingested materials or gas, a symptomatic colic results.

Warning Signs of Impaction Colic

Advance warning signals include mild depression, decreased appetite, lying down frequently, and scanty, hard, and dry fecal balls, if any. The normal number of bowel movements per day averages 8 – 12. Fecal passage may diminish over a period of days before a problem is evident.

The earlier an impaction is recognized, the better the prognosis for successful medical treatment using oral laxatives, restorative intravenous fluids, and pain control. Occasionally, surgery is necessary to remove the obstruction. Excess pressure on the bowel or stagnant blood flow causes gangrene in a loop of intestine. Surgical removal prevents septic shock and death.

Preventing Impaction Colic

Prevention seems simple: ample water, high quality feed, and exercise. A special effort should be made to ride in the winter, or to find a large turnout area. Induced exercise by longeing, or playtime in a herd is preferable. Vary the daily routine so confined or exercise-restricted horses do not become bored and eat bedding or foreign objects.

Fresh, ice-free water should always be readily accessible. Tank heaters keep water at an acceptable temperature in the harshest winters. Make sure the heater does not short out and shock the horse every time it tries to drink. If a dominant herd member hogs the trough, add another water tank to ensure equal opportunity.

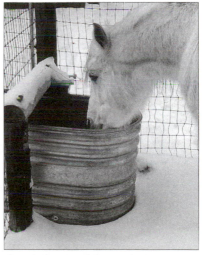

Feed good quality hay that is neither excessively coarse nor fine. A bran mash does not act as a laxative due to the unique structure of the equine intestines, but a mash will encourage water consumption. Adding 1 – 2 tablespoons of salt to the mash further encourages drinking, but do not give extra salt to a horse that is drinking poorly, as salt worsens dehydration.

Fig. 13–6. A tank heater prevents water from freezing.

Careful observation of the number and quality of bowel movements each day, the amount of water consumed, and the horse's general attitude help prevent serious impaction colic.

Gaseous Colic

Any change in normal movement patterns in the intestines can cause problems. When bowel movements cease altogether, it is called an *ileus*. Fermentation continues, but gas does not move towards the rectum. As gas builds within the intestines, the overdistention results in pain. Bacterial overgrowth occurs in the stagnant gut, and bacteria begin to die. The death of certain types of bacteria release endotoxins that can result in shock, laminitis, or death.

Building gas in a stagnant gut compromises the blood supply by exerting excess pressure and tension on the blood vessels. Portions of the bowel may be displaced as the segments balloon with gas and attempt to fully occupy the abdominal cavity. The left side of the large intestine normally floats freely in the abdomen with no supporting attachments to the body wall or other organs. The large intestine is therefore prone to great movement within the abdomen.

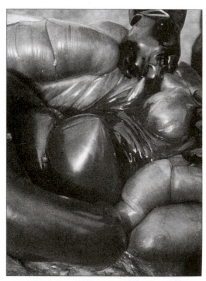

Fig. 13–7. A rotated intestine, with gas distention and gangrene where the blood supply was cut off.

Intestinal Torsion

Abnormal contractions, aided by gravity, may cause an actual rotation of the intestine, and result in an intestinal twist *(intestinal torsion)*. The free suspension of the left large colon, coupled with gas distention, abnormal peristaltic waves, or an ileus (ceased bowel movements) can result in a torsion.

It is largely myth that a horse rolling around in pain will cause twisting of the intestines. Twisting can happen, but intestines can twist even if a horse is standing. Allow a colicky horse to lie quietly if it will, but prevent the horse from rolling so it does not hurt itself or the handlers. Forcing the horse to walk or trot may be beneficial for 10 – 15 minutes, or may keep a restless horse moving until veterinary help can arrive. However, hours of forced movement only exhausts a horse and handler. Prolonged, forced walking depletes valuable energy and calories needed to combat the illness.

Diet

Many colics are caused by inappropriate dietary management. An overabundance of excessively rich feeds (grain, alfalfa hay, lush pasture) stimulate excess gas production within the stomach or large intestines.

Sudden changes in feed are detrimental to the bacterial microflora in the gut and predispose to overproduction of gas or endotoxins. Moldy food, or rapid introduction of large amounts of grain or legume hay will upset the system.

Feeding After Exercise

Feeding immediately after vigorous exercise can be dangerous. At this time, blood is still circulating in the muscle tissue, and shunted away from the stomach. This lack of blood flow delays emptying of food from the stomach, promoting excess fermentation. After the horse is cool, the blood supply is diverted back to the intestines and then it is safe to feed. The time required to cool down the horse depends on its condition, the environmental temperature and humidity, and the demands of the workout.

Cold Water After Exercise

Drinking excessively cold water after exercise may set off spasms at the *pyloric sphincter* located between the stomach and the small intestine. Pyloric spasms delay movement of ingesta out of the stomach. Overdistention of the stomach with gas is quite painful, causing a sudden and violent colic.

Cribbing

Cribbing is a behavioral vice that is a liability for a performance horse. Cribbers do so out of boredom, then out of habit. A horse that

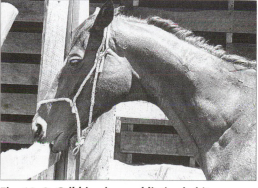

Fig. 13–8. Cribbing is an addictive habit.

cribs grabs onto a firm object like a fence rail or post, a water tank, or a stall door. It then pulls back on the object and sucks air into the stomach with each pulling exertion. Not only does a cribbing horse turn away from eating and drinking to nurture its addictive habit, but it is at risk of developing gaseous colic. It is hard to keep weight on a "cribber," and performance suffers. This vice also causes management problems because the horse's teeth wear down fencing, stall doors, etc.

It is easy to identify a cribbing horse by examining the incisors for abnormal wear. The incisors will be excessively worn and rounded. A cribbing collar limits the behavior by causing pain as the horse pulls back and flexes its throat and upper neck. The collar bites into its flesh, making cribbing physically uncomfortable.

A surgical option is available, but it has limited success of less than 60%. It involves cutting the nerve supply to the muscles under the neck that enable a horse to crib.

Colic From Lipomas

An overweight horse is predisposed to *lipomas,* which are tumors of fatty tissue. As fat accumulates in the body, it builds into lumps within the mesentery. Gravity may pull these lumps of fat into one large mass with a stalk attaching it to the mesentery. It is possible for a loop of small intestine to become entrapped around this stalk, and strangulate.

Colic From Parasites

Internal parasites create areas of inflammation and irritation as they migrate through the intestinal lining or the blood vessels supplying the intestines. Bloodworms interfere with blood supply and intestinal movement, while roundworms form obstructions within the cavity of the bowel *(lumen).* Interrupting blood flow diminishes oxygen to bowel loops, and interferes with nerve input to the intestines. Waves of contractions then become disorganized, or may cease altogether. Other internal parasites damage and erode the bowel lining, causing leakage of fecal contents into the abdomen. The re-

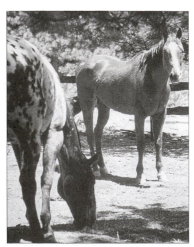

Fig. 13–9. Horses are reinfested with parasites by eating manure.

sulting infection and inflammation are called *peritonitis*. This condition is painful and potentially lethal.

The role of parasites in colic cannot be overstated. Adequate cleaning of corrals and stalls, along with an aggressive parasite control program at least every 2 months, markedly reduces this cause of serious colics. *(See Chapter 14 for more information.)*

Sand Colic

Over time horses can consume a large amount of dirt or sand, which can weigh heavily in the gut and severely abrade the intestinal lining. Due to the insidious nature of this sanding syndrome, a long period may be required before it progresses to the point of overt abdominal pain.

Sand colic is not solely a problem in specific areas, such as the West Coast, Eastern seaboard, Mississippi delta, or the sandhills of North Dakota. Anywhere there is sand, decomposed granite, or just plain old dirt, sand colic can arise. Many people cover paddocks or arenas with sand or road base to improve footing, so even if these soils are not naturally found in the environment, they can be delivered to it.

Mechanics of Sand Colic

The design of the equine large colon, with its narrowing segments, encourages deposit and trapping of sand in constrictive areas. If excessive sand accumulates in the large colon, it obstructs passage of food materials. This unmovable impaction causes gas to build behind it, with associated pain as segments of bowel distend and swell. Pain reflexes and spasms around an impaction may shut down movement. Abnormal peristaltic contractions in the gut can lead to a displaced or twisted intestine.

At the site of the impaction, the heavy and abrasive material can erode through the intestinal lining. Pressure necrosis on that portion of bowel causes the intestinal contents to leak into the abdominal cavity. Inflammation and infection of the abdomen *(peritonitis)*, *endotoxic* and/or *septic shock*, and death can result. A similar situation occurs if a swollen or weakened bowel ruptures.

Symptoms of Sand Colic

Several symptoms are tip-offs to a problem from excess sand ingestion. Often a persistent diarrhea develops (in about 35% of afflicted horses) before the onset of painful symptoms. Because it abrades the lining of the intestinal tract, sand impairs absorption of nutrients and fluids. As intestinal movement slows, diarrhea intensifies.

In some individuals the only signs may be depressed appetite and weight loss. Performance may suffer because of chronic discomfort or reduced nutrient efficiency. Other horses experience low grade, mildly painful bouts of colic that appear as intermittent, but recurrent episodes. Sometimes a colic crisis starts during or after riding, possibly because the sandpaper-like abrasion stimulates painful spasms of the intestine. Imagine a sausage of concrete lining the gut, as it is subjected to extreme physical exertion.

Any horse that experiences chronic diarrhea or recurrent episodes of mild colic should be examined by a veterinarian. The key is to diagnose the problem early, before it becomes too advanced to rectify.

To give a mental picture of how serious sand accumulation can be, consider results of necropsies on horses that died due to sand colic. Up to two-thirds of the intestinal space was full of sand, wall to wall. In some places this material could be crumbled between fingers; in others it was so tightly packed that it could not be manually broken up.

Managing Sand Colic.

Feeding Systems

Feeding off the ground may simulate natural grazing, but consider what happens when hay is thrown on the ground. The horse spreads it around to pick out the tastier morsels. It may step in it, grinding it into the dirt. When it finally gets down to the leftovers, a still-hungry horse consumes the rest, sand included. If alfalfa is fed, the leaves drop out, and the horse snuffles around in the dirt to get every last tasty leaf. Tipped over feed buckets spill grain onto the ground and, with attempts to pick up each piece, dirt is also ingested. Horses foraging on overgrazed pastures will eat cropped grasses and roots, with soil attached.

Horses on a pellet diet quickly finish their feed. Either lack of fiber or boredom may cause them to eat manure (with dirt), board

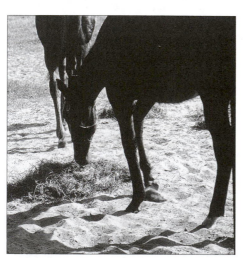

Fig. 13–10. Feeding hay off of sand offers a high potential for causing sand colic.

fences, or dirt. Also, a fiber deficiency limits normal stimulation of the large colon, resulting in sluggish intestinal movement that allows sand to separate out into the intestine.

If the only available water source is a shallow, muddy, or sandy pool, soil in the water will separate out inside the horse.

Diagnosing Sand Colic

Gut Sounds

Occasionally, a veterinarian can listen to the abdomen in front of the naval with a stethoscope and hear sounds similar to what one hears in a conch shell, that is, surf on sand. These sounds may also resemble the sound made by slowly rotating a paper bag partially filled with sand. Not hearing these sounds does not mean that sand is not present. For "sand sounds" to be heard, the bowel must be heavy enough to be lying next to the abdominal wall, and the bowel must be moving.

Sand in the Feces

Any sand or grit in the fecal material is significant. Lack of sand does not guarantee that it is not present in the gut. A simple test can be performed to monitor sand build-up. Take six fecal balls from the center of a fresh pile of manure where it has not contacted the ground. Mix the feces in a quart of water. Once the solid material separates out, measure the amount of sand in the bottom of the vessel. More than one teaspoon per six fecal balls is abnormal.

Rectal Examination

Rectal examination of the intestinal tract does not always reveal definitive information. If a large amount of sand is present in the gut, it may pull the intestines downward to the bottom of the abdomen, and out of reach.

Belly Tap

A belly tap (*abdominocentesis*) involves inserting a needle into the abdomen to determine fluid character and volume. This technique is not generally used to diagnose sanding, but if such information is accidentally obtained this way, it clarifies a tentative colic diagnosis. Sand may be obtained through such a tap because the weight of the sand pushes the intestines along the belly wall, and the needle may inadvertently penetrate the intestine.

X-Ray Films

X-ray films of the abdomen can positively diagnose sand in the intestines. This procedure requires powerful x-ray equipment, often available only at a University veterinary teaching hospital.

Treating Sand Colic

Water

Medical therapy of a "sanded" horse must ensure adequate hydration, by oral and intravenous fluids, of the intestinal contents to help the horse pass the sand. Ample water moves material through the gut and prevents dehydration and a resultant impaction.

Laxatives

Laxatives are administered by stomach tube. The best medication is *psyllium hydrophilia mucilloid,* commonly known as Metamucil®. Psyllium was once thought to move sandy material out of the gut by lubricating it in a gelatinous material. Now it is thought to stimulate movement of the bowel, and to pull fluids into the intestine.

A study at Colorado State University radiographically illustrated that only 2 days of psyllium therapy resolved chronic diarrheas caused by sand. However, because sand builds up over a long time, it may require a lengthy period to pass it out. Treating seriously "sanded" horses includes stomach tubing with psyllium for 2 – 5 days, followed by feeding ½ pound twice a day to adult horses, or ¼ pound twice a day to foals. This regimen is carried out for 4 – 5 weeks. Sand is inconsistently found in the feces during psyllium therapy, so treatment should not be prematurely discontinued.

Pain Relievers

Pain relievers, such as non-steroidal anti-inflammatory drugs, help resolve a sand impaction. They reduce spasms around the impaction, and allow gas to escape so water can enter and soften the obstruction. By relieving pain from abrasion, water and food intake improve.

Hay

If a sanded horse has only mild pain and is still having bowel movements, high quality hay promotes movement of sand out of the intestinal tract.

Surgery

Surgery for sand colic may be necessary if:

- there is a limited response to medical treatment within 48 – 72 hours
- vital parameters such as heart rate, capillary refill time, and mucous membrane color deteriorate
- pain persists and worsens

Surgery may be the only alternative — to physically remove the sand from the gut. How aggressively the horse is treated affects its chances for survival. A University of Minnesota study determined that horses undergoing surgery for sand colic experience a 50% survival rate. A study at the University of Florida revealed that those cases treated surgically had a survival rate of 92%, because of the aggressive treatment before the bowel became gangrenous and necrotic.

Bran

Contrary to popular myth, bran is neither therapeutic nor preventive. Due to peculiar equine intestinal anatomy, by the time the relatively small amount of bran reaches the large intestine of the horse it can hardly exert any laxative effect. The equine gastrointestinal system is radically different from a human's. Bran encourages water consumption, which indirectly improves intestinal movement and passage of material through the bowel. If peristaltic contractions move feed along normally, then fecal contents will not stay in the bowel long enough for sandy material to separate out.

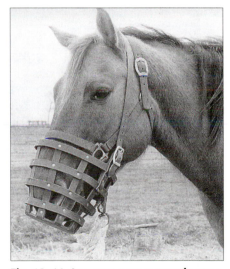

Preventing Sand Colic

Monitor each horse for differences in eating habits, especially those that eat anything, or that search the ground all day. To prevent sand colic in these horses, feed more roughage, or feed more often, and provide more exercise to curtail boredom. A rare individual may need a muzzle to prevent it from eating dirt.

Fig. 13–11. In a rare case a muzzle may be needed to prevent a horse from eating dirt.

Changing Feeding Practices

By recognizing an evolutionary need for horses to frequently eat small amounts of good quality fiber, feeding practices can be modified to not only prevent sand colic, but to improve the health of the digestive system, and the horse's mental happiness. A horse performs better if the natural urge to constantly nibble is satisfied. This urge is satisfied by free choice grass hay, and supplementing only hard-working individuals or difficult keepers with alfalfa and grain. Feeding enough hay, or feeding at frequent intervals can also eliminate behavior such as licking the ground or eating dirt. By not overstocking pastures, ample forage is available so horses do not consume dirt. A diet of free choice grass hay, salt, and adequate water limits sand and dirt ingestion.

Using Feeders

Removing the hay from the ground is essential for prevention. Using racks, hay nets, or tire feeders minimizes spillage. Feeding on rubber mats or concrete pads may be an alternative in special cases. Overhead feeding arrangements present another problem. A horse with an overhead feeder is prone to respiratory problems. It cannot clear foreign material and mold spores from the respiratory tract, because the head is held up in an unnatural position. Also, hay is pulled out of overhead feeders and scattered on the ground. Rubber tire feeders better ensure that the feed material stays put. They allow head down feeding, and are relatively safe.

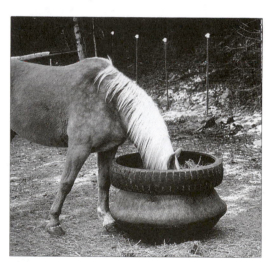

Fig. 13–12. Tire feeders limit sand intake.

Be aware that young foals can get trapped inside such feeders and be injured. Youngsters (and some adults) also like to chew on the rubber feeders, eating white walls or rubber material, and may develop a severe impaction colic.

Providing Clean Water

Check water tanks to see if sand is in the bottom of the tank. Sand in the water tank is a signal that the horses' mouths are full of sand. Clean, fresh water encourages drinking which promotes intestinal health and normal peristaltic movement.

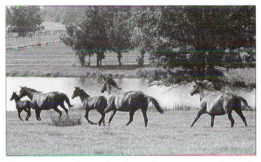

Fig. 13–13. Clean, fresh water promotes intestinal health.

Preventative Medications

Along with changes in feeding practices, preventative medication with psyllium products can prevent sand colic. Feed 1 cup a day of psyllium for 5 consecutive days each month. Lengthy treatment is unnecessary because the laxative effects slightly disturb normal electrolyte and fluid balances. For stubborn cases, or horses attended by a veterinarian, long-term psyllium treatment may be necessary.

Choke

Horses can choke on their food, but rather than an obstruction blocking the airway as in people, food is lodged somewhere along the esophagus, making it impossible to swallow.

The first impression as a horse suddenly turns away from its food and stops eating is that it is colicking. Initially, a horse appears distressed and agitated, exhibiting colicky type behavior. It stretches the neck to relieve the pressure, or paws, sweats, or rolls on the ground. Saliva foams from the mouth, but with a choke there is a greenish froth coming from the nostrils, often accompanied by gagging and coughing.

Problems Associated With Choke

Aspiration Pneumonia

Choke is a true emergency, requiring immediate veterinary attention. Food, mucus, and saliva that are regurgitated from the mouth and nostrils can be inhaled into the lungs as a horse struggles to relieve the esophageal obstruction. Material inhaled into the lungs and airways rapidly leads to an *aspiration pneumonia*.

Electrolyte and Fluid Loss

A choked horse suffers serious electrolyte imbalances, as well as dehydration. Not only does an esophageal obstruction prevent drinking, but the horse loses saliva as it drools from the mouth. Saliva contains large quantities of sodium and chloride, and is essential for recycling these salts through the intestinal tract where they are reabsorbed by the body. A horse experiencing a prolonged episode of choke is unable to swallow the saliva, and needs intravenous fluids and electrolytes.

Treating Choke

With immediate veterinary attention, the majority of chokes are easily resolved without complications. While awaiting a veterinarian, it is helpful to place the horse on an incline with the head facing downhill. Such a small change in position helps drain regurgitated material out of the mouth and nose and minimizes the chances of it being inhaled into the airways. Remain calm and talk soothingly to help control the horse's anxiety. If the ball of food is visible on the left side of the neck as a bulge, *very* gentle massage may help break it down.

Sedatives administered by a veterinarian position the head and neck

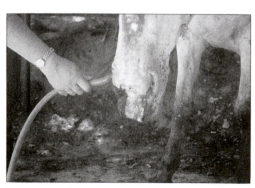

downward, and relax the muscles spasming around the food mass. A stomach tube is passed into the esophagus to the level of the obstruction, and a gentle stream of water breaks it up. Non-steroidal anti-inflammatory drugs minimize scar tissue formation once the obstruction is dissolved. Broad spectrum antibiotics prevent infection of the esophageal lining.

Fig. 13–14. During a choke, green–tinged saliva froths from the nostrils.

Feeding After a Choke Crisis

Follow-up care after a choke crisis is critical. Withhold food from a sedated horse until it is fully recovered, because both the cough reflex and swallowing apparatus are depressed under the influence of sedatives. In some cases, it is necessary to entirely withhold food for the first 24 – 48 hours. For a horse to safely swallow food, it must be adequately chewed and softened liberally with saliva. Pre-soaking pellets in ample water for 20 – 30 minutes breaks apart and softens them. This gruel slips easily down an irritated esophagus, allowing the esophagus to heal, and inflammation to subside. When it is safe for the horse to eat again, feed the gruel in small amounts, several times daily for up to 2 weeks after the episode. During this time, a horse is highly susceptible to a recurrent episode of choke, so care must be taken to remove all coarse or dry feed from the diet.

Preventing Choke

Implementing certain management procedures prevents choke, or prevents a reoccurrence in a previously choked horse. Most chokes are caused by large pelleted concentrate, or by coarse hay. These feeds are easily eliminated from the diet. If pellets are fed, they should be the small variety. Grass pasture and hay cubes rarely cause a choke, however, competition with herd-mates may make a horse bolt its feed. Such a horse should be separated at feeding time to encourage it to eat slowly. If a greedy horse seems to "inhale" grain or pellets, place smooth rocks (2" minimum size) in the feed tub with the concentrate. The rocks slow intake because the horse must rummage around them.

Inadequate water intake can result in a choke. Drinking plenty of fresh water ensures ample saliva, and adequate water for intestinal digestion. During transport, it is important for a horse to drink enough to limit dehydration. Some horses stressed by trailering may snatch and gobble hay or grain. It is best to withhold feed from anxious horses.

Dental problems may cause a horse to swallow food before it is chewed properly. Teeth should be checked and floated regularly.

Introduction of new or palatable bedding materials, such as straw or wood shavings, should be monitored carefully to ensure a horse does not eat them.

Some instances of choke are unpreventable if caused by tumors, space-occupying abscesses, or scar tissue from an old injury. These problems functionally decrease the diameter of the esophagus. If there is suspicion of such a malady, a veterinarian can diagnose it with an endoscope or by contrast radiography. With contrast radiography, a radio-opaque material is injected into the esophagus and x-ray films are taken of the area.

Diarrhea

Inflammatory conditions of the large intestine can lead to diarrhea. The performance of an equine athlete suffers from diarrhea because it loses valuable electrolytes and fluids in the feces. Persistent diarrhea also leads to weight loss or colic. With careful management practices, many cases of diarrhea in the mature horse can be quickly resolved.

Causes of Diarrhea

Poor Dental Care

Poor tooth care is a common case of diarrhea, especially in the aged horse. If feed is not properly ground, it irritates and inflames the intestine. Coarse food or chronic sand ingestion creates a similar irritation leading to diarrhea. Regular tooth care, premium hay quality, and not feeding on sandy soil are easy ways to eliminate these sources of diarrhea.

Overfermentation in Bowel

A horse that is fed an abnormally high grain ration or moldy food may develop diarrhea due to overfermentation of bacteria in the bowel. Bacterial endotoxin or fungi inflame the bowel. An inflamed bowel cannot absorb nutrients, water, and electrolytes, so they are lost through the feces. Feeding at least half of the ration as roughage ensures normal intestinal function. Discard all spoiled feed.

Nervousness

A nervous horse, or a horse verging on exhaustion may have temporary diarrhea due to changes in intestinal activity. These horses may benefit from electrolyte supplements during transport or competition. It is equally important that they have frequent access to fresh water to restore fluid losses.

Parasites

Infectious organisms also contribute to diarrhea in horses. Parasite infestation of the intestines creates inflammation in the intestinal lining, the intestinal blood vessels, and the abdominal cavity. A heavily parasitized horse often has loose stools along with an unthrifty appearance and a loss of performance.

Other Causes

Intestinal bacterial and viral organisms infrequently infect adult horses and lead to diarrhea. A veterinarian should evaluate such ailments so effective treatment can be instituted. Liver disease, intestinal cancer, heart failure, and poisoning by medications, plants, or heavy metals are rare causes of diarrhea.

Potomac Horse Fever

A potentially fatal diarrheal disease has emerged over the last decade that is a major concern to performance horses: *Potomac Horse Fever.* Its mode of transmission is still unknown, but it is thought that the *Ehrlichia risticii* bacteria may be transferred to a horse by a tick or insect. The disease does not seem to be transmitted between horses. Most cases are seen in late spring, summer, and early fall.

Horses infected with this bacteria rapidly develop severe diarrhea, accompanied by fever and depression. If not promptly treated, the horse can lapse into shock and die, or complications of severe laminitis may develop if the horse recovers.

A vaccine is available to protect horses against this disease. Two intramuscular injections are given, 3 – 4 weeks apart. Any horse living in an area with a confirmed incidence of this disease or any horse traveling to a known area of this disease should be vaccinated against Potomac Horse Fever.

14

INTERNAL PARASITE CONTROL

A key feature of equine health management is effective control of internal parasites. Horses continually reinfest themselves with parasites while eating on ground contaminated with manure. Given the opportunity, most horses will defecate in an area separate from their feed supply. Heavily populated pastures do not provide horses enough space to separate a pasture into roughs (ungrazed grass around feces) and lawns (grazing area). Studies in England and Ohio have shown that twice weekly removal of feces from pastures or corrals is an even greater method of parasite control than dewormer treatment at 4 – 8 week intervals. Combining manure removal and dewormer medication promotes a healthy and minimally parasitized horse. If left unchecked, the impact of intestinal worms on the horse's health is dramatic.

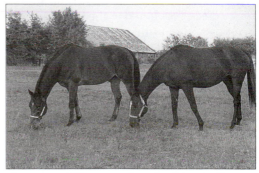

Fig. 14–1. Without good pasture management, grazing horses can easily be reinfested with parasites.

TYPES OF INTERNAL PARASITES

An understanding of the various species of worms and their life cycles helps eliminate infection within an individual and a herd. In general, horses obtain infective larvae through contaminated feed or water, manure eating *(coprophagy)*, or contaminated pastures. Adult worms are rarely seen in the feces unless a horse is severely parasitized. The various egg stages of the worms can only be viewed through the microscope.

Large Strongyles
Bloodworms

One common internal parasite is the large strongyle. The three most common species of large strongyles affecting the horse are *Strongylus vulgaris, Strongylus equinus,* and *Strongylus edentatus.* These bloodworms are examples of the complex life cycle of intestinal worms.

Life Cycle

An infected horse passes eggs in its feces, and it is there that the eggs hatch. A hatched egg develops into a first stage, then a second stage larva, and finally the infective third stage larva. If a horse ingests the third stage larva, the larva penetrates the wall of the large intestine. For about 7 days it remains there, developing into a fourth stage larva. Then the fourth stage larva wanders through the bloodstream for about 8 more days.

By 2 weeks after infection, the worms are in the cranial mesenteric artery and adjacent vessels. These vessels provide the main blood supply to the intestinal tract. The larvae remain there for 3 months. As they develop to fifth stage larvae, damage to these blood vessels reduces blood flow to the intestines and surrounding tissues.

Once developed to the fifth stage, the larvae return to the large intestine and mature to egg-laying adults, and the cycle repeats. The period from ingestion of infective larvae to egg-producing adults is called the *prepatent period.* For *Strongylus vulgaris* this period requires 180 – 200 days. Whatever strongyle larvae a horse acquires today will not complete its cycle or associated damage until 6 – 7 months later. Since strongyle larvae require 4 – 7 days to reach the infective stage, cleaning up manure deposits twice weekly reduces the risk of a horse consuming them.

Prepatent periods for *Strongylus equinus* and *Strongylus edentatus* are 9 months and 10 – 11 months, respectively. These large strongyles migrate through the abdominal cavity, liver, and pancreas, causing damage to these internal organs.

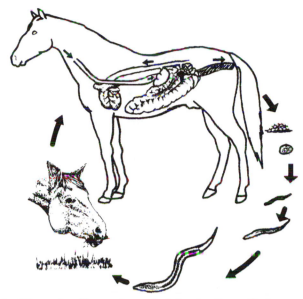

Fig. 14–2. The life cycle of large strongyle takes 6 – 7 months to complete.

Symptoms

Clinical signs of strongyle infestation are:

- diarrhea
- colic
- weight loss
- poor hair coat
- unthriftiness, depression, poor appetite, or dullness
- anemia, resulting in reduced athletic performance or growth
- changes in intestinal movement resulting in impactions, intestinal twists, or death
- obstructions of the blood vessels, leading to death

Small Strongyles

Another group of parasites that has recently received much attention is the small strongyles. Their life cycle and biology are similar to that of the large strongyle except the fourth stage larvae do not invade the blood vessels of the intestinal tract. Instead, they move to the lining of the large intestine, causing diarrhea and/or constipation, and ill-thrift.

Normally, the prepatent period for small strongyles is 2 – 4 months, however, a larva may remain as a *cyst* in the tissues for up to 2½ years. Frequent deworming controls these parasites.

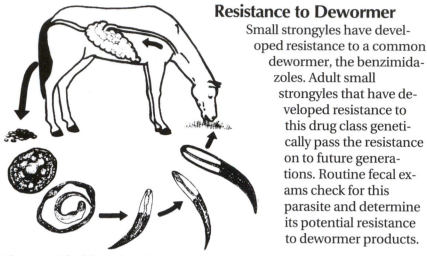

Resistance to Dewormer

Small strongyles have developed resistance to a common dewormer, the benzimidazoles. Adult small strongyles that have developed resistance to this drug class genetically pass the resistance on to future generations. Routine fecal exams check for this parasite and determine its potential resistance to dewormer products.

Fig. 14–3. The life cycle of the small strongyle.

Ascarids

The most important parasite infecting the small intestine is the Ascarid (roundworm). Ascarid eggs are extremely resistant to environmental conditions and persist in the environment for years. Usually, they require 2 weeks to hatch to infective second stage larvae.

Life Cycle

After ingestion of infective larvae, the journey through the body begins in the small intestine, and continues through the circulatory system reaching the liver, heart, and the lungs. As Ascarid larvae mature, they travel up the airways of the lungs and trachea into the mouth. There they are swallowed, and again pass into the small intestine where the larvae mature into the adult egg-laying stage. The prepatent period (time between ingestion of infective larvae to egg-producing adults) for the Ascarid is 10 – 12 weeks.

Symptoms

Clinical signs of Ascarid infestation include an unthrifty, poor-doing horse with a rough hair coat. Diarrhea and gas, alternating with constipation, are fairly common. Many Ascarid-infested youngsters have a potbelly and fail to gain weight.

Not only do the migrating larvae damage the lungs, but viruses and bacteria can invade the damaged respiratory lining. Respiratory infections induced by migratory, immature forms often occur, particularly if the horse is 1 – 2 months old.

If many adult worms ball up in the small intestine, the obstruction leads to colic, peritonitis (inflammation or infection of the abdominal cavity), or death.

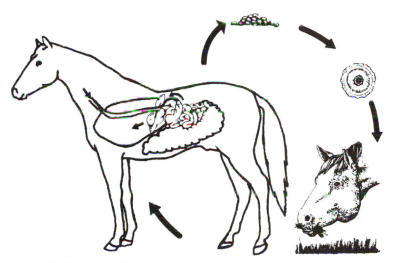

Fig. 14–4. The life cycle of the Ascarids.

Roundworms in Young Horses

The age of a horse greatly affects Ascarid infection. Horses develop an acquired immunity with age until about 15 years old. Ascariasis is a problem in young horses less than 2 years old, and in older horses over 15 years old.

Not only are foals extremely susceptible to Ascarids, but foals tend to consume the mare's manure (coprophagy). If the manure is loaded with Ascarid eggs, a foal becomes heavily infected. Both mare and foal should be dewormed often, and the environment cleaned of feces. Mature horses are rarely heavily infected unless the immune system is compromised by disease or stress.

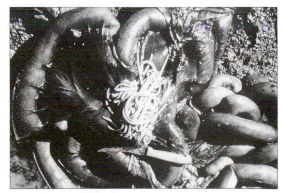

Fig. 14–5. Ascarid impaction in the small intestine.

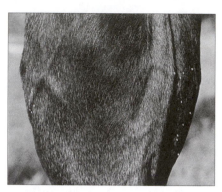

Fig. 14–6. Bot fly eggs attached to leg.

Bots

Bot "worms" are not actually worms at all, but are the larvae of the bot fly, *Gastrophilus sp.* (all species of the genus, *Gastrophilus).*

The bot fly lays its eggs on the leg and chest hairs. When the horse licks or rubs the hairs, the eggs are transferred to the horse's mouth. Unhatched bot eggs can survive for up to 6 months on the hairs.

Life Cycle

Once in the mouth, hatched larvae burrow into the tongue and tissues of the mouth and esophagus. While in the mouth tissues, the bot larvae may cause pain with chewing, or may impede swallowing because of throat swelling. After about 3 weeks, the larvae travel to the stomach.

The larvae attach to the stomach lining, and can cause ulcers, food impaction, colic, or peritonitis (inflammation of the abdominal wall).

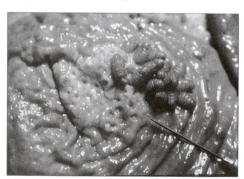

Fig. 14–7. Bot fly larva on the stomach.

Although rare, the stomach may rupture and cause death. Bot larvae require about 10 months to develop once they enter the mouth. Certain species of bot larvae attach to the rectum as they pass to the anus. Their presence causes irritation and tail rubbing, and is often mistaken for pinworm infestation.

Stomach Worms

Life Cycle of Habronema sp.

Stomach worms, *Habronema sp.*, pass their eggs through the feces, and then fly larvae ingest the eggs. The horse either ingests the fly larvae and stomach worm egg, or infected adult flies deposit their larvae around the mouth and lips of the horse. From there they pass directly into the stomach and develop to the egg-laying stage, repeating the cycle. Larvae in the stomach may stimulate an immune response, forming large, tumorous masses. Although these disappear once the larvae are gone, areas of glandular stomach tissue are replaced with scar tissue.

Summer Sores

The most significant damage caused by the *Habronema sp.* is summer sores. If a horse's skin is broken from a wound or abrasion, flies feeding on the injury may infect it with larvae. The larvae do not grow or develop here, but they cause a pronounced tissue response. A non-healing sore persists that is easily invaded by bacteria. Deworming a horse kills the larvae, reducing its chances of contracting this parasite.

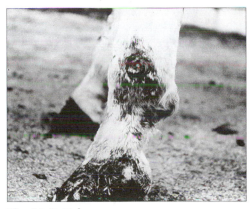

Fig. 14–8. Habronema causes summer sores.

Life Cycle of Trichostrongylus axei

Another stomach worm is *Trichostrongylus axei*, a common parasite of cattle and other ruminants. Infective larvae develop similarly to large strongyles, but only require 3 days to become infective. Horses infected by this worm exhibit a loss in condition, with diarrhea and/or constipation, protein loss, and anemia. A chronic inflammatory response develops in the stomach.

Other Worms

There are a variety of less important parasites to consider that may affect the health and well-being of a horse.

Pinworms

Pinworms, or *Oxyuris equi*, ingested from feed contaminated with manure, develop in the cecum (part of the large intestine). Then, a fertilized, adult female enters the rectum, passes through the anus, and deposits her eggs around the anus and/or vulva. These eggs

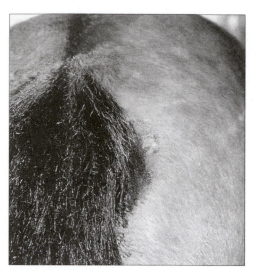

Fig. 14–9. This horse rubs its tail head due to pinworms.

drop onto the ground or food (that has been placed on the ground), with the entire prepatent period being a rapid 52 days. An affected horse itches and rubs the tailhead with an associated loss of hair.

Intestinal Threadworms

Intestinal threadworms, *Strongyloides westeri*, are primarily a problem in foals and have been implicated in foal diarrhea and scours. The infective stage of the larvae is passed through the mare's milk, or penetrates the skin. As with Ascarids, immunity to infection increases with age; by 4 – 5 months of age, foals are resistant to infection. Because of the association of foal scours with the life cycle of this parasite, deworming of scouring foals is recommended.

Lungworms

Although their natural host is the donkey, lungworms can infect horses. Usually donkeys do not show clinical problems, but will pass larvae in their feces. Horses pastured with donkeys are at high risk of infection, but it is possible for horse-to-horse transmission to occur. Associated problems due to lungworms include a chronic cough, pneumonia, and pleuritis.

Tapeworms

Tapeworms are becoming more common in the horse population of the United States. Their life cycle depends on a mite which the horse ingests while eating pasture or hay. Development in the mite requires 2 – 4 months, while in the horse the adult tapeworm takes another 6 – 10 weeks to develop. Heavy infestations lead to intestinal perforations, peritonitis, colic, or intestinal inflammation *(enteritis)*.

MANAGING INTERNAL PARASITES

A century ago, during the rise of the industrial age, crowding of horse populations within increasingly urban areas resulted in enormous worm infestations and ill health in horses. An excerpt from Miles' "Modern Practical Farriery" (1896) comments: "Whoever will take the trouble to visit a knacker's, and to turn over the dunghill in its yard, will find it to be composed quite as much of worms as of excrement."

Parasite control methods diminish the number of infective larvae available to a horse. Twice weekly removal of manure from pasture and corrals is a very effective method. Deworming medications are the other ingredient to a comprehensive parasite management program.

Less than two decades ago, veterinary medicine only offered an arsenal of fairly potent chemicals to kill adult worms. These chemicals were not without hazard. Many of them were toxic to the horse, in some cases lethal, and they needed to be given in large quantities to be effective. The best way to administer the medication rapidly was to give it by stomach tube. Before safe paste formulas, and with extreme risk of drug toxicity reactions, stomach tube deworming was the only way to go.

Horses living on the uncrowded, open range may have only needed a drench once or twice a year. However, in these days of concentrated housing where horses are at continual risk of reinfesting themselves, they should be dewormed at least every 6 – 8 weeks. Deworming at this interval interrupts the damaging life cycle of internal parasites.

Ideally, aggressive deworming programs of monthly treatments between April and October (in average United States climatic conditions) will kill most internal parasites. During the winter, due to dormancy and reduced maturation of worms in the body, deworming every 2 months is usually enough.

Deworming Products

The pressures of urban living have promoted intensive research over the last decade into newer, more efficient, and safer dewormers in the form of pastes and powders.

Everyone says: rotate, rotate, rotate. Many conflicting ideas on what rotate exactly means further confuse the issue. Every time a deworming product is given, the horse is being administered a drug. It is important to know what the chemical is, and what its purpose is. Learn about the nature of the chemicals in these compounds, taking note of the active ingredient listed under the brand name.

Dewormer Classification

There are so many anti-parasite products available on the market to-day for a horse, it is no wonder that confusion exists. By simplifying the list of dewormers, a strategy can be devised to limit the parasite burden of a horse by reducing the number of infective larvae. Our chemical arsenal revolves around six different classes of dewormers.

Benzimidazoles

The benzimidazoles, include products with chemical names of oxibendazole, oxfendazole, mebendazole, fenbendazole, thiabendazole, cambendazole, to name a few.

Febantel

A second drug class, called the pro-benzimidazoles, includes only one drug, febantel. Febantel has similar effects as the benzimidazoles. For the sake of convenience, these two drug classes are considered as one, the benzimidazoles.

Pyrantel

A third drug class called the tetrahydropyrimidines is commonly known as pyrantel (Strongid®). Pyrantel comes in pellets, pastes, and liquid.

Ivermectin

A fourth class called avermectins describes the drug, ivermectin (Eqvalan® or Zimecterin®), produced by fermentation of a certain bacteria.

Organophosphates

Organophosphates are a fifth drug class, with active ingredients of either dichlorvos or trichlorfon. This drug class is specifically targeted at bot fly larvae in the stomach.

Piperazine

Piperazine belongs to the sixth class, and is effective against Ascarids. Although the organophosphates and piperazine are effective against their specific target worms, these two classes are obsolete due to the development of safer, broad spectrum products found in the other drug classes which are effective against all parasites.

From six classes, we have simplified to three:

- Benzimidazoles
- Pyrantel
- Ivermectin

Each drug kills intestinal worms by a different mechanism of action; for example, ivermectin interferes with neuromuscular coordination of the worm, causing a flaccid paralysis. Pyrantel also interferes with neuromuscular activity, but causes a spastic paralysis of the worm. Benzimidazoles interfere with energy metabolism, and the worms die of starvation.

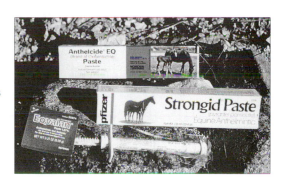

Fig. 14–10. Various brands of dewormers.

Preventing Resistance

Specific strategies can be used to maximize the effect of dewormers. Currently, it is feared that by exposing parasites to a rapid rotation of different drug classes every few months, we may inadvertently select parasites that develop resistance to many of these chemicals. Resistance allows the worm to tolerate dewormer doses that previously killed them.

Based on current research, an optimal strategy is one of slow rotation of dewormers at 1-year intervals. More frequent rotation may result in multiple drug resistance to several different classes at once. Ideally, one product should be used during the season of maximum egg transmission. In this way, a single generation of parasites (of 1 year) is not exposed to different and multiple drug classes. By slowly rotating at yearly intervals, each generation is only subjected to one mechanism of action by a drug, and is subsequently less likely to develop drug resistance. The next year another drug class is used, the third year a third drug class, the fourth year returns to the first year's product, and so on.

Resistance to Benzimidazoles

To date, many of the 40 species of small strongyles have developed resistance to the benzimidazoles. Not only are adult worms able to develop resistance, but they genetically pass resistance genes along to future generations. Of the benzimidazoles, the only drug currently available that the small strongyles cannot resist is oxibendazole (Equipar® or Anthelcide-Eq®).

Ivermectin

As yet, no parasite resistance has developed to either pyrantel or ivermectin. Using ivermectin twice a year at 6-month intervals in addition to daily pyrantel should eliminate damaging migratory forms of the parasites. Ivermectin can also be incorporated into a system of slow rotation, but should not be used exclusively so resistance does not develop.

Recommended Deworming Schedules

Different climatic conditions dictate how a management program should be approached. For instance, in the northern United States, peak *strongyle* egg counts occur in the spring and summer with release of larvae from the intestinal walls. There is vast contamination of pastures and corrals at this time of year. Moisture and warm temperatures speed larval development into an infective stage.

The infective larvae are at their peak between April and October when temperatures range between 45° – 100° F. They can survive freezing temperatures, emerging in the spring with warmth and moisture.

In southern climates, warm and moist environmental conditions encourage persistent development of infective larvae year-round. Overcrowding or excessively unsanitary conditions may also require the deworming schedule to be increased. Each horse's immune response is different. A sick or unthrifty horse may have trouble ridding its body of parasites even with the aid of dewormers, especially if it is continuously re-exposed to infective larvae in mounds of uncollected manure.

Daily Pyrantel Pellets

A formulation of pyrantel, called Strongid® C, comes in a pelleted alfalfa feed. By feeding a measured volume of these pellets each day to the horse, ingested worm larvae are killed before they reach migratory or invasive stages. Before beginning a course of such treatment, deworm the horse in a standard manner with a paste formula.

Once a horse's system has been cleaned out and daily administration of Strongid® C begun, any larval worms in the intestines are eliminated by the pelleted pyrantel. The drug is extremely safe, causing rapid excretion of worms from the body.

Use of this pelleted formulation of dewormer requires conscientious management. Horses on this plan must receive it daily according to manufacturer's recommendations, or some larval forms can slip by and invade the deeper tissues or blood vessels. There, they are unaffected by the daily medication.

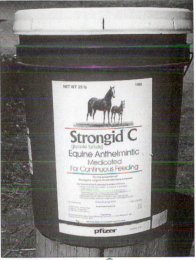

Fig. 14–11. Strongid® C is a pyrantel dewormer.

Advantages of Daily Pyrantel

An advantage to continual daily feeding of pyrantel pellets is the prevention of intense infection from living in a highly contaminated environment. Overstocked and over-grazed pastures, confinement with horses that receive inadequate deworming, or location on a farm that has previously experienced poor parasite management are high risk factors that create problems for any horse. Feeding Strongid® C builds a "protective bubble" around a horse exposed to these conditions.

Deworming Schedule With Daily Pyrantel

For the northern United States, Strongid® C can be used February through September, with administration of a boticide, like ivermectin, in June and December. Ivermectin eliminates bots and any worm larvae that may have slipped by the pelleted pyrantel preparation. In the southern United States, it is best to maintain horses on a year-round, daily dosing of pyrantel pellets because of constant transmission of infective larvae with warm temperatures and high humidity. Again, ivermectin is used in June and December to kill bots.

Deworming Without Daily Pyrantel

If a horse is not at high risk from environmental factors, or if a daily therapy program of pyrantel pellets is not chosen, an example of an effective deworming program is as follows:

Deworming Without Daily Pyrantel	
YEAR	**TYPE AND FREQUENCY OF DEWORMER USE**
Year 1:	Ivermectin every 2 months.
Year 2:	Oxibendazole, but use ivermectin in June and December to kill bots. Deworm every 2 months.
Year 3:	Pyrantel, but use ivermectin in June and December to kill bots. Deworm every 2 months.
Year 4:	Back to ivermectin every 2 months.

Fig. 14–12.

This program is an example of a deworming strategy that will achieve effective and safe parasite control, but should **not** be construed as the only possible approach.

Administering Dewormers

The individual horse, management and hygiene practices, and expertise at handling and restraining a horse determine how consistently the deworming task is performed. The method by which a dewormer is given is not nearly as important as the frequency, the drug used, and the assurance that the **entire dose** is received. If uncertain, discuss with the veterinarian about what would be best for the horse. Deworming with a medication spray "gun" ensures that a liquid drug is given at the appropriate dose and that all of it reaches its destination, the stomach. Yet, pastes or powders can be used with equal effectiveness.

Effective Deworming Technique
Dosages

Effective deworming depends on knowledge of body weight. Read package inserts about the toxic levels particular to a drug. Adjust upwards of suspected weight, but **keep out of the toxic range**. A wide therapeutic index indicates the safety margin that protects a horse from toxic levels, but is a strong enough dose to kill the parasite. As examples of safety margins, oxibendazole can be given up to 60 times the recommended dose before toxic effects are seen. Pyrantel has a safety factor of 20 times, while ivermectin has a safety margin of 6 times the recommended dose.

There is **no reason** to administer such a walloping amount. Usually, overestimating an adult horse's weight by 200 – 300 pounds when determining the correct dose will not produce any adverse effects, **except** if using organophosphates. *(Even the recommended dose for organophosphates can be toxic to a horse.)*

Be sure to check specific products for safety claims regarding use in pregnant mares or foals. If in doubt, consult a veterinarian about what amount and which product to use.

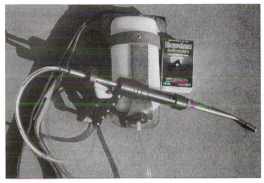

Fig. 14–13. An oral spray applicator for ivermectin allows very precise dosages.

Paste Dewormers

If a paste dewormer is correctly administered, it is absorbed in the stomach and alters biochemical pathways necessary for parasite survival but not to the host horse. There is no reason to deworm on an empty stomach as was done in the old days. In fact, feeding enhances absorption of a drug from the stomach.

However, when paste is given, be sure all food is out of the mouth, then place the syringe on the back of the tongue. Gently hold the horse's head up while depressing the plunger. Stimulate the tongue to move back and forth so the horse swallows the paste.

To avoid mistakes, it is helpful for a veterinarian to give instructions in paste administration. Paste deworming should be executed with confidence, and with certainty that the drug has been received by the horse. If a horse is particularly fractious, a veterinarian can perform the necessary task every 6 – 8 weeks.

Powder Dewormers

If dewormers are given in powder form on feed, the total dose must be consumed within 8 hours to be effective. Powder is an uncertain method of delivery. It is ineffective if feed spills from a bucket, food is spit or dribbled onto the ground, or if the powder is filtered out by the horse and pushed to the side. Mixing powdered medication with molasses or corn syrup into a small amount of grain or bran improves chances of consumption of the entire dose. Watch the horse eat to be confident of success, or aware of failure.

Ineffective Deworming Technique

Deworming failure occurs if an inappropriate dose is given, or if a horse does not actually receive all, or any, of the medication. With paste dewormers, a common error occurs when a horse suddenly moves as the plunger is depressed, and part of the medication shoots out of the side of the mouth. Another way a horse will not receive an appropriate dose is if it has food in its mouth at the time of paste administration. As the dewormer syringe is removed, the horse might spit out the food and paste. A drink at the water trough immediately after deworming causes loss of a considerable amount of medication.

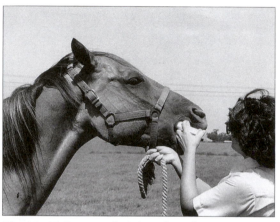

Fig. 14–14. Proper administration of a paste dewormer.

Although an owner may deworm every 2 months with an approved product, a horse may still show obvious signs of parasitism: poor hair coat, potbelly, and unthriftiness. In some instances, a horse may fail to gain weight, or performance may suffer. These problems disappear within weeks of a *proper* deworming — an adequate dose is given and received by the horse. Such horses respond magically; they bloom and flourish.

Underdosing Causes Drug Resistance

Consistent underdosing can lead to larger problems than not deworming at all. Constant exposure to doses not large enough to kill, but large enough to stress the worm promotes the worm's drug resistance. When finally exposed to adequate levels of a drug, resistance capabilities prevent the worm from dying. Moreover, it genetically passes on such resistance to its offspring. Despite the deworming, a horse retains an overwhelming parasite load.

Egg Count

If a horse does not respond to a regular parasite control program, a fecal exam analyzed 2 weeks or more after deworming determines the number of parasite eggs, or egg count, per gram of feces. Parasites such as the *Ascarids* may produce 100,000 eggs per day, while large strongyles may only produce

5,000 eggs per day. Pinworm eggs are not normally seen in the feces, but are obtained by pressing cellophane tape against the anus.

Large numbers may mean the worms are resistant to a dewormer product. Fecal analysis by a veterinarian allows close monitoring of a parasite load within a horse, and observations of hair coat, body condition, weight gain, attitude, and performance provide other clues. A veterinary exam may reveal other metabolic, nutritional, or dental problems contributing to a horse's unthrifty health. Not all illness can be blamed entirely on worms.

Efficacy of Dewormers

Another important characteristic of dewormers is described as efficacy, which is the effectiveness in achieving the desired result (greater than 85% kill of a particular parasite). Oxibendazole has 95% – 100% efficacy against both large and small strongyles, 90% – 100% against Ascarids, and zero effect against bots. Pyrantel has 92% – 100% efficacy against *Strongylus vulgaris*, 86–100% for mature Ascarids, 100% for immature Ascarids, but is only 50% – 70% efficacious against pinworms, 65% – 75% against *Strongylus edentatus*, and zero for bots. Ivermectin possesses 95% – 100% efficacy against large and small strongyles, pinworms, Ascarids, and bots.

Efficacy of Dewormers		
OXIBENDAZOLE	**Large Strongyles**	95% – 100%
	Small Strongyles	95% – 100%
	Ascarids	90% – 100%
	Bots	0%
PYRANTEL	**Large Strongyles:**	
	S. vulgaris	92% – 100%
	S. edentatus	65% – 75%
	Ascarids:	
	Mature	86% – 100%
	Immature	100%
	Pinworms	50% – 70%
	Bots	0%
IVERMECTIN	**Large Strongyles**	95% – 100%
	Small Strongyles	95% – 100%
	Ascarids	95% – 100%
	Pinworms	95% – 100%
	Bots	95% – 100%

Fig. 14–15.

Immunity to Parasites

Normally over time, a healthy horse develops some degree of immunity to certain parasites, and can fend off massive infestation.

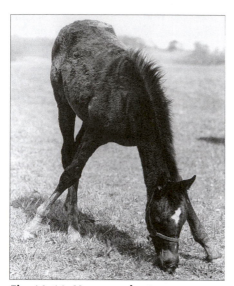

The body's immune system recognizes the parasite's proteins (antigens) as foreign and launches an immune attack by forming antibodies. The more antigens are in the horse's body, the more antibodies are formed. Dewormer efficacy of 100% may not be advantageous, because it eliminates the source of the antigens. Then, a horse's uneducated immune system cannot defend against future parasite infection.

Foals and young horses under 2 years old that have not yet developed immunity may succumb to overwhelming parasite loads by Ascarids or large strongyles if not regularly dewormed.

Fig. 14–16. Horses under 2 years can have an overwhelming parasite load.

Allergic Reaction

When a horse with an overwhelming infection is dewormed for the first time, the destruction and breakdown of the worm expose the horse to foreign proteins. This exposure can result in an allergic reaction, or severe inflammation in the intestine where the parasite attaches, causing edema and thickening of the intestine. These reactions decrease absorption of nutrients and fluids, and may be accompanied by temporary diarrhea. An overwhelming infection produces a similar response, resulting in chronic diarrhea or colic, common signs of intestinal parasitism.

It is far better to have a consistent deworming program than to subject a horse to continual internal damage, or to side effects associated with deworming an older horse for the first time. The objective is to allow a horse's normal immune system to deal with a very small load of parasites.

Preventive Management

By minimizing an internal parasite burden in the horse, health and performance flourish, and gastrointestinal disturbances are averted. Controlling internal parasites with dewormers is an essential part of management, but should be combined with intelligent husbandry.

Introducing New Animals to a Herd

New individuals should not be introduced to the herd immediately, but should be isolated. Before allowing them to join the herd, deworm new arrivals 2 or 3 times, at 3 – 4 week intervals. This practice protects those horses that have received excellent deworming management from reinfection.

Concurrent Deworming Schedules

All members of a herd, including foals, should be dewormed at the same time. It serves little purpose to deworm only a small percentage of a herd, because untreated horses continue to excrete eggs in their feces, recontaminating not only themselves, but the treated horses as well.

Maintaining Pasture

Contaminated forage results in reinfection with worm larvae. Careful pasture management prevents overgrazing that would otherwise encourage manure deposits to outstrip available forage. Removing manure manually by shovel or pitchfork twice weekly will control parasite populations. Chain dragging a pasture spreads the manure and prevents overgrazing of certain areas, while also breaking parasite life cycles. If economically feasible, mechanical removal of feces by pasture vacuums provides excellent parasite control. Harrowing spreads the larvae throughout the grazing area and damages the forage, therefore it is not advised.

Collected manure should be composted before spreading it on a pasture. Heat within the compost pile kills infective larvae and prevents pasture contamination.

Maintaining Pens and Paddocks

Manual cleaning of manure from pens and paddocks twice a week removes parasite larvae before they become infective. By cleaning pens, the frequency of treatments between April through October is reduced to every 2 months instead of the recommended monthly administration.

The more often a dewormer is given, the greater the possibility for drug resistance to develop.

Monitoring With Fecal Analyses

To monitor the parasite control program's effectiveness, fecal analyses can be performed, comparing a fecal sample before deworming treatment with a fecal sample obtained exactly 2 weeks after treatment.

Most dewormers result in decreased egg shedding of strongyles for 4 – 6 weeks after treatment, while ivermectin depresses egg shedding for up to 8 weeks. Because large and small strongyles create such havoc and danger within a horse, a primary goal in any deworming program is to concentrate efforts on removal of these particular parasites.

15

SKIN AILMENTS: AVOIDING & CURING

The condition of a horse's coat is a reliable reflector of internal body health. External parasites, fungal infections, scratches, skin growths, or saddle sores can mar any coat and create performance problems.

EXTERNAL PARASITES
Flies and Gnats
Horse Flies

Flies cause troublesome skin irritations. One such culprit is the horse fly, *Tabanus*. Its bite is painful and causes nodules on the skin. The most commonly affected areas are along the neck, withers, back, and legs.

Stable Flies

The stable fly, similar to the common house fly, also pierces the skin with its mouthparts, irritating the horse and leaving behind nodular swellings. Stable flies are poorly named because they really prefer light and sunny areas, only going inside during rainy weather. They lay eggs in decaying urine-soaked straw and manure. Adequate manure removal and stall cleaning, along with the use of insecticides, controls the stable fly population to a manageable level.

Blackflies

Blackflies (Simulium), commonly known as ear gnats, feed on blood drawn from the flat surface inside the ear *(pinnae)*. Blackflies are found throughout the U.S., particularly near running water, which is a breeding ground for the pest. Adults travel great distances, up to 100 miles, therefore control is nearly impossible.

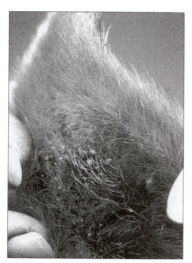

Fig. 15–1. Blackflies feed in the ears.

Blackflies are also known as *buffalo gnats* due to their humpbacked appearance. These tiny insects reach a maximum length of 5 millimeters, about the size of an apple seed.

As the blackflies feed on the delicate lining of the ears, toxins secreted in their saliva increase permeability of capillary beds, improving access to blood meals. Oozing and blood-encrusted scabs form where blackflies have fed. The discomfort from an intense inflammatory response causes the horse to become head-shy. What begins as an instinctive response to avoid pain and discomfort can develop into a habit of head-shyness even after the ears are healed.

Allergic Reaction

Some horses respond to blackfly bites with a severe allergic reaction. Horny growths, or *plaques*, develop inside the ear. These cauliflower-like plaques peel away easily by rubbing with a thumbnail or a piece of gauze (if the horse allows them to be touched). Their easy removal distinguishes them from more tenacious sarcoid tumors often found in the ears.

Once blackfly plaques are removed, applying a topical corticosteroid ointment reduces the severity of the allergic response. A horse can be encouraged to accept daily topical medication inside the ears by quickly applying ointment while it is distracted with a bucket of grain.

Effects on the Ears

Pigmentation Loss

A persistent inflammatory response to blackflies causes a horse to permanently lose skin color inside the ears. This white patch is only of cosmetic significance, and does not interfere with the skin's return to function or health.

Treatment

Immediate recognition of a problem helps to correct it before poor behavior or white patches develop. Normally, hair in the ear protects the deeper ear canal from collecting dirt or debris, and keeps insects or ticks from crawling into the ear canal.

Hair Removal

If a horse has blackflies, trimming or shaving away all fine hairs lining the ear pinnae helps restore health to the ear. Wads of cotton should be inserted into each ear before clipping to prevent particles of hair or debris from falling into the deep ear canal where they can stimulate an infection. It may be necessary to have a veterinarian tranquilize or sedate a head-shy horse. A sedative encourages the horse's head to droop, and allows thorough cleansing of afflicted skin in the ears. After shaving, be sure to remove the cotton wads.

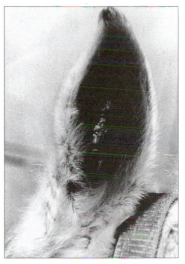

Fig. 15–2. A large blackfly plaque resembles a cauliflower.

Removal of hair inside the ears allows thorough inspection of scabs or sores. Without hair for scabs and oozing serum to cling to, the tender skin inside the ears heals quickly. Without the presence of blood to attract blackflies to a "banquet," it is easier to provide relief for the horse. Anti-inflammatory corticosteroid creams or topical roll-on insect repellants are easily applied to hairless skin. Spray insecticides into the ears with caution, taking care not to accidentally spray an irritating substance into an eye.

Once ear hair is removed, smearing the inside of the ears with a light layer of a petroleum-based salve also deters blackflies from reaching the skin for feeding. Only products intended for use in the ear should be used, or a veterinarian should be consulted. Body heat causes salves to melt into the deep ear canal.

Prevention

Ear Nets

To prevent blackfly irritation, ear nets can be purchased as part of a netted face mask. Mosquito net material forming the mask covers the face, eyes, and extends over the poll and ears to keep insects off all structures of the head.

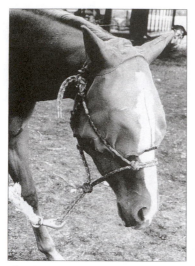

Fig. 15–3. An ear net protects from insects.

Blackflies feed mainly during the day, so in areas of high blackfly populations an allergic horse can be stalled indoors during those hours. Yet, other insects, like *Culicoides* gnats, emerge at dusk.

Culicoides Gnats

The bite of the Culicoides gnat may cause an allergic reaction, called *Culicoides hypersensitivity*, Queensland's itch, sweet itch, or summer eczema. The gnats feed along the topline of the horse, and the horse self-mutilates to appease an intense itching *(pruritis)*. It starts by rubbing the mane and tail down to raw and bleeding skin. As the syndrome worsens, all body areas itch, and the horse traumatizes its neck, chest, and belly. In a delirium of itching, it pauses over bushes to rub its belly, abuses fence posts, stall doors, and sides of barns.

Not only does a horse destroy its hair coat and skin with this behavior, producing a scruffy appearance, but the horse becomes depressed and irritable. It may become belligerent to handlers. Even if it is ridable (depending on the degree of skin damage), its performance suffers.

There is a hereditary predisposition to Culicoides hypersensitivity. Usually it surfaces in horses over 2 – 3 years old, and the allergic response worsens with age.

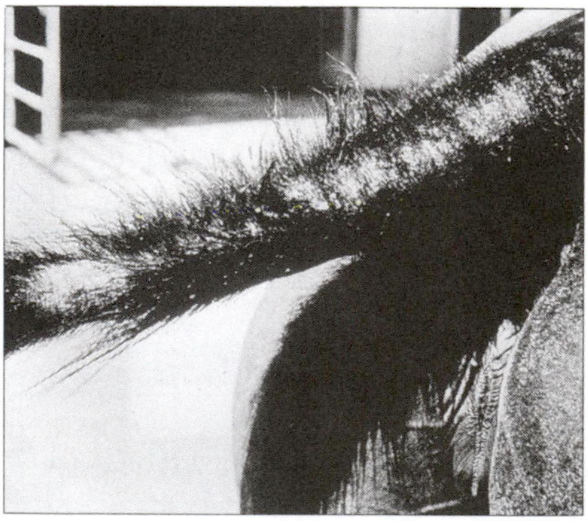

This ailment is seasonal, showing up from late spring through late fall as it coincides with warmth and the fly season. The Culicoides gnat prefers areas of high humidity such as damp pastures, edges of ponds, or areas around wet, decaying plants. The gnats are evening feeders, particularly around dusk, so management control of this syndrome is best aimed at stabling the horse from dusk to dawn.

Fig. 15–4. This horse has rubbed away all its tail hair due to itching.

Mosquito netting or screening over the stalls keeps Culicoides out, and a protective "fly sheet" minimizes bites. Frequent and repeated applications of insect repellants are advantageous, and automatically timed mist sprayers in the barn help kill the gnats and flies.

Unless a horse is relocated to a different environment that is not a favorable breeding ground for the gnat, it is almost impossible to entirely protect an allergic horse from bites. Corticosteroid medications, at a dose recommended by a veterinarian, reduce the allergic response to a manageable level throughout the fly season.

Ailments Similar to Culicoides Hypersensitivity

It is important to differentiate pinworms and bot fly larvae from the more dramatic Culicoides hypersensitivity reaction. These parasites cause similar symptoms.

Pinworms

Initially, Culicoides hypersensitivity is confused with pinworms due to the horse's tendency to rub away the hair on the tailhead. However, Culicoides hypersensitivity progresses along the topline of the horse, whereas pinworms or a normal estrus cycle causes a horse to concentrate on rubbing the rear end only.

By applying scotch tape to the skin around the anus, and then sticking it onto a microscope slide, a veterinarian can microscopically examine the sample for pinworm eggs.

Bot Flies

As bot fly larvae mature and travel from the stomach of the horse to the rectum and anus, they spend a short time attached to the lining of the rectum. These parasites also can cause itching of the tailhead.

If there is any doubt about the possibility of infection with either bots or pinworms, it is simple to administer an appropriate deworming paste, and see if the itching disappears in about a week.

Horn Flies

To make matters even more confusing, another fly bite hypersensitivity reaction—which is easily confused with Culicoides hypersensitivity—is called *focal ventral midline dermatitis*. As the name of this problem suggests, it is found only under the belly. The skin around the navel is scaly, crusty, ulcerated, and lacks hair *(alcopecia)* and color. This reaction is due to the horn fly, *Haematobia*, which prefers to obtain a blood meal along a narrow strip on the abdominal midline. The horn fly can be recognized by its peculiar feeding position with the head pointing towards the ground. Use of fly repellants and corticosteroid-antibiotic

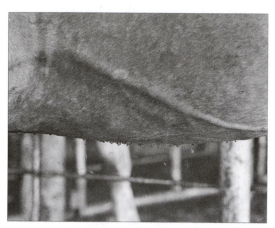

Fig. 15–5. Horn flies on the abdominal midline.

combination creams minimize inflammation and any secondary bacterial infection.

Warbles

If a large single nodule on the horse's back has an opening, it is most likely the breathing pore of a warble called *Hypoderma*. The warble, also called a heel fly, lays eggs on a horse's hairs. Once these eggs hatch, the *Hypoderma* larvae migrate through the skin, arriving at the back about 4 – 5 months later during the fall and winter months. On rare occasions, the warble could migrate to the brain instead of the back, resulting in severe neurological problems. Warbles are common to cattle, so horses pastured with or near cattle are at risk.

Other Causes of Nodules

If there is no breathing pore, the nodule may instead be a nodular *necrobiosis*, which is the result of cell death and scar tissue build-up. This nodule is caused by reaction around a particle of synthetic material from a saddle pad, or from a mini-infection from a recent fly bite. These firm lumps are easily seen and felt in areas along the withers, back, thorax, or belly. They are not usually painful and there is no skin ulceration or reddening over the lumps.

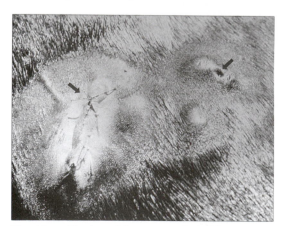

Fig. 15–6. The breathing pores of warbles.

Applying a topical corticosteroid cream may cause the knot to disappear. If not, it can be treated by a corticosteroid injection into and under the lump. The nodule regresses within about 3 weeks. During the healing period, it is important that no tack pressure is placed over the lesion. If the nodule persists, or if it is constantly aggravated by tack, it may be necessary to surgically remove it. The nodule does not grow back, but healing takes longer than treatment with corticosteroids.

Fly and Gnat Bites and Their Symptoms	
Horse Flies	**Nodules on the neck, withers, back, and legs.**
Stable Flies	**Nodules on the entire body.**
Blackflies	**Oozing, blood-encrusted scabs, inflammation, perhaps loss of skin color or cauliflower-like plaques inside the ear canal.**
Culicoides Gnat	**Itching starts at the tail and mane, then spreads to the entire body.**
Horn Flies	**Scaly, crusty, ulcerated lesions, lacking hair and color around the navel.**
Warbles	**Large nodules with a breathing pore on the back.**

Fig. 15–7.

Mites

Mange Mites

Many other parasites cause intense itching in the horse. *Mange mites* stimulate severe itching around the head and neck and can progress over the entire body. There are many species of mange mites, most of which are difficult to see. Mites are usually transferred by direct contact of horse to horse, or by contaminated grooming tools, blankets, and tack. Treatment with ivermectin twice at a 2-week interval usually controls these parasites.

Scabies

Scabies or *Psoroptic* mites prefer areas of skin folds, the throat, and even the ears. Intense itching may cause the skin to thicken and the horse to self-mutilate affected areas. In the United States, it has been more than 30 years since equine scabies has presented a major problem.

Sarcoptic Mites

Sarcoptic mites can be a moderately serious skin ailment in the horse, beginning around the head, neck, and shoulders, accompanied by intense itching. This type of mange mite is contagious to humans.

Demodectic Mites

Demodectic mites are extremely rare, producing nodular lesions of the head, neck, and withers. They burrow deeply into the skin to the base of the hair follicles. Consequently, a very deep skin scraping is necessary for microscopic identification. Demodectic mites may inhabit the skin of up to 50% of normal horses, but usually elicit no disease symptoms unless a horse suffers from immune suppression or deficiency.

Chorioptic Mites

Chorioptic mites are a problem in winter, involving the abdomen or the lower limbs, especially the hind legs. Due to the cracked, greasy appearance of the skin of the lower leg, a case of chorioptic mites may be confused with "scratches" or "grease heel." Normally, scratches is *dermatitis* caused by a skin irritant, or a bacterial and/or fungal infection around the back of the pastern. Dermatitis is inflammation of the skin. Its symptoms include painful, itchy, weeping, red, and inflamed skin. Some or all of these symptoms may be present, depending on the cause. If a case of dermatitis does not respond to conventional treatment with antifungals, antibiotics, and anti-inflammatory topical ointments, chorioptic mites may be the cause.

Straw Itch Mites

The *straw itch mite* causes small raised areas of edema *(wheals)* on a horse's skin. They are non-itchy, crusty eruptions. The straw itch mite normally parasitizes grain insect larvae and is commonly found in alfalfa hay or straw. Humans are also affected by this mite, with intense itching. The problem usually recedes within 3 days without special treatment.

Chiggers

Infestation with *chiggers,* or harvest mites, is called *trombiculiasis.* In the southern Midwest and eastern states, chiggers can be a problem in late summer and fall. Horses pastured in fields and woods may develop crusty *papules* (elevated areas with a defined border) on the face, neck, thorax, and legs. Commonly, the lips and face are involved, with scaly, scabby areas lacking color. It is easy to mistake affected lesions around the muzzle as areas of *photosensitization.* (Photosensitization, discussed later this chapter, is an abnormal reaction of the skin to sunlight, causing sunburn and dermatitis.) Chigger sites may or may not itch.

Mites and Their Symptoms	
Mange Mites	Itching starts at the head and neck, then spreads to the entire body.
Scabies	Itchy, thickened skin in skin folds, throat, and ears.
Sarcoptic Mites	Itching starts around the head, neck, and shoulders.
Demodectic Mites	Nodular lesions on the head, neck, and withers.
Chorioptic Mites	Cracked, greasy lesions on the abdomen and lower limbs, especially the hind legs.
Straw Itch Mites	Small, crusty, non-itchy wheals.
Chiggers	Crusty, scaly, scabby, colorless papules on the neck, thorax, and legs.

Fig. 15–8.

OTHER EXTERNAL PARASITES
Onchocerca Worm

External parasites come in all shapes and sizes, and inflict damage in a variety of ways. Some parasites may be transmitted to a horse by a biting insect. The microscopic *Onchocerca* worm lives along the crest of the neck in the nuchal ligament. Adult Onchocerca produce larvae *(microfilaria)* that migrate just under the skin to the abdominal midline, to the head and face, or into the deep tissues of the eye.

The *Culicoides* biting gnat serves as a vehicle for spread of the Onchocerca among horses. A horse with an Onchocerca infection often has scaling, crusty lesions around the face and eyes, under the belly, along the neck, and over the topline. The lesions are hairless and usually lack color.

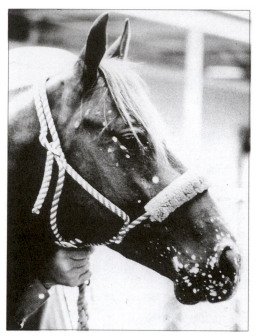

Fig. 15–9. Onchocerca lesions are scaly, crusty, and lack color.

A mild allergic reaction causes the involved areas to become itchy. As a horse rubs the itch, the areas inflame further. This skin problem is common during warm weather due to transmission by Culicoides gnats, and a more active microfilaria production by the Onchocerca adults, as they are stimulated by longer daylight hours.

Diagnosis of *Onchocerciasis* is made by microscopic examination of affected tissue obtained by surgical biopsy, or skin scraping. Seeing microfilaria through the microscope positively identifies the skin ailment.

Moonblindness

If the microfilaria migrate through the eye, *periodic ophthalmia,* or "moonblindness," can result. Moonblindness is accompanied by chronic attacks of *anterior uveitis,* which is an inflammation of structures surrounding the pupil. Uveitis is painful, and symptoms include tearing, squinting, and sensitivity to bright light *(photophobia).* Corneal ulcers develop subsequent to swelling of the eye's internal structures.

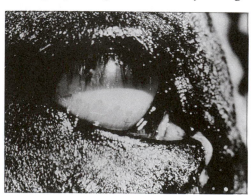

Fig. 15–10. A horse with moonblindness.

Fortunately, the incidence of onchocerciasis has dramatically diminished due to the drug ivermectin which effectively kills the parasite. Ivermectin has reduced the reservoir of the Onchocerca worms, and today it is rare to see well-maintained horses with this skin problem. However, there may be horses with eye damage from previous exposure to migrating microfilaria.

Pelodera strongyloides

The symptoms of a microscopic parasite that affects the skin of the thighs and belly, called *Pelodera strongyloides*, may be mistaken for urine or manure scald. This parasite causes *rhabditic dermatitis* which is itchy and painful. Usually, sanitation of the environment controls this problem. Diagnosis often is only accomplished by a skin biopsy.

Lice

Onchocerca and *Pelodera strongyloides* are invisible to the naked eye. But carefully brushing the hairs the wrong way may lead to the discovery of more obvious skin predators, such as *lice*.

Infestation with lice is called *pediculosis*. Typically, this parasite is a problem in winter, because the eggs *(nits)* thrive in the deep layers of a fuzzy winter hair coat. Lice are host specific, meaning that a horse louse will not infest a person, dog, or cat.

The louse spends its entire life cycle on the host. They can be seen along the topline and look like "walking dandruff." The nits are cemented to the hairs, and should not be mistaken for bot fly eggs. Nits are white and more oval than the yellow bot fly eggs normally found on the legs. Using a magnifying glass aids identification.

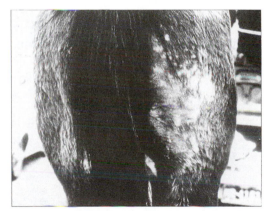

Fig. 15–11. The hair coat of a horse infested with lice appears moth-eaten.

Lice cause intense itching, and a horse self-mutilates to satisfy the itching. The hair coat may appear moth-eaten in places, and large areas of hair will be rubbed out, especially over the buttocks, thighs, neck, and head.

Poor sanitation, overcrowding, and undernutrition cause lice infestation. They are transmitted directly from horse to horse, or by brushes, blankets, and tack. Specific louse shampoos are necessary to treat the horse, while tack and equipment should be soaked in a Clorox® solution of at least 4:1 dilution (4 parts water to 1 part Clorox®).

Ticks

Spinous Ear Tick

The spinous ear tick, *Otobious*, inhabits the ear canal. These ticks remain attached for up to 7 months, feeding off lymph secretions,

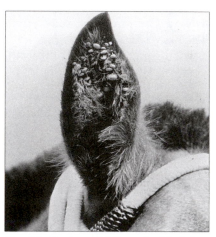

Fig. 15–12. An ear infested with ticks.

and causing irritation and head-shaking. Sometimes a horse may droop a particularly affected ear, or rub incessantly on a post. The intense inflammation caused by these ticks makes their attachment sites susceptible to bacterial infection. It is often necessary to sedate the horse to properly examine the ear canals and remove the ticks.

Hard Ticks

Another type of tick, *Amblyomma*, is a hard tick common to the southeastern U.S. It prefers to feed on blood deep within the ears. Their bites are quite painful. These ticks are also found along the mane and tail, withers, and flank. Ticks irritate soft-skinned areas around the groin, under the tail, around the anus and vulva, and under the throat and belly, so look carefully in these areas.

Ticks burrow their heads into the superficial skin layers. Secondary bacterial infections around these bites can occur, and occasionally edema and soft tissue swelling result even after the tick has dropped off.

It is important to remove the head by grasping the tick and slowly easing it out of the skin. Burning it with a match while still on the horse, or applying alcohol or turpentine are not advised methods for tick removal. These techniques do not induce the tick to release itself, and may irritate or chemically burn tender skin.

Ticks can transmit serious diseases, such as Lyme Disease and protozoal diseases, and may be responsible for Potomac Horse Fever infection. Providing they do not carry a disease, ticks generally cause little harm to the horse, although a heavy infestation may signal a suppressed immune system. A horse could easily develop anemia from blood loss if a heavy enough tick load occurs.

Summer Sores

A syndrome caused by abnormal larval migration of the stomach worm, *Habronema*, is called *summer sores* or *cutaneous habronemiasis*. During the warm months when house or stable flies are active, larvae from the stomach worm are passed in the feces and ingested by larvae of these host flies. Once the fly larvae hatch and begin feeding on the horse, they are deposited at feeding sites. If worm larvae are deposited in areas other than around the mouth, such as the mucous membranes of

the eyes and prepuce, or on wounds or traumatized skin, they migrate underneath the skin, causing a severe allergic hypersensitivity reaction.

The lesions that develop appear ulcerated, raw, and bleeding, and are very painful and itchy. A horse may bite at and traumatize the lesions. Although they may regress during winter, the lesions reoccur the next year at the same time and in the same place.

Summer sores resemble proud flesh, *fibroblastic sarcoids*, or a *squamous cell carcinoma* tumor. Biopsies must be performed to differentiate from these other problems. Surgically cutting away dead and dying tissue, along with non-steroidal anti-inflammatory

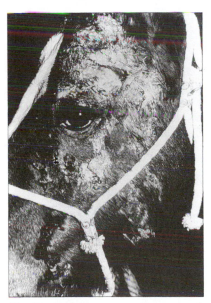

Fig. 15–13. Summer sores are caused by habronema larvae.

drugs and antibiotics, helps control tissue proliferation. Ivermectin is effective in killing the worm larvae.

Black Widow Spider

An unusual creature that can bite the horse is the *black widow spider*. The horse responds quickly to the spider's poison, developing a severe and enormous swelling, along with considerable pain, illness, fever, depression, lack of appetite, and perhaps hives.

Normal wound management such as cold or hot soaking and administration of antibiotics and anti-inflammatory drugs are the only treatment for the noxious bite.

Other External Parasites and Their Symptoms	
ONCHOCERCA WORM	Scaly, crusty, hairless, colorless lesions on the face and around the eyes, under the belly, on the neck and topline. If the microfilaria migrate through the eye, moonblindness can result.
PELODERA STRONGYLOIDES	Painful, itchy dermatitis on the thighs and belly.
LICE	Intense itching, "walking dandruff" especially around the mane and tail.
TICKS Spinous Ear Tick	Irritation, head shaking, drooping, or rubbing of ears; found inside ear canal.
Hard Tick	Feed inside ears, around mane, tail, withers, flank, groin, under throat and belly.
SUMMER SORES	Ulcerated, raw, bleeding, painful, itchy lesions in old wounds or on mucous membranes of the eye, mouth, and prepuce.
BLACK WIDOW SPIDER	Severe and enormous swelling with pain, illness, fever, depression, and lack of appetite, perhaps hives.

Fig. 15–14.

FUNGAL INFECTIONS

A fungus is a living organism invading the hair coat. Small, firm, pea-sized bumps in the skin, skin flaking, or hairlessness signals the beginning stages of fungal infection. A fungus cannot grow in living tissue, but produces toxins to create an environment in which it can thrive.

These toxins cause an inflammatory reaction in the skin, with resultant edema, necrosis (tissue death), or an allergic hypersensitivity reaction. Because the fungus weakens the hair shaft, the hair easily breaks off.

Ringworm

Fungal infections called *ringworm* or *girth itch*, often result in circular patches of hair loss, with scabby or flaking skin beneath, and broken hairs visible in the lesions. In horses under 2 years old, the immune system is less developed, and the entire body may be overwhelmed by the disease.

The fungus can persist in the environment for up to a year, and it is transferred by brushes, blankets, clothing, rake handles, etc. Ringworm is extremely contagious from horse to horse, and to small children. Wash hands thoroughly with povidone-iodine after handling an infected horse, and soak

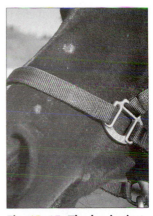

Fig. 15–15. The beginning signs of a fungal infection.

all tack and equipment in a diluted 6% Clorox® solution (approximately 17 parts water to 1 part Clorox®), straight povidone-iodine, or a 3% Captan solution (approximately 33 parts water to 1 part Captan 50% Powder). (Captan 50% Powder can be found at nurseries as an orchard spray.)

Sunshine helps to rid the environment of a fungus, which is why many dark, damp barns provide a perfect environment for fungal growth. Fungal infections are common in fall and winter when sun rays diminish, dampness prevails, and horses are housed inside.

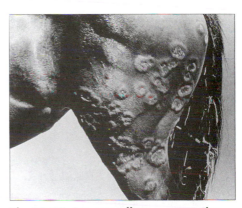

Fig. 15–16. An unusually severe reaction to ringworm.

Diagnosis and Treatment

A veterinarian can diagnose a fungal skin infection by obtaining a scraping of an affected area, and growing it on "dermatophyte test media," which is a gel-like nutrient medium especially for fungus. Results usually require 4 – 14 days to confirm the presence of a disease-causing fungus.

Normally, fungal infections resolve by themselves within 1 – 3 months, unless a horse has an immune deficiency, another debilitating disease, malnutrition, or stress from overcrowding or poor sanitation. Such horses are unable to rid their bodies of the fungal infection, or may be persistently reinfected.

Treatment requires shampoos using povidone-iodine, followed by a rinse with Captan 50% Powder, mixed at 2 ounces per gallon of water. On localized spots, specific anti-fungal ointments may be used. If the entire body is involved, or if a case does not respond to topical treatment, then griseofulvin powder may be prescribed by a veterinarian. (Do not use griseofulvin on a pregnant mare.)

Fungal Infections and Their Symptoms	
General Fungal Infection	Small, firm, pea-sized bumps, skin thickening and roughening, scaling and crusty skin, hair loss.
Ringworm	Circular patches of hair loss, scabby or flaking skin, broken hairs.

Fig. 15–17.

SCRATCHES

White markings on a horse's legs add flash to its overall appearance. Beneath the white fur lies pink skin, which under most circumstances poses few problems as the hair coat protects pink skin from sunburn.

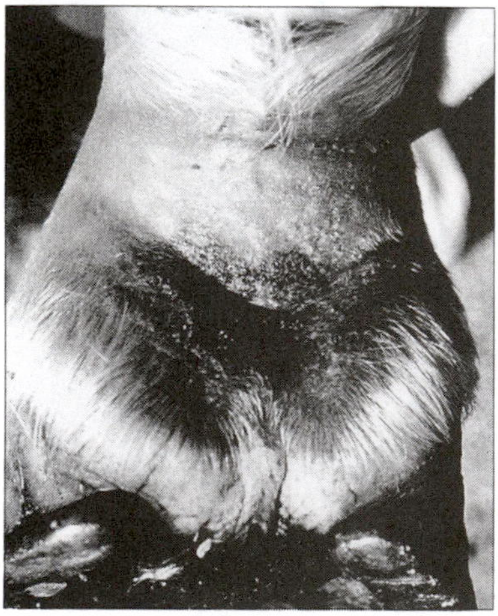

Fig. 15–18. Scratches occur at the back of the pastern.

Yet, legs marked with white socks or stockings are prone to irritation. Irritation creates a skin inflammation (dermatitis) of vulnerable tissues at the back of the pastern. The syndrome has many names, each a description of either the cause or symptoms of the problem. Commonly called *scratches*, other descriptive terms include *grease heel, mud fever, cracked heels, white pastern disease*, and *dew poisoning*.

Under the right conditions, any horse can develop scratches. Like chapped hands, the skin is painful and is often accompanied by localized swelling and lameness. Initially, there is no visible evidence of an inflammatory crisis, but in a short time hair loss occurs, along with weeping, red skin at the back of the pasterns. Constant motion of the pastern causes the skin to crack and form fissures. Ulcerated and raw sores persist beneath the scabs.

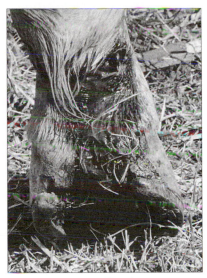

A cracked skin surface that is caked with dried and moist serum appears greasy, hence the name grease heel. Over time, inflamed skin overreacts by growing thickened, horn-like proliferations called "grapes." These growths must be removed surgically to treat the underlying skin.

Typically scratches is confined to a small area with swelling beginning directly around the lesions, but some cases may be

Fig. 15–19. Grease heel.

aggravated by sun exposure and are called *photoaggravated vasculitis. (Vasculitis is inflammation of blood vessels.)* Ultraviolet radiation may trigger cases during the long days of summer.

Usually only white-marked limbs are affected, and swelling and lameness are out of proportion to the mildness of the skin lesions. As a case of scratches progresses, swelling may encompass the entire lower limb. Lesions weep and ooze serum. Sores develop not just on the back of pasterns, but also on the sides and fronts of pasterns and fetlock. If pink skin ascends the leg, the dermatitis may spread to the cannon area.

Causes of Scratches

Rough stubble in a field, sand, soil, and grit of training surfaces, and muddy pastures irritate the skin on the lower legs. Unsanitary conditions of urine-soaked and dirty bedding cake on the feet and pasterns of stalled horses, creating chemical and bacterial irritation to skin.

In horses with particularly long hairs down the back of the legs, such as the feathering common to certain draft breeds, scratches occurs even under the best conditions. Long hair traps moisture and debris, which are prime conditions for dermatitis.

Other Related Problems

Skin irritation is not the only cause of "scratches." Infectious organisms, mites, or *photosensitization* can cause dermatitis or can complicate an existing case.

Fungal Infection

Fungus proliferates in dense hairs and the unsanitary skin environment common to the lower limbs and may be mistaken for scratches. However, a fungal infection may also occur on a darkly marked limb or on other parts of the body. Skin scrapings grown by a veterinarian on a special nutrient medium can identify a fungus.

Chorioptic Mange Mite

Another organism that invades long hairs around the pastern is a *chorioptic mange mite*. Draft horse breeds are particularly susceptible. This mite causes an intense itching in the invaded area, causing horses to stomp or bite at their legs in agitation. This mite is diagnosed by analyzing a skin scraping under a microscope.

Rain Scald

In moist areas of the United States like the southeast, or during warm and rainy spring months in any region, a common problem is infection with the *Dermatophilus* bacteria. Spores are continually present in the environment and are activated by moisture. Commonly seen along the back, loins, and croup, Dermatophilus is also called *rain scald*. Activated spores infiltrate skin traumatized by flies. Lower limbs are affected in areas of moist terrain, earning it the name *dew poisoning*. Dermatophilus dermatitis which is limited to pastern areas is often mistaken for scratches. Daily antiseptic cleansing of afflicted skin assists a normal immune system to defeat infection by Dermatophilus.

White Pastern Disease

Bacterial organisms can cause or complicate a case of white pastern disease. Specifically, a *staphylococcal* bacteria infection is the most common cause. A veterinarian can diagnosis and treat these infections. Unlike scratches, only one limb may be affected.

Photosensitization

Photosensitization occurs when the skin overreacts to sunlight, causing sunburn and/or dermatitis. It is difficult to distinguish from scratches, especially the more severe photoaggravated vasculitis. Photosensitization is caused by a breakdown product called *phylloerythrin*, which is released from plant chlorophyll.

Certain plants, such as ragwort (groundsel) and horsebrush, cause liver disease. Liver disease prevents normal body excretion of phylloerythrin, and the chemical accumulates in the skin. A horse with either plant-induced or metabolic liver disease can develop photosensitization.

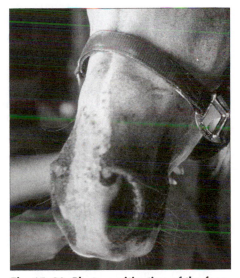

Fig. 15–20. Photosensitization of the face and muzzle.

Phylloerythrin accumulates in skin tissues where it absorbs ultraviolet light. Sunburn results, leading to tissue edema, inflammation, and cracked, peeling skin that weeps serum. The matted, crusty appearance of the skin and hair closely resembles the symptoms of scratches. As scabs peel away, ulcerated, raw areas are revealed underneath.

Other plants, such as St. John's Wort and buckwheat, contain excess amounts of a chemical, which accumulates in the skin. The chemical causes the skin to absorb UV rays of the sun, and photosensitization results.

Because sunburn only affects pink skin, photosensitized horses react on areas of the legs with white markings. Distribution is similar to that of scratches, but photosensitization reactions may also include other white areas, including the face and muzzle. One way to distinguish scratches from liver disease is that with liver disease, the mucous membranes of the gums and eyes are jaundiced.

Differentiating between a dermatitis that involves all four limbs and possibly the muzzle, and a photosensitization reaction to a plant (with or without liver disease) can be difficult. Dermatitis can be caused by parasites, bacteria, or fungus. Photosensitization can be caused by certain plants or liver disease. Biochemical analysis of liver enzymes in the bloodstream can diagnose liver disease.

Treating Scratches

Various home remedies are concocted to treat scratches, including sauerkraut poultices. People struggle for months using home remedies trying to rid a horse of scratches, to no avail. There is no substitute for cleaning affected legs and shaving away the hair so topical salves and bandages can be applied.

The first step in treating scratches is to soften and remove matted hair and crusts. Gently soap the area with warm water and an antiseptic scrub, such as tamed iodine (Betadine®) or chlorhexidine (Nolvasan®). An antiseptic scrub also treats any superficial bacterial infection.

Once all of the crusts and mats are loosened and the hair is toweled dry, clip all hair away with electric clippers. Residual particulates, crusts, and contaminants are removed along with clinging hair. Many horses resist scrubbing and clipping. Veterinary help and sedatives may be necessary for treating objecting horses.

If crusting tissue adheres tightly to underlying, ulcerated skin, removing the scabs forcefully causes more harm than good. Instead, coat matted areas with a salve and bandage them for a day or two. Then, crusts, mats, and scabs easily peel away from the skin without further trauma.

Once the crusts and hair are removed, apply a topical antibiotic-corticosteroid combination cream or ointment. Not only is this preparation soothing, but it restores pliability to cracked tissue. A light bandage over the wounds keeps them clean and protects pink skin from ultraviolet rays. Also, a bandage supports damaged tissues and promotes healing.

If a case of scratches has developed beyond a local irritation to a grease heel, apply zinc sulfate (contained in white lotion) or calamine lotion to suppress serum production and weeping. After a day or two, apply an antibiotic-corticosteroid cream and bandage as above. The tissues should never be dried out with astringent products such as copper sulfate or lime, because they worsen the dermatitis and substantially slow healing.

NSAIDs

Inflammation and tissue swelling impair circulation to the area, and must be controlled for healing to advance. This goal is accomplished with non-steroidal anti-inflammatory drugs, like flunixin meglumine (Banamine®) or phenylbutazone ("bute"). In photoaggravated vasculitis cases, corticosteroid medications may be necessary.

Preventing Scratches

It is of little benefit to address the symptoms of the problem without also addressing the cause. Unsanitary housing conditions should be improved. A horse pastured in irrigated fields, moist grass, or mud should be removed from this environment until the legs are healed, or until the environment dries up. If sunshine aggravates the condition, the legs should be covered with bandages, or the horse should be housed indoors during the daytime.

For light or Warmblood breeds, shaving the back of the fetlocks maintains cleanliness. If feathering down the legs is desired for draft breeds, diligent attention to hygiene is essential. Careful daily inspection of all limbs identifies a beginning problem before it gets out of hand.

Scratches and Similar Ailments	
Symptoms of Scratches	Dermatitis, consisting of painful, inflamed, cracked, weeping, red lesions at the back of the pastern. Also, hair loss and "grapes."
Problems Similar to Scratches	Fungal Infection Chorioptic Mange Mite Rain Scald White Pastern Disease Photosensitization

Fig. 15–21.

ALLERGIES
The Role of the Immune System

The world teems with invisible organisms. Under the right conditions, these microbes colonize the body, afflicting an animal with disease symptoms. Normally, the immune system keeps the organisms at bay.

These disease-producing organisms are made partly of proteins. Inflammatory cells recognize these proteins, called *antigens*, as foreign, and wage invisible battles when they attempt to invade the body. Antigens then stimulate the body to launch an immune response.

The immune system responds by manufacturing other proteins, called *antibodies,* which are weapons against a specific antigenic target. Pre-programmed antibodies set off a cascade of biochemical events. Localized inflammation starts within minutes.

Normally the immune system works in harmony with other biochemical responses to keep a horse disease free, healthy, and vital. Occasionally however, the body rebels and an immune response is blown out of proportion. This hypersensitivity response is called an *allergy.* It can range from a serious, life-threatening reaction within the respiratory tract to mild, but disagreeable skin reactions, called *hives* or *urticaria.*

Hives

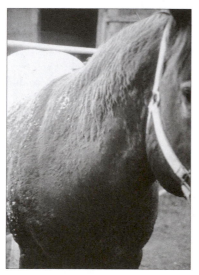

Fig. 15–22. Large, round bumps are characteristic of hives.

Hives are areas of edema (swelling of cells with fluid) that begin as small lumps. Then they grow together into large, elevated, round, flat-topped bumps with steep sides, about the size of a fingernail. Pressing one leaves an impression of a fingertip, and is called *pitting edema.*

They initially form on the neck and shoulders and along the thorax. If the symptoms are not stopped early, the entire body may become involved, especially the upper hind limbs. An affected horse appears droopy and depressed as the immune system wages a silent war.

Hives usually appear 12 – 24 hours after exposure to the foreign protein, and resolve as quickly. Because hypersensitivity reactions take months or years to develop, a sudden onset of hives is *not always* a result of a very recent change, making it difficult to locate the source of the problem.

Causes of Hives

Most hives are caused by an allergic response to a plant, food, or drug, although the specific cause is isolated less than half of the time. Blood transfusions, ingestion of certain plants, or feed additives can be responsible for hives. Liver disease is sometimes associated with recurrent hives; in those cases once the liver heals, hive episodes abate.

Drug Allergies

Medications such as non-steroidal anti-inflammatory drugs like flunixin meglumine (Banamine®) or phenylbutazone, and procaine in procaine penicillin may cause allergic reactions. Hives can also occur after administration of equine influenza vaccine or tetanus antitoxin.

Food Allergies

Certain food substances, particularly those with high protein contents, cause hives in some horses. This allergic reaction is accompanied by small, raised areas, or wheals, that itch intensely and cause the horse to rub its tail.

Pollen and Mold

Inhaled allergens, such as pollen or molds, are common sources for hives. Antigens inhaled into the lungs stimulate swelling in the respiratory tract, similar to asthma in people.

Topical Applications

Not all incidents of hives are caused by intake of a foreign substance. Localized, topical application of tamed iodine scrub, liniments, insecticides, or contact with bedding may also spark an allergic reaction.

Insect Bites

Insect bites often stimulate an outbreak of hives. Isolated groups of bumps that appear rapidly, especially in thin-skinned areas, may be allergic reactions to mosquito bites, Culicoides gnat bites, or Onchocerca parasites. Most insect bite reactions resolve with no treatment within 12 – 72 hours. These wheals are mildly tender and flat. Insect bites rarely cause hives on the entire body unless it is overwhelmed by the bite toxin. Usually the wheals are confined to one area.

Other Forms of Hives

Ehrlichia equi

An odd form of hives develops secondary to some bacterial or viral infections, and specifically to *Ehrlichia equi,* an organism similar to that responsible for Potomac Horse Fever *(Ehrlichia risticii). E. equi* is not as severe as *E. risticii,* and horses do not usually die from it. Infection causes fever, depression, weakness, and poor motor coordination rather than the life-threatening intestinal diarrhea experienced with Potomac Horse Fever.

E. equi forms unique "target" lesions, called *erythema multiforme,* that remain for weeks or months in a fairly symmetrical distribution. These hive-like lesions have an area of central clearing, and look like dough-nuts or bull's eye targets.

Purpura Hemorrhagica

An unusual allergic response to the bacteria responsible for strangles *(Streptococcus equi)* can cause *purpura hemorrhagica.* A month or two after a bout of strangles, a Streptococcal respiratory infection, or influenza, the horse appears stiff from muscle soreness. It is unwilling to walk or move its sore neck. The limbs are stocked up, and edema extends into the belly and prepuce.

Hives appear on the entire body in a case of purpura, due to a breakdown in blood vessel walls. The breakdown occurs because of an immune response to the *Streptolysin O* toxin remaining from the *Strep equi* infection. Small blood spots are visible on the mucous membranes of the gums, eyes, and inside the vulva. As the syndrome progresses, swelling increases in the legs, and the skin begins to ooze serum.

To combat an allergic response to the Strep toxin, massive quanti-ties of penicillin and potent anti-inflammatory agents (corticoster-oids) are administered for weeks until the symptoms abate.

Angioedema

Profound hypersensitivity allergies occasionally result in a syn-drome called *angioedema.* This reaction is more severe than simple hives. The head and respiratory tract swell, and respiratory swelling moves downwards. The wheals are infiltrated with cellular compo-nents, turning soft, pitting edema lesions into firm bumps.

Anaphylaxis

Angioedema is a life-threatening condition—it can rapidly progress to *anaphylaxis* and death. Anaphylaxis begins with muscle tremors and patchy sweating. The horse appears anxious or colicky. Respiratory distress quickly follows, due to pooling of blood and fluid in the lungs. The horse collapses and may go into convulsions before death.

Anaphylaxis can occur rapidly and progress to an irreversible con-dition within a few minutes. Hives is a precursor to angioedema which is a precursor to anaphylaxis, so it is important to summon a veterinarian if a horse has hives. There is not always the luxury of seeing an allergic response before it becomes a death warrant to a horse. If a horse's specific drug allergy is not known, accidental ad-ministration of an offending medication can cause immediate disaster.

Preventing Hives

When buying a horse, question the seller about previous allergic responses the horse may have experienced. Inform the veterinarian, trainer, and barn manager about these allergies. A big sign written in red should be placed outside the horse's stall describing known allergies.

Determining Cause of Hives

If a horse erupts in hives, discontinue new medications or food supplements immediately. To determine if the hives is a result of a food allergy, change the grain and hay ration for at least 2 weeks. Slow reintroduction of an original feed may stimulate reappearance of the hives, which will determine the food that sparks an allergic response.

If hives occur as an isolated incident, the cause may never be discovered. However, if hives is a recurrent problem, tracking down the source includes intradermal skin testing for pollen (plants, bushes, and trees), molds, grasses, weeds, dust, and farm plants such as corn, oats, wheat, and mustard. After identifying the source, hyposensitization injections may prove successful over the long-term. Treatment must be continued for life.

Allergies and Their Symptoms	
HIVES	Small, elevated, flat-topped, lumps that grow together into large lumps. Appear first on the neck, shoulders, and thorax, eventually spreading to the entire body, especially the upper hind legs.
Ehrlichia equi	"Target" lesions, with fever, depression, weakness, poor motor coordination.
Purpura Hemorrhagica	Stiffness, stocking up, then edema extends to the belly and prepuce, until the skin oozes fluid. Hives on the entire body, with blood spots on mucous membranes.
Angioedema	Hives are firm, the head and respiratory tract swell.

Fig. 15–23.

Most horses affected with a case of hives usually recover uneventfully with little cause for concern. Pay attention to recent changes in diet, environment, medications, vaccinations, or stress factors that may cause the immune system to overreact.

SKIN GROWTHS

Skin growths are a form of cancer, and may be either *benign* or *malignant*. Benign means the growth is only of cosmetic significance, and it does not spread to other organs. Rarely, skin growths become malignant, which means the cancer spreads to internal organs. Cancers of the skin are rarely life-threatening in horses as they are in dogs or people, but skin growths do detract from a horse's appearance. However, any skin growth that appears suddenly or enlarges rapidly should be examined by a veterinarian.

Sarcoids

One of the common skin growths found on horses is the *sarcoid*. It is a benign tumor unique to equine skin. The term tumor is misleading since a sarcoid growth is usually localized to a small area and does not invade underlying tissues or lymphatic vessels. Unlike malignant and life-threatening growths, sarcoids do not spread to internal organs. They remain an external, cosmetic blemish, but may occasionally interfere with tack or skin mobility and if traumatized, a sarcoid can become ulcerated or infected. Over 50% of horses with a single sarcoid ultimately develop multiple sarcoids.

Sarcoids are thought to develop from an infective virus that enters a break in the skin, or as a transformation of cell components in an abnormal response to trauma. Areas of skin subjected to trauma are predisposed to sarcoids. These tumors can be transmitted from one part of a horse to another by biting, rubbing, or contaminated tack.

Almost half of all sarcoids are found on a horse's limbs, while 32% are located on the head and neck, especially the ears, eyelids, and mouth. Other locations for sarcoids include the chest and trunk, the abdomen and flank, and the prepuce.

Verrucous Sarcoids

Verrucous sarcoids are wart-like, dry, horny masses, resembling a cauliflower. They are usually less than 2½ inches in diameter. Verrucous sarcoids can appear spontaneously without any prior trauma or wound of the skin. They are difficult to distinguish from warts except that verrucous sarcoids tend to lack hair, partially or totally, while warts have hair growing up to the edges, and often regress spontaneously. Verrucous sarcoids do not regress as do warts. Warts are usually seen in young horses under 2 years old, particularly around the muzzle, but they can also appear on the legs, prepuce, ears, or abdomen.

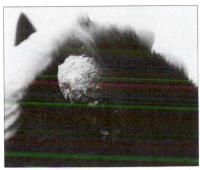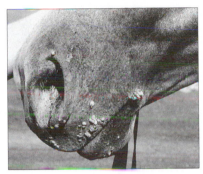

Fig. 15–24. On the left, a verrucous sarcoid in the ear. On the right, warts.

Fibroblastic Sarcoids

If a verrucous sarcoid is traumatized, it can develop into a *fibroblastic sarcoid*. Fibroblastic sarcoids often develop subsequent to a wound, and are difficult to distinguish from normal granulation tissue. These masses are like proud flesh, and may enlarge and expand to greater than 10 inches in diameter. A fibroblastic sarcoid may remain as a small lesion for years, and then suddenly erupt into a nasty-looking sore. Or, it can start as a rapidly and aggressively growing tumor. A wound that refuses to heal and is repeatedly ulcerated and infected may actually be a fibroblastic tumor.

Mixed Sarcoid

Both the verrucous or fibroblastic types are further classified as broad-based (sessile), or with a stalk (pedunculated). A mixture of verrucous and fibroblastic forms represents the third type, a *mixed sarcoid.*

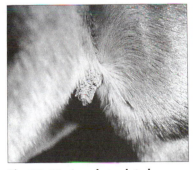

Fig. 15–25. A pedunculated sarcoid on the flank.

Occult Sarcoid

Flat tumors represent the fourth type, the *occult sarcoids.* They are usually flat or very slightly raised, the skin is thickened, and the surface

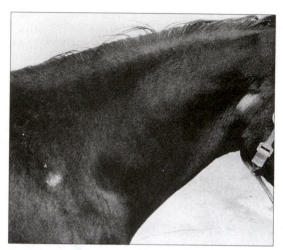

Fig. 15–26. Occult sarcoids are often found on the neck.

roughened. They may even resemble ringworm, or skin crusting from a bacterial infection or poor skin health. Occult sarcoids typically appear around the head, especially the ears and eyelids. If aggravated by a surgical biopsy, they may revert to the fibroblastic form. Rubbing or traumatizing an occult sarcoid can also stimulate conversion to a fibroblastic sarcoid.

Recognizing Sarcoids

It is virtually impossible to determine the exact nature of a growth based on appearance. Fibrosarcomas, neurofibromas, neurofibrosarcomas, and squamous cell carcinomas are all malignant tumor types easily confused with a sarcoid. Fibromas, although mistaken for sarcoids, easily shell out and are well-defined, while a sarcoid infiltrates around its margins, without a neat border. Summer sores caused by *Habronema* fly larvae also develop ulcerated masses not readily distinguishable from sarcoids. Keloids are made of collagenous, connective tissue that may resemble a sarcoid.

Often, it is difficult to identify the exact nature of a growth without a complete or partial biopsy of the enlargement. The biopsy will show any abnormal cells. However, a biopsy or surgery may stimulate an occult sarcoid to revert to the fibroblastic form, therefore occult sarcoids should be left alone.

Treating Sarcoids

Unless a sarcoid obstructs performance or tack, is an ugly and ulcerated mass, or its location causes a horse to become head-shy, it is best to leave it alone. Carefully monitor the sarcoid for any growth or change.

If treatment is necessary, various techniques are available for different types and locations of a sarcoid tumor. The most difficult sarcoids to remove are those on the limbs. If multiple sarcoids are present, a complete cure is less likely.

Along with a treatment, most of a growth must be surgically removed. With surgery alone, 50% recur within 3 years, often within 6 months. By combining surgery with another treatment, such as cryosurgery, immunotherapy, or hyperthermia, greater success may be achieved.

Cryosurgery

The most successful therapy to use along with surgical removal is *cryosurgery.* It is up to 80% effective if performed correctly. The lesion is frozen rapidly to -20° C and then allowed to thaw slowly to room temperature, whereupon it is refrozen, followed by a slow thaw. It may even be frozen a third time.

Before a cryosurgical site has healed, it normally develops a noticeable inflammatory reaction with swelling, edema, and discharge. This reaction may last for a week. Complete healing may take up to 2 months for the body to reject all the dead tumor tissue.

Drawbacks

Although cryosurgery is a preferred treatment, it does have some drawbacks. It is not useful in locations around the head and ears, the eyelids, thin-skinned areas directly over a protruberant bone such as the hip, or points on the lower limbs over joints. In these locations, there is risk of injuring tissue beneath the sarcoid with freezing.

Usually, scarring is minimal. The area loses hair color due to hair follicle and pigment-producing cell *(melanocytes)* destruction by freezing.

Immunotherapy

An alternative treatment is *immunotherapy.* The success of immunotherapy demonstrates that the health of the immune system plays a large role in the development and regression of the sarcoid tumor. Two different methods of immunotherapy have been used, BCG injection, and sarcoid tissue insertion.

BCG Injections

The first and most successful treatment involves a tuberculosis vaccine called Bacillus Calmette-Guerin, or BCG. BCG is made from the cell wall of the organism which causes tuberculosis, the *Mycobacterium.* Success depends on the horse's ability to develop a delayed hypersensitivity response to activate the cellular immune system.

Method of Action of BCG

BCG mobilizes specialized white blood cells that "reject" a sarcoid, much like bacteria and viruses are rejected from the body. BCG is injected directly into a tumor. The normal immune response removes this foreign protein while at the same time recognizing the tumor cells as foreign. Tumor cells are then destroyed.

Following injection of BCG, a local inflammatory reaction and swelling occur within the first 24 – 48 hours. Sites of BCG injection usually worsen before they improve. To achieve adequate regression of a tumor, 3 – 6 injections of BCG are required at 2 – 3 week intervals. BCG injection of a head or ear sarcoid may also stimulate regression of other sarcoids on the legs or flank.

BCG is best applied to tumors less than 2½ inches in diameter. With multiple or excessively large lesions, injecting excessive amounts of BCG vaccine may be necessary to achieve the desired results. These excessive amounts can cause adverse systemic reactions, such as hives or anaphylaxis. Current products of BCG on the market are highly purified protein derivatives of tuberculosis bacteria. Purification decreases the risk of adverse systemic reactions.

Success rates of 50% – 80% are achieved with BCG application combined with surgical removal. Over 90% of flat sarcoids on the head or neck regress with BCG therapy.

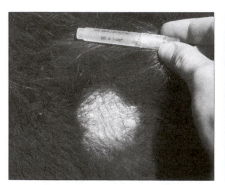 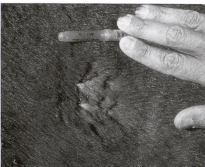

Fig. 15–27. On the left, an occult sarcoid before BCG immunotherapy. On the right, the same sarcoid after four BCG injections.

Sarcoid Tissue Insertion

Another way to stimulate an immunotherapeutic response is to implant match-size slivers of sarcoid tissue just under the skin of the neck. These slivers should be frozen before implantation to prevent new sarcoid formation at an implant site. This method typically takes 6 months to achieve sarcoid regression.

Hyperthermia

A less common therapy for sarcoids is *hyperthermia*, which uses a radio-frequency current to heat the tissue to 50° C for about 30 seconds. This technique may be repeated up to 4 times at 1 – 2 week intervals, depending on the size of the tumor. A cosmetic advantage of hyperthermia is that the hair follicles remain functional after treatment, and a natural hair color grows back.

In general, sarcoids do not pose a major health hazard to a horse. Because it is a common ailment of the equine skin, monitor any skin growths so benign tumors can be differentiated from dangerous ones.

Melanomas

As horses tend to live outside under all sorts of conditions, skin pigmentation is advantageous to their survival. Melanin is a substance produced by pigment-secreting skin glands; it protects against "sunburn" of the skin from ultraviolet radiation. Horses with black hides are rarely bothered by the sunlight. However, black skin can harbor a tumor of abnormal pigment-producing cells *(melanoblasts)*. The tumor, called a *melanoma*, forms when melanoblasts increase their metabolism and reproduce in localized areas of the skin. The black skin of a gray horse with excessive skin pigment can develop melanomas.

Of gray horses over 15 years old, 80% ultimately develop some form of melanoma. Most melanomas begin as slow-growing, encapsulated, and relatively benign growths. The tumors develop just under or above the skin with hair at first obscuring them until they become large enough to be visible. It can take years (as long as 10 – 20) for a melanoma to become hyperactive to the point of concern. Once a melanoma displays an accelerated growth rate, the malignant cells rapidly invade surrounding tissue.

Tissue around the tumor cannot keep pace with the consumptive tumor cells so tissue dies and ulcerates. Then the horse has bleeding or infected skin sores that fail to heal. Surrounding normal tissue may be displaced or replaced with the invasive melanoma.

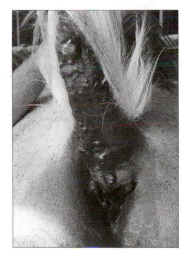

Location of Growth

Melanomas develop around the anus, tailhead, vulva or prepuce, and occasionally are found around the parotid salivary gland, head, and neck. However, they can be found anywhere on the body, with a rare report of location within a hoof.

Fig. 15–28. These melanomas may or may not be malignant.

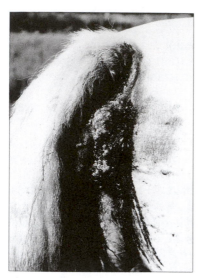

Fig. 15–29. A melanoma can grow to severe proportions.

Normally, melanomas take a long time to spread to internal body organs, such as the spleen and lungs. It usually takes years to wreak detrimental changes on the body and metabolism. It is not usually life-threatening, but when a tumor rapidly invades tissue around the anus or urinary tract, it may interfere with a horse's quality of life. In these cases, the humane option is to euthanize the horse to end pain and discomfort caused by ulcerated skin masses or obstructed bowels.

Treating Melanoma

If the tumors are isolated and single, it is advisable to leave them alone. Treatment by surgical removal tends to "anger" the skin. Not only do many of the tumors regrow, but they become more aggressive than before. Multiple melanomas spread over much of the body are not only a cosmetic problem. These melanomas are difficult to manage if they interfere with saddling, or the ability of a mare to breed or foal without discomfort.

Cimetidine

A new form of chemotherapy offers an exciting possibility for treatment of melanomas. The oral drug cimetidine (Tagamet®), commonly used for treating stomach ulcers, has successfully stimulated remission of melanomas in horses. The medication can be used by itself or along with surgical removal to halt progression or recurrence of melanomas.

Method of Action

It is thought that cimetidine modifies the immune system to control the cancer. Under normal circumstances, white blood cells called *suppressor T-cells* stop the attack of other white blood cells once an infection or "foreign" protein is defeated. This cellular check-and-balance system prevents an immune response from raging out of control. Cancer patients have an excessive number of suppressor T-cells that suppress the anti-tumor defense mechanism.

Role of Histamine

Histamine is a chemical that activates the suppressor T-cells. Therefore, histamine reduces the host's defenses against cancer. In an anti-stomach ulcer medication, cimetidine blocks histamine pathways responsible for excessive secretion of gastric acid. By blocking histamine pathways, cimetidine may also indirectly block activation of the suppressor T-cells. Then normal anti-tumor defense mechanisms can function. *Macrophages* (specific white blood cells) battle against "foreign" cancer cells to eradicate them from the body without being suppressed by the suppressor T-cells.

Squamous Cell Carcinomas

Horses with too little pigment in their skin can also develop skin cancer. *Squamous cell carcinomas* are cauliflower-like growths that tend to be ulcerated and bleed easily. They occasionally spread to other organs, like the lymph nodes. Pink-skinned horses, like Appaloosas and Paints, are predisposed to squamous cell carcinoma around mucous membranes where there is no hair, and no melanocytes to protect the skin from ultraviolet rays.

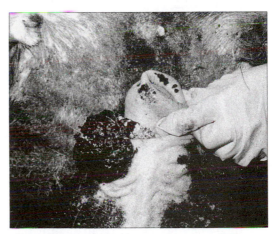

Fig. 15–30. Squames commonly occur on the prepuce.

"Squames" mostly occur around the anus, vulva, prepuce, or eyes of pink-skinned horses. Ultraviolet radiation may cause normal cells to change into tumorous cells, but squamous cell carcinoma also develops in areas never exposed to the sun.

The only cure is surgical removal, or cryotherapy (freezing the tissue). Horses with pink skin around the eyes may benefit from fly face masks to reduce the penetration of ultraviolet radiation. These mosquito-netted masks can reduce ultraviolet rays by 70%. Zinc oxide or sun-blocking agents can be applied to the face, reducing sunburn that may ultimately create tumors on the lips or muzzle.

Skin Growths and Their Symptoms	
SARCOIDS	Non-malignant. Appear on the limbs, head, ears, eyelids, mouth, neck, chest, trunk, abdomen, flank, and prepuce.
Verrucous	Dry, horny, wart-like, hairless, cauliflower growths.
Fibroblastic	Lesions resembling proud flesh, growing to greater than 10 inches in diameter.
Mixed	Mixture of verrucous and fibroblastic sarcoids.
Occult	Flat or slightly raised, thick, rough lesions.
MELANOMAS	Benign or malignant, slow-growing, encapsulated just under or above the skin surface. Appear around the anus, vulva or prepuce, parotid salivary gland, head, and neck.
SQUAMOUS CELL CARCINOMAS	Cauliflower-like growth on pink skin, appearing around the anus, vulva or prepuce, and eyes.

Fig. 15–31.

DIAGNOSING SKIN DISEASES

In the field of veterinary dermatology sometimes the disease cannot be positively identified, but rarely are skin diseases life-threatening. When a blemish is discovered, it is best to get veterinary advice for rapid treatment. Diagnosis of any skin disease requires more investigation than a simple glance. Try to identify the type of lesion found.

- How many are there, and how big are they?
- On which parts of the body are they found?
- Is the skin scaly or scabby or crusty?
- Are the hairs broken, or do they pull out readily?
- Do the hairs mat together?
- Is there hair at all?
- Is there a firm nodule, or a soft swelling?
- Is there any redness?
- Is there a lack of color?
- Is the affected area moist or dry?
- Is the skin of normal texture, or thickness?
- Is there granular material? What color is it?
- Does the horse itch and scratch?
- Are the areas sensitive when touched or pressed?

Consider also whether the horse is pastured or stalled, what sort of diet or medication it may have received, and its age and breed. By examining the horse carefully, and noting these particulars on the checklist, an owner or trainer can help portray a clinical picture to a veterinarian about the progression of a skin problem.

A careful veterinary examination combined with further diagnostic aids facilitates a rapid diagnosis of the skin problem. To track down the source of a skin malady the veterinarian may take skin scrapings for microscopic examination to identify mites and ticks, cultures and antibiotic sensitivities to define bacterial infections and specific treatment, fungal cultures to identify ringworm, and skin biopsies to identify Onchocerca, summer sores, or allergic reactions.

See that manure and soiled bedding are removed to reduce breeding grounds for flies. Deworm regularly to reduce internal parasites, such as pinworms, bots, and stomach worms that could infect a horse's skin.

Keep brushes and tack separate for each horse so a communicable disease will not reach epidemic proportions if transferred from horse to horse. In summer, bathing with insecticide shampoos not only deters bites and skin irritation, but removes dirt and sweat from the skin, allowing the coat to bloom and shine. Massage from currying, brushing, and shampoos enhances the luster of the fur.

SADDLE SORES

Sometimes it is hard to detect problems that occur with saddle fit until an obvious soreness or wound develops. Not all horses provide clues that tack is ill-fitting. If a horse shows progressively poor behavior such as tail wringing, back humping, crankiness, or sluggishness when asked to move forward, look for saddle sores. Some self-preserving individuals have less subtle behavior changes. They stop in their tracks, refusing to move until an offending article is removed.

Even with a custom-fit saddle, problems can arise. Uphills and downhills in steep terrain cause a saddle or girth to shift, creating

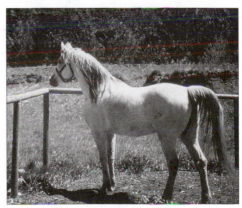

Fig. 15–32. Thin-skinned Arabians are prone to saddle sores.

friction points. Changes in physique accompany changing seasons. A summer fat or winter lean frame changes saddle fit.

A tired horse may subtly alter its gait. Then, imperfectly fitting tack chafes in unlikely places.

Different breeds of horses are prone to saddle sores. Thoroughbreds are known for their thin, tender skin. Thin-skinned Arabians are also at risk of saddle sores.

Signs of Saddle Sores

There is no substitute for well-fitted equipment and diligent monitoring for problem spots. Signs of impending saddle sores include subtle behavioral changes, and raised swollen areas of the skin. Swelling is caused by a serum leak beneath the skin, along with edema due to poor circulation beneath a pressure or friction point. These spots often are tender to finger pressure, and are red, inflamed, or ulcerated.

Other warning signs are isolated spots of missing hair with a pinkish tinge to the skin, indicating mild abrasion at a friction point. Note isolated dry areas under the saddle after a workout. Dry heat builds under pressure points where the skin cannot sweat and breathe.

Hair follicles and pigment-producing cells (melanocytes) may succumb to localized heat production, resulting in growth of black hairs on a gray horse, or white hairs on any other colored horse. This destruction of melanocytes results not only from heat injury to the skin, but from any form of physical trauma.

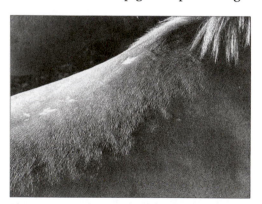

Fig. 15–33. Hair may grow back white on a colored horse and black on a grey horse.

If sweat and caked-on mud remain on a horse after a workout, it irritates the skin, creating conditions that favor bacteria. Commonly, Staphylococcal organisms that normally live on the skin invade irritated tissues. Initially, a small nodule is felt. The nodule develops into a painful pustule that ruptures.

Leaking pus and serous material forms small crusts and scabs, further matting down the hair. Low grade bacterial infections are easily avoided by rinsing hair and skin after a workout to remove accumulated sweat and debris.

Preventing Saddle Sores

To prevent saddle sores, many factors should be considered, including selecting the right saddle and accessories, and grooming and stretching the horse. Also, rider expertise is important. When a horse carries an unbalanced rider, the tack should be checked frequently. A rider sitting off center may grip more with one side of the body than another, or may dig in with calves or heels. Sores may be found under the leg skirts or stirrup leathers.

Selecting the Proper Saddle

The type of athletics pursued is critical when selecting a saddle. Using a dressage saddle on a long distance horse invites problems with sore backs, for both horse and rider. Although a heavy duty roping saddle may fit a horse's back well, its added weight can hasten fatigue in a long distance athlete. When a horse is putting out a great work effort for many hours, a heavy saddle also contributes to heat build-up.

Grooming

Before saddling, carefully curry and brush the horse so grit does not embed in the skin. Dirt particles abrade protective hair from the skin, contributing to skin chafe. Saddle blankets should be cleaned of matted hair and sweat-caked dirt before the next use, so no friction points develop under the saddle.

Saddle Pads

Moisture and salts from sweat need to be removed from the skin by an absorbent saddle pad that can breathe and release accumulated moisture. Wool has always been a favored material for this purpose.

Saddle pads should be uniformly thick and smoothed out so there is no material bunching up. When saddling, put the saddle blanket on the horse's neck, and slide it backwards into position in the same direction that the hairs lay. This method flattens the hairs beneath the pad.

Gunny Sacks

A simple trick prevents saddle sores from developing. Burlap gunny sacks (that peanuts used to come in and bran still does come in) serve as girth sleeves, saddle pads, or as padding over hobbles. Gunny sack material is absorbent, soft, and breathes, making it an excellent way to prevent a mild chafe from worsening. This trick is particularly helpful for long camping trips or for ranch work where the horse remains saddled for up to 12 hours a day.

Stretching the Legs

Some horses develop fat rolls or loose skin around the girth area. Once the saddle is on and the girth or cinch tightened, pick up each forelimb, and stretch it forward to relieve pinching of loose skin rolls.

Girth Sleeves

Fleece-like girth sleeves can be fitted over an English or Western girth to absorb moisture, and prevent pinching of the skin between the elbows and the girth. Cord girths configure more exactly to skin contours as a horse moves, and an English figure eight girth also conforms better than a straight piece of leather.

Rubberized, elastic pieces at the top of an English girth connect to the billets to allow greater flexibility in the girth. Flexibility is helpful for a horse that negotiates trails and hilly terrain. Elasticized rubber gives as the abdomen and thorax expand when a horse travels uphill. The horse breathes better, and saddle sores are avoided.

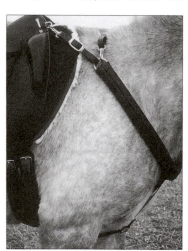

Fig. 15–34. Neoprene breast plate and girth.

Neoprene Equipment

Recently, tack has been made of rubber neoprene to prevent chafing in areas commonly rubbed by conventional equipment. Neoprene breastplates and girth covers are used for horses worked under saddle for many hours. The skin beneath the neoprene does not overheat from contact with the equipment. Neoprene tack slides over sweaty skin and fur with ease. Cleaning neoprene tack is a horse owner's dream — it is hosed off after each use to remove sweat and mud, and hung up to dry.

Healing Saddle Sores

Most superficial skin abrasions heal rapidly within 10 – 21 days provided reinjury does not occur. If a girth or saddle sore is discovered and treated immediately, it remains only in the outermost tissue layers, capable of healing in 1 – 2 weeks. If deeper tissues are injured, the wound may not fully heal for up to 3 – 6 weeks.

Cleansing the wound with a dilute tamed iodine/salt water solution removes superficial bacteria. The wound should be softened with an antiseptic ointment, and the scab removed daily, or bacteria trapped beneath the scab will reproduce in a moist, warm environment.

The main objective in encouraging healing is to prevent further trauma to the area. The saddle should be locked in the tack shed, and not brought out again until the wound is healed. In a mild case, a doughnut shape can be cut out of a thick Cool-Bak® or felt pad to prevent saddle contact. Any pressure around a sore limits circulation necessary for wound healing.

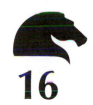

16

WOUND MANAGEMENT

Of all the medical incidents with which a horse owner or trainer is confronted, the most common are skin wounds. In most instances, a veterinarian is not present at the time of injury, and hours may pass before a veterinarian is summoned and can arrive.

INITIAL TREATMENT

Initial treatment greatly influences the outcome and duration of wound healing. Many people assume that applying a topical salve is sufficient while waiting for the veterinarian, but this erroneous notion can do more harm than good.

When the protective skin layer is broken open, environmental and skin contaminants are introduced into the wound along with dirt, gravel, and foreign materials like wood, paint, or hay. Certain soils, clay, and organic matter inhibit the immune action of white blood cells, antibodies, and antibiotics, and also interfere with the normal antibacterial activity of serum. A wound should be cleansed of all foreign material as rapidly as possible to prevent bacteria from gaining a foothold and deeply invading the tissue. Normal immune mechanisms at a local tissue level effectively deal with up to 1 million bacteria per gram of tissue. More than 1 million per gram will overwhelm the immune system, creating infection. Antiseptic ointments, creams, or sprays cannot reach deep into a wound if devitalized tissue and foreign debris obscure it.

Debridement

Once the skin surface is broken, underlying tissues lose their protective barrier to bacterial invasion. Without the skin as a protective barrier, airborne, environmental, and skin bacteria contaminate the wound. Wound margins are colonized with bacteria within 2 – 4 hours after injury. If the immune system at the wound site is overwhelmed by high bacterial numbers, they proliferate and flourish, resulting in tissue invasion and infection.

A wound that has been present for more than 1 – 3 hours is probably already so contaminated that a topical antibiotic does little to fend off infection. Extensive cleansing and *debridement* (cutting away devitalized tissue with a scissor or scalpel) of the wound is necessary for successful treatment.

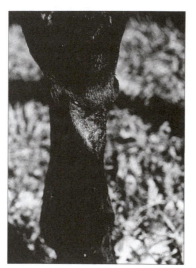 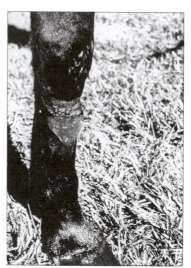

Fig. 16–1. On the left, a non-healing wound. On the right, the same wound after debridement, which will allow the wound to heal.

Shaving

If possible, hair should be removed from the edges of a wound to prevent it from acting like a foreign body or harboring bacteria or dirt. Hair obscures drainage, and prevents thorough examination of the extent of the wound. Before shaving, cover the wound with a water-soluble, sterile K-Y® lubricating jelly or moist gauze sponges to prevent shaved hairs from falling into the wound.

Scrubbing

Vigorous scrubbing with an appropriate cleaning compound is essential to prevent infection. Scrubbing a wound accomplishes several things. The mechanical action loosens and removes dirt, debris, large particles, and dead tissue. Use of appropriate scrub solutions delivers an antiseptic layer to live tissue. To kill bacteria, a wound should be vigorously scrubbed for a minimum of *10 minutes*, alternately scrubbing and rinsing until it glistens and bleeds with healthy pink tissue.

If a horse does not permit vigorous scrubbing of the wound, hose the wound for 5 or 10 minutes while waiting for the veterinarian to arrive. Gentle water pressure mechanically loosens debris and grit that has adhered to the area. This action substantially reduces the numbers of contaminating bacteria at the wound site.

Cleaning Compounds

While certain compounds are beneficial to healing, others are useless as antiseptics. Some may even slow healing by irritating the wound or causing cell death.

It is best to use a mild salt solution when scrubbing equine tissue. Plain tap water is better than distilled water, but both of these salt-free solutions have a lower electrolyte content than the wound tissues. Consequently, the tissue will "drink up" the salt-free water. The cells swell, contributing to localized edema and cell death.

If physiologic sterile saline or Lactated Ringer's solution is unavailable, a home-made salt solution can be made to wash the wound. To approximate the physiologic salt content of a horse's tissues, dissolve ½ tablespoon of table salt into 1 liter of water. Add an antiseptic to the solution, such as povidone-iodine (Betadine®) or chlorhexidine (Nolvasan®).

Povidone-Iodine

To commercially make povidone-iodine of a 0.5% preparation, tincture of iodine (7%) is combined with a polyvinyl substance to decrease staining, stabilize the iodine, and reduce its irritability to tissues. Tincture of iodine is an excellent antibacterial agent, but it is **too strong** for wound cleansing.

To make a scrub for wound cleansing, povidone-iodine (PI) solution is added to the salt water to a concentration that visually approximates weak tea. To achieve this concentration, add 10 milliliters (ml) or less of the PI solution to 1 liter of salt solution. For the horse, the best antibacterial and least tissue-toxic effect of PI occurs at concentrations of less than 1%. At a low concentration of less than 0.03%, white blood cells of

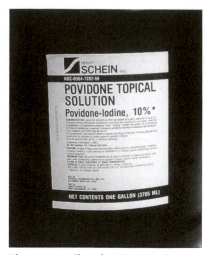

Fig. 16–2. Diluted PI is a good cleaning compound.

the immune response are stimulated to migrate to the wound to perform their clean-up function. Conversely, at concentrations of 5% – 10%, iodine dramatically hinders the immune function of white blood cells, increasing a wound's susceptibility to infection.

The antibacterial activity of PI lasts for only 4 – 6 hours in the wound without any residual effect. Because a horse is so large, absorption of iodine into the body is insignificant. Humans, however, who must frequently apply this solution should wear rubber gloves to avoid absorbing iodine in toxic amounts.

Chlorhexidine

Chlorhexidine (Nolvasan®) is an excellent cleaning solution, effective against bacteria, viruses, and fungus. An ideal concentration of 0.05% for wound cleansing is prepared by mixing 25 ml with 1 liter of salt water, or 1:40 dilution. Not only does chlorhexidine work against a broad spectrum (many kinds) of bacteria, but its effects persist in the tissues because it binds to skin proteins. Therefore, its antibacterial effects outlast those of PI.

Both PI and chlorhexidine are available as antiseptic scrubs, and should be diluted with a salt water mixture when scrubbing the wound. Adequate rinsing removes sudsy cleanser from the wound once it has been thoroughly cleaned and investigated.

Ideally, anything that is put into a wound should be so mild that if it were instilled into the eye it would not irritate mucous membranes or the eye itself. Following this principle avoids trouble.

Compounds That Slow Healing

Using other types of soaps in a wound slows healing, and increases the susceptibility of a wound to infection. Detergents and soaps are toxic to the cells, causing them to swell and break which adds to devitalized tissue. Only wound-specific, soapy antiseptics should be applied to equine tissue, such as chlorhexidine scrub, or PI scrub. If these are unavailable, Phisohex® soap (containing chlorhexidine) can be used with ample rinsing.

Tincture of Iodine

Tincture of iodine (7%) is a strong antibacterial agent, however, it is so destructive to tissue that the only safe application is to the soles and frogs, to control thrush or toughen the feet. It should not be applied to intact skin because it will irritate, causing a rash or skin inflammation. Healing tissues are also negatively affected by tincture of iodine.

Hydrogen Peroxide

People commonly pour 3% hydrogen peroxide into a wound. Peroxide is useful on human skin for wounds with *anaerobic* (oxygen-free) bacterial growth, because the foaming action increases the oxygen tension in a wound, which destroys anaerobic bacteria. Yet, hydrogen peroxide is toxic to equine cells, especially to migrating fibroblasts that produce collagen to repair a wound. Peroxide also causes blood clots in microvessels, interfering with oxygen supply to the tissues. Reduced oxygen results in more devitalized tissue, and delayed healing. Hydrogen peroxide should be reserved only for cleaning off blood that has splattered the hair *below* a wound.

Alcohol

Alcohol (isopropyl or rubbing) should never be applied to open wounds because it destroys protein in the open tissues. It can be used to wipe *around* a wound perimeter to loosen debris, but should not contact open skin.

Evaluation

While scrubbing, evaluate the wound and determine its depth and seriousness. It is possible for soft tissue planes to separate, leading into a tunnel much like a puncture wound. Sometimes these "punctures" pass unnoticed at the time of the injury unless veterinary care is obtained.

Exudate

Initial examination of a wound identifies its smell, if any, and the amount and character of the discharge *(exudate)*. The exudate may be nothing more than shedding dead and dying tissue, and white blood cells. It does not necessarily include bacteria. However, an odd or foul odor, or a large amount of exudate is highly suspect of infection, requiring immediate veterinary care.

A veterinarian should be summoned for such wounds, or if a wound is deeper than a superficial laceration. Foreign bodies in the wound need to be extracted, and skin flaps removed or sutured by the veterinarian to maintain adequate blood supply.

Once a wound has been scrubbed and debrided to healthy-looking tissue, the next step is to maintain it in a moist and clean environment. Appropriate antiseptic ointments and bandages promote tissue healing.

PROMOTING WOUND HEALING

Healing begins with fibrous connective tissue collagen, or fibrin strands, which are made of proteins. *Fibroblasts*, which manufacture the fibrin, migrate into the wound by the third day. Budding blood vessels appear after the fibroblasts.

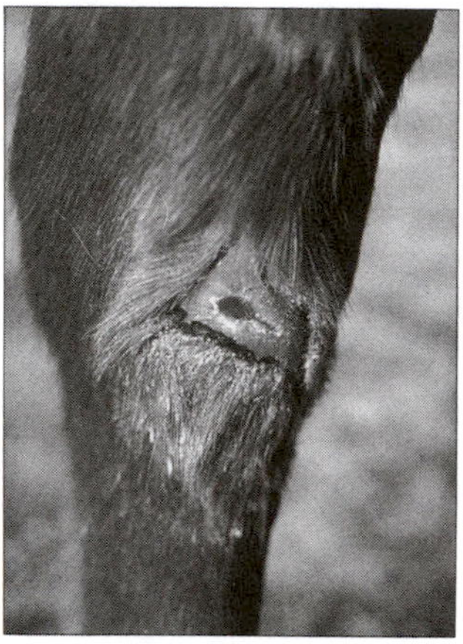

As *granulation tissue* (made of capillaries and fibroblasts) fills in the wound, it provides a surface along which *epithelial cells* (new skin cells) will migrate. Regrowth of skin between the wound margins is called *epithelialization*. Not only does bacteria slow healing, but it produces potent enzymes that destroy fragile and newly formed skin cells.

Fig. 16–3. Epithelial tissue surrounds the granulation tissue in the middle.

Contraction

Wound size reduces through a process known as *contraction*. Adjacent, full-thickness skin at the wound margins is pulled in towards the center of a wound by the action of *myofibroblast cells* (specialized cells that convert from fibroblasts to act like muscle cells).

In a chronic wound, granulation tissue consists more of fibrous connective tissue, and is relatively sparse in myofibroblasts. Debulking with a scalpel removes a stagnant granulation bed, or proud flesh. Fresh tissue replaces it, including myofibroblasts capable of reducing wound size over time.

Factors Affecting Contraction Rate

Contraction rates of 0.2 millimeters per day during the first few months can only reduce a scar to half the original size. Continued remodeling of a scar over the next 6 – 12 months further reduces its size.

Skin Tension

The size of a wound does not affect contraction rate, but skin tension does. Lower leg wounds tend to have taut skin edges and contract slowly. Also, dry wounds are tighter and therefore contract slower than moist wounds.

Any excess tension, edema, or movement of a wound interferes with function of the myofibroblasts. Then, contraction is limited, and may cease prematurely before the wound edges meet.

Hydration and Warmth

Because the mammalian body is made of almost 70% water, skin dehydrates if a wound is left open to the air. Dehydrated tissue eventually becomes devitalized tissue and compromises healing.

The skin on the lower limbs of a horse inherently lacks blood supply and warmth as compared to the skin of humans or many other animal species. For the processes of skin repair and wound closure to advance, a wound needs to be maintained in a warm, moist environment, especially during the early stages of tissue repair.

The length of time from when the injury occurred to when it receives professional attention affects the extent of tissue dehydration and onset of infection. While awaiting professional medical evaluation, apply a water-soluble dressing and a light bandage to the cleaned wound to limit tissue dehydration. A bandage maintains a moist environment, and retains a moderate amount of body heat at the wound site; both features enhance the early stages of healing.

Sutures

Since initial evaluation of a wound does not always determine if a wound can be surgically repaired and sutured, assume that a wound will be sutured, and proceed accordingly. If a wound is to be sutured, no ointments, sprays, or creams should be applied. Medications that are not water-soluble stick to the tissue, preventing the edges from touching when they are stitched together. Insoluble substances are also difficult to remove from the deeper tissues of a wound, which interferes with how well a suture will hold. The decision to stitch a wound depends on:

- location of the wound
- skin tension at that site
- configuration of the wound
- degree of tissue damage
- tissue contamination

Facial wounds or wounds on the torso respond well to suturing efforts even if discovered days after an injury. However, a limb wound may not be amenable to sutures even if evaluated within a few hours of injury.

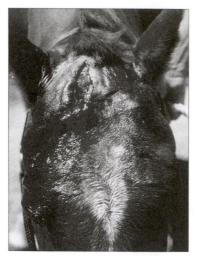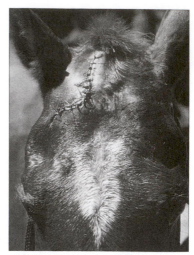

Fig. 16–4. On the left, a clean, shaven head wound before suturing. On the right, the wound after suturing.

Topical Ointments

No matter what is applied to an equine skin wound, little can be done to accelerate healing. However, the natural healing process can be delayed by infection or tissue dehydration.

Blunt trauma, such as a blow from a kick, fall, or collision with a solid object damages the surrounding tissues considerably, making the wound edges jagged. Such wounds are at significantly greater risk of infection due to compression of blood vessels, an increased area of devitalized tissue, swelling, and edema. They also do not suture well. All these factors contribute to an environment right for bacteria.

If a wound is so traumatic that suturing will not work, or so mild that veterinary care is not needed, topical ointments prevent a wound from drying out. Each veterinarian has his or her special recipe or topical medication for treating wounds.

Water-Soluble Ointments

Only water-soluble ointments should be applied to a wound that is to be sutured, or on open, contaminated wounds until the wound has filled completely in with granulation tissue.

The list of commercially available wound preparations is exhaustive. A short list of some examples of the antiseptic products proven to be safe and effective includes these medications:

- Silvadene® Cream is a broad spectrum, topical antibiotic that is water and tissue-soluble. It increases the rate of new skin growth (scientifically tested on pigs) by 28%, and has proven to be reliable on horses.
- Nolvasan® ointment is another water-soluble, broad spectrum, topical cream that thwarts infection in deep wounds.
- Any triple antibiotic ointment that contains polymixcin-B sulfate, neomycin sulfate, and bacitracin provides broad spectrum antibacterial activity. They are non-toxic to fibroblasts, and increase new skin growth (in pigs) by 25%.
- Povidone-iodine ointments are broad spectrum and tissue-soluble, and enhance rapid formation of granulation tissue to hasten repair of a deep wound.
- Morumide® is a non-irritating wound salve, which is a mixture of a sulfa drug with a vitamin A and D ointment. Vitamin A supports skin cell health, and it counteracts the delaying effects of steroids on wound healing, making it a useful addition to topical corticosteroid application.

Many other wound preparations are available with beneficial effects and it is best to consult a veterinarian before applying them to a wound.

If a wound has been present for more than 1 – 3 hours, antiseptic ointments are unlikely to prevent infection. Oral antibiotics or antibiotic injections, along with vigorous wound cleansing and debridement, are imperative for managing these wounds.

USP-Petrolatum-Based Ointments

Petrolatum-based ointments are used on the normal skin around a weeping wound. They protect the skin from skin scald, caused by the protein-rich serum that drains from a productive injury.

A variety of these products are available, yet when applied directly to a wound, certain topical ointments interfere with healing if their pH or ingredients are inappropriate. Their *antimicrobial* agent has little actual effect on wound healing, and the carrier base compound dramatically **slows** healing. Any product that contains a USP-petrolatum ingredient slows skin growth, and delays wound healing. It is best to use tissue-soluble compounds that are not lethal to the cells. Consider the chemical compositions of antibacterial ointments that are purchased at feed and tack stores. Those products with a USP-petrolatum ingredient irritate the tissue and slow healing.

Amount of Ointment

Only a very thin layer of antiseptic ointment is necessary to achieve the desired effect. Too much ointment has adverse effects, including:

- encouraging excessive exudate and wound debris by impairing normal drainage
- reducing air circulation to the tissues
- attracting dirt and soil to a wound, which negates all positive effects achieved by a previous scrubbing

Antiseptic powders or sprays also obstruct natural drainage, leading to accumulation of exudate. These substances dry out the skin margins, inhibiting normal skin cell growth.

Antibiotic Absorption

The penetration of antibiotics in a wound is influenced by different factors. Inflammation causes an increased blood supply. Increased circulation enhances antibiotic (both injected and topical) penetration to a wound site.

Dead and dying tissue and white blood cells cause an acidic pH in the wound site. The presence of pus and serum, along with an acidic pH inhibits the antimicrobial action of many antibiotics, such as the sulfa drugs. After healing begins, fibrin or blood clots in the wound further block antibiotic penetration.

Ointment Contamination

When using large jars of ointments, be careful not to contaminate them with dirt, hair, and debris so bacteria are not placed into a wound. Use tongue depressors, clean rubber gloves, or gauze to remove medication from a jar, keeping the ointment clean for future use. Pay attention to the expiration dates on products containing antibiotics, and discard outdated ointments, because time renders them ineffective.

Bandaging

A study done at the Kansas State College of Veterinary Medicine compared 4 types of treatment regimens on equine skin wounds.

- Group 1 received daily irrigation with physiologic saline for the first 11 days, and then a 5-minute tap water lavage from day 12 on. No medication or bandage was applied to these horses.
- Group 2 received daily application of a nitrofurazone ointment only.

- Group 3 received nitrofurazone ointment plus a bandage.
- Group 4 received a bandage and the wound was lavaged with tap water every third day.

The results showed marked differences between treatment regimens. Wounds from Groups 1 and 2 formed hard, thick scabs that were persistently contaminated with dirt and bedding, resulting in increased inflammation of the wounds. In contrast, the bandaged wounds had less inflammation, less dehydration, and less contamination than the unbandaged wounds.

Healthy granulation tissue formed faster under a bandage, with those wounds healing faster (63 days) than the wounds left open to the air (96 days). Faster healing may have been caused by reduced contamination or inflammation in the earlier healing phases.

Yet, once the bandage was removed, the wounds from Groups 3 and 4 seemed prone to trauma and loosening of the fragile new skin. In the unbandaged wounds, the collagen organized faster than under a bandage, possibly due to tension forces in surrounding skin that resulted from mild dehydration by air exposure. Though the unbandaged wounds healed slower, they were not as prone to reinjury.

Despite these results, many bandaged wounds often progress faster and more successfully than wounds that are left open to the air. In many cases, healing progresses slowly without the protection and moisture-retention achieved from a bandage. Although more granulation tissue formed under bandages than on unbandaged legs, bandaged wounds had less scar tissue, and an improved scar contraction.

Bandaging Recommendation

These results indicate a wound should be kept bandaged until an intact, healthy granulation bed is present. Once a layer of granulation tissue has filled in a wound, a bandage may do more harm than good by reducing oxygen to the wound, and by trapping an accumulation of inflammatory cells (pus). A lack of oxygen causes tissue to die. The dead tissue and an accumulation of pus leads to an acidic pH.

To counteract these conditions, a wound produces more capillary buds to compensate for an oxygen deficit, while fibroblasts are stimulated by the acid environment to produce more collagen. The result is production of proud flesh.

Benefits of Bandaging

Retaining Moisture

Covering a wound with a bandage reduces evaporative fluid loss from

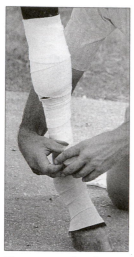

Fig. 16–5. A bandage keeps a wound warm and moist.

the surrounding and involved tissues. If a wound surface is moist and oxygen-rich, new skin growth proceeds at up to 0.2 mm per day on the lower limbs. On the torso, progress may be as rapid as 2 mm per day. If a wound dehydrates, the decreased circulation deprives the wound of the internal oxygen source. Then cellular migration proceeds at less than 0.1 mm per day in any area.

Bandaging does reduce the wound's uptake of atmospheric oxygen. But keeping the wound moist, and therefore allowing the circulation to flow freely, compensates for a relatively minor deprivation of atmospheric oxygen. Bandaging with cotton pads and Elastikon® bandages also helps a wound to absorb atmospheric oxygen.

Protection From Distortion

A bandage also provides a stable support for migration of new skin cells across a wound. Distortion of a wound surface due to excessive movement, edema, or trauma disrupts myofibroblasts and epithelial cells that are moving across to bridge the gap. Collagen fibers and capillary buds are also broken by such distortions. A bandage protects a wound from further trauma and excessive movement and reduces edema swelling. The slight pressure exerted by a bandage reduces the development of proud flesh, provided the bandage is not wrapped so tightly as to interfere with limb circulation.

Retaining Body Temperature

Temperatures of approximately 86° F promote wound healing, while temperatures less than 68° F result in a 20% reduction in tensile strength. Possibly, cooler temperature at a wound site constricts superficial vessels to the skin, resulting in reduced blood and oxygen supply to the wound and its healing connective tissue components. Applying an insulating bandage over a wound retains body temperature to provide the healing benefits of warmth.

Removing a Bandage

The appropriate time to remove a bandage is determined by examining the color of the skin cells. While the newly-formed skin is still a thin layer, there is an apparent color difference between the thicker, outer margin and the thin skin layer covering the granulation bed. Once the skin has uniformly thickened, it is the same color, indicating that it may be appropriate to remove the bandage.

Slow Healing

If a horse persists in traumatizing a wound, or a wound remains subject to irritation from manure, mud, or flies, a protective wrap allows healing to continue to completion.

Wounds over movable surfaces, such as joints, heal slowly and produce greater amounts of proud flesh. Proud flesh slows wound healing because skin cells do not migrate up and over a mound of proud flesh. Instead, it layers itself at the base of the mound. Healing ceases at this point, and the layer of proud flesh grows without restraint. In such cases, a light pressure bandage may temporarily stop the build-up of proud flesh.

Controlling Proud Flesh
Steroids

Corticosteroid added to a salve aids healing by controlling proud flesh. Steroids stabilize the release of enzymes from local white blood cells that begin an inflammatory response, therefore granulation tissue formation is slower. Also, corticosteroids inhibit new capillary growth, so by decreasing surface blood vessels, granulation tissue production is reduced.

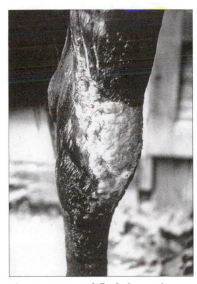

However, steroids inhibit skin cell growth and stop a healing process if applied for too long. Steroids should never be placed in a deep wound before the granulation bed has formed, because they depress normal function of the immune system and can promote infection.

Nitrofurazones

Certain compounds contribute to the formation of granulation tissue. Nitrofurazones, used on deep wounds, delay new skin growth by 30%. A thick scab forms over the wound surface, preventing healing

Fig. 16–6. Proud flesh formation.

from the "inside out." However, on superficial skin abrasions, nitrofurazones keep the skin moist and supple, so hair quickly grows back.

Damaging Chemicals

Other substances have been used to stop development of proud flesh, such as copper sulfate, bleach, lye, and similar caustic chemicals. By chemically cauterizing proud flesh, they also damage the migrating skin cells, and ultimately slow healing if used to excess.

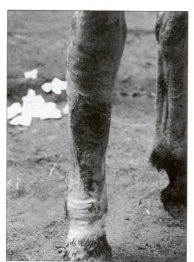

Fig. 16–7. Lye and bacon grease damage a wound.

An old timer, but destructive "remedy" applies a mixture of lye and bacon grease to wound surfaces. In principle, the salty bacon grease may "pull" swelling from a wound, as would a poultice. Lye is destructive to bacteria, and grease keeps a wound soft and pliable. However, lye is also toxic to fragile skin cells and deeper tissues. Too much salt dehydrates the tissues. Grease attracts dirt and grit to the wound surface. The result is a non-healing, open wound which develops profuse amounts of proud flesh.

Surgical Removal

It is better to surgically remove proud flesh than to resort to chemical irritants. Caustic substances cause tissue death, with redevelopment of proud flesh that persists as a non-healing, grotesque wound.

For a non-complicated wound that is clean and uninfected, healing proceeds in spite of our ministrations. In many cases, time and cleanliness are the best remedies.

Remodeling of the Tissue

The ultimate tensile strength of a wound allows tissue to sustain normal mechanical stress so it does not tear or break open. Complete remodeling and contraction of a scar from a skin injury occurs rapidly for 3 – 6 months, reaching maximum tensile strength up to 1 year after injury. Collagen, rapidly manufactured by fibroblasts during the first 2 – 4 weeks, is responsible for tensile strength of a wound as it organizes. By

40 – 120 days, skin regains 50% – 70% of its original strength. Collagen continues to remodel for 1 – 2 years. Epithelial cells and fibroblasts produce enzymes to break down existing collagen. Newly deposited collagen fibrils more tightly interweave, with a corresponding increase in tensile strength and flattening of the scar.

Despite a horse's apparent tendency to self-destruct, regeneration and repair of skin wounds can return an injury to not quite, but almost, as good as new. Usually, wounds that do not penetrate all the way through the skin form tissue identical to the original skin, without scar formation. In actuality, however, large connective tissue and collagen components may not regrow to their original pattern. Although "healed" epithelial tissue appears identical to original skin, the new connective tissue is functionally less efficient. Even under ideal conditions, the scar tissue ultimately remains 20% weaker than the original tissue.

Managing a skin wound with rapid and aggressive veterinary treatment significantly reduces the time required for healing. Risk of infection is diminished, and a wounded area heals with an acceptable cosmetic appearance and return to function.

PUNCTURE WOUNDS

In the most carefully managed stabling operation, horses are often surrounded by man-made objects, such as fences that splinter or crack, nails, gates, latches, stable tools, and farm equipment. A horse can accidentally snag itself on any of these objects.

A superficial-appearing abrasion can disguise a deeper, penetrating hole through the skin. Long hairs, mud, and dirt mask the extent of an injury. Bacteria introduced into a wound can quickly grow to enormous numbers. Numbers of greater than 1 million organisms per gram of tissue overwhelms the local immune response, creating infection.

Anaerobic Bacteria

If left unattended, puncture wounds have serious consequences, despite a mild appearance. Of the many kinds of bacteria introduced into a wound, the potentially life-threatening organisms include those that live in an environment lacking oxygen (anaerobic).

When the skin is punctured, germs are introduced beneath the flesh. The small portal of entry through the skin often seals over, providing an oxygen-depleted environment ideal for growth of anaerobic spores. As a wound festers, devitalized and dead tissue in the wound encourages the anaerobic bacteria to prosper.

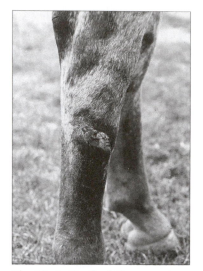 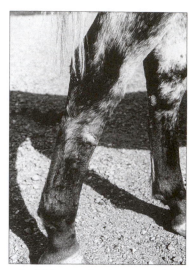

Fig. 16–8. On the left, a puncture wound which remained untreated for 10 days. On the right, the scar would be smaller if treatment had been sought immediately.

Clostridia is one family of anaerobic bacteria. With only 20 minutes exposure to oxygen, these bacteria can be inactivated. The *Clostridial* family are common inhabitants of the digestive tract. They are passed as spores into manure, soil, and decomposing organic matter. The spores can survive in the soil for years, so any wound is at risk of contamination.

Tetanus

One of the most common anaerobic bacteria associated with equine wounds is *Clostridium tetani*, the organism responsible for *tetanus*. In the decades before vaccines were available, tetanus infected an alarming number of horses, causing a prolonged and painful death.

As the tetanus bacterium dies, an *exotoxin* is released. The exotoxin reaches the brain through the bloodstream, or migrates up peripheral nerves to the central nervous system. It slows normal nerve transmission by preventing release of a chemical neuro-transmitter, *acetylcholine*, and by preventing release of an inhibitory transmitter, *glycine*, at the neuron. Rapid paralysis descends from head to toe.

Symptoms begin in the head and forequarters, as spastic contraction of skeletal muscle results in "lockjaw." Facial muscles become rigid. The horse cannot acquire, chew, or swallow food. Nostrils flare, the third eyelid descends over the eye, and the ears remain rigid and upright due to persistent spasms of the facial muscles.

As exotoxin progressively paralyzes the body, the horse assumes a stiff "saw-horse" stance with legs extended. If the horse goes down, it is unable to rise due to the rigidity of legs and neck.

Afflicted animals are hyper-responsive to external stimuli or noise, convulsing as muscles spasm and contract incessantly. Eventually, paralysis of the diaphragm or complications of aspiration pneumonia cause a horse to suffocate. Or, it may succumb to dehydration or malnutrition.

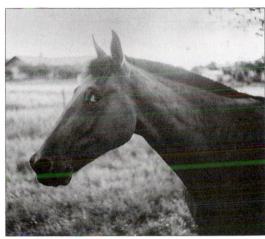

Fig. 16–9. A horse with tetanus.

Today, such an unfortunate demise from a wound is rare. If a horse is injured, and has not been on a regular immunization program that includes a yearly booster of tetanus toxoid, it should receive prophylactic, or preventative tetanus therapy. This tetanus antitoxin neutralizes exotoxin circulating outside the nervous system. If the horse has not received a tetanus toxoid booster in the past 8 – 12 months, boosting it stimulates sufficient immunity in the face of an increased risk.

Malignant Edema

Another life-threatening anaerobic bacteria is *Clostridium septicum,* which is responsible for a syndrome known as *malignant edema.* This organism produces a large amount of gas in muscles, creating a crackling feel *(crepitation)* beneath the skin over the wounded area. The wound site is hot and painful, and swollen with edema and gas. An accompanying fever may spike to 106° F. Toxins released from the bacteria rapidly spread through the body, capable of killing a horse in less than 2 days.

Although infection with tetanus or malignant edema is uncommon, such possibilities cannot be ignored. Penicillin injections kill anaerobic bacteria, and anti-tetanus prophylaxis protects the horse.

Treating Puncture Wounds

Initially, hair is clipped or shaved away from the wound edges so it will not interfere with healing. The puncture opening is then vigorously scrubbed with antiseptic to prepare for examination. Thorough wound cleansing prevents infection from contaminating organisms, removes devitalized tissue, and flushes away exudate that interferes with healing.

Puncture wounds are irrigated with antiseptic, electrolyte solutions under mild pressure to loosen hair and dead tissue. It is important to cleanse wounds of soil particles, because certain soil types inhibit the immune response. Immediate veterinary attention is also essential for any puncture wound.

Evaluating the Wound

If it is difficult to see if the skin has been punctured, prepare the wound for further evaluation by scrubbing thoroughly around the injury so no contaminants will be carried into a deep wound. Gently insert an antiseptic-soaked cotton swab into the wound to see if a hole or pocket is present. Do not attempt to completely probe the hole with the cotton swab; cotton fibers or broken swabs discourage healing.

This procedure evaluates if a wound is more than a superficial abrasion. A veterinarian should be summoned if any swelling, pain, or heat accompanies a wound. Because a hole is often too small to scrub deeper tissue, a small, seemingly superficial wound may require professional care.

A puncture into a joint, tendon sheath, or bone requires immediate professional expertise to prevent crippling consequences. The extent of tissue damage can be assessed by a veterinarian. The wound is probed for foreign bodies such as wood, plastic, glass, or metal fragments, and it is determined if tendon sheaths or joint capsules have been penetrated, or if a wound tract leads down to muscle or bone.

Drainage

If a pocket has formed below a puncture, it is often necessary to establish a drainage hole at the low point of the wound so serum does not accumulate. A serum pocket slows healing because it prevents tissue connection and harbors bacteria. Accumulated serum flows from the pocket once there is an opening at the lowest point of the wound.

The original puncture may also need to be enlarged so a wound can heal from the inside out, without obstruction to drainage. Similarly, any scab that forms over the top of the wound should be removed. If a wound seals too quickly, trapped bacteria rapidly infect it.

Local antibiotics are infused into a wound; these liquid antibiotics do not obstruct drainage from the puncture. Covering the hole with thick ointments or creams obstructs drainage and attracts dirt and manure to the wound.

If a wound is left unbandaged, a petrolatum-based ointment can be applied to normal skin *below* the wound to prevent scalding of skin and hair loss from irritating serum that drains from the opening.

Bandaging

A puncture wound on the lower limb is usually bandaged to protect it from contaminants and further trauma. The bandage should not be applied too tightly or it will impair drainage. Some puncture wounds develop localized or gravitational swelling that is relieved by a light pressure bandage. As edema decreases, drainage improves so healing can proceed faster.

Poultice

Application of a poultice or "sweat" to a puncture site draws away the swelling or pulls the infection out for further cleansing of the wound. Warm Epsom salt soaks, 2 – 3 times daily, serve a similar purpose.

Wound dressings should be absorbent and should not block drainage. Change bandages frequently to assess healing and to remove encrusted material. Initially, bandages are changed every 2 – 3 days, or more frequently, depending on the seriousness of an injury.

Identification of Bacteria

Most puncture wounds heal uneventfully within 1 – 2 weeks after treatment is begun. If a wound remains undiscovered for even a day or two, it may be valuable to obtain a bacterial culture and antibiotic sensitivity. Before cleaning a wound, a sterile swab placed into the wound soaks up secretions, and then it is replaced into its sterile sleeve. The swab is sent to the lab for cellular examination and bacterial growth.

Accurate identification of bacteria defines appropriate antibiotic treatment. For the next 2 – 3 days, while the lab is growing the culture, the horse receives broad spectrum antibiotic injections, which are selected by a veterinarian according to the greatest likelihood of success.

Kick Wounds

Kick wounds are similar to puncture wounds because blunt impact from a hoof causes a small break in the skin. Deeper connective tissue separates from the blow, leaving a tunnel along which bacteria can travel. If the blow is over a muscle, the wound heals with few complications when appropriately treated. If the kick is over ill-protected bone, a crack can form in the bone, a piece can be chipped off, or inflammation of the bone may interfere with its blood circulation.

If a kick wound is deep or traumatic enough to affect underlying bone, a *sequestrum* may develop. A sequestrum is a fragment of bone that has broken off with the initial impact of trauma, or has become devitalized due to reduced blood supply from infection. This dead bone fragment acts like a foreign body. The wound may initially heal, only to break open again. A chronic, draining tract persists until a sequestrum is surgically removed.

Tendon or Joint Punctures

If a puncture endangers a tendon sheath or joint space, special x-ray films can show the extent of injury. Injection of a sterile, radio-opaque dye into a wound is immediately followed with radiographs to outline the entire depth of the puncture tract with the dye. Such films are called *fistulograms.* Dye also passes around foreign bodies such as wood, plastic, or glass that do not show on regular survey films because of their similar density to soft tissue.

ROPE BURNS

A horse's hide is a tough but resilient structure, providing a thin, protective armor against perils in the environment. A common hazard to horses is a rope. As a rope entwines around a horse's leg, it often causes the horse to panic. The horse fights to get free of the entrapment, and as it kicks and struggles—without regard to any injury it inflicts upon itself—living hide disappears, revealing muscle and sinew beneath.

Characteristics of Rope Burns

Rope burns exhibit some unique characteristics. They are initially difficult wounds to manage, and require prolonged healing time. The friction can generate enough heat to burn, or thermally injure the tissues.

Although rope burns are similar to lacerations, they are considered burns due to the heat created by rope sliding across skin. If tissue is heated to more than 140° F, thermal injury results.

A large amount of heat is necessary to raise tissue temperature high enough to damage tissue proteins. However, considerable time is required for heat to dissipate from the burned tissue. Because of this time lag to restore an area to normal temperature, injury continues despite removal of the rope from the leg.

Classes of Burns

Instead of classifying rope burns as first, second, or third degree, it is more informative to assess thermal injury in terms of depth of skin and tissue damage. Rope burns are classified as:

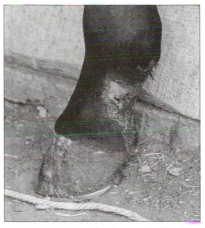

Fig. 16–10. Rope burns are difficult wounds to manage.

- superficial
- partial-thickness
- full-thickness

Superficial and Partial-Thickness Burns

A *superficial* (minor) burn reveals reddened, thickened skin only. A *partial-thickness* burn is accompanied by edema beneath the skin, intense inflammation, and pain. Damage to lymphatic vessels, along with increased leaking of capillaries, causes seepage of protein-rich fluids into the subcutaneous tissues. This material provides the structural basis for fibrin clots to stop bleeding, repair a wound, and provide a scaffold for healing. However, a high protein concentration in damaged tissue also serves as a nutrient medium for bacteria, with the potential for infection.

Full-Thickness Burn

A *full-thickness* (major) burn results in profound limb swelling, and tissue appears "tanned" and leathery. Because pain fibers are disrupted in a deep wound, the area is numb.

Although many rope burns are relatively minor and do not often progress beyond a partial thickness depth, any minor rope burn can become a full-thickness wound if inappropriate topi-

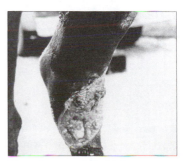

Fig. 16–11. A full-thickness rope burn.

cal medications are applied, or if a bacterial infection overwhelms the healing process.

Treating a Rope Burn

Wounds that appear minor may disguise extensive tissue damage caused by crushing and thermal injury when the horse struggled against the rope. The deeper the "burn," the longer the healing time, and the greater the likelihood of tendon or ligament involvement. From the onset, rope burns should receive aggressive medical treatment to aid healing and limit scarring.

Immediate application of ice (wrapped in a towel) to the injury arrests persistent heat damage. Even a seemingly mild rope burn should be treated in this manner. What appears as a relatively superficial friction burn early presents a serious appearance days later, accompanied by swelling and lameness.

Because most rope burns tend to worsen dramatically before they improve, it is impractical to suture them. Instead, they are allowed to heal by *second intention*, that is, as an open wound that will fill in with granulation tissue. The same principles applied to any open wound also apply to second intention healing of rope burns.

Cleaning the Wound

Soil, manure, and hair ground into the wound encourage rapid bacterial colonization of dead and dying tissue. To keep injured tissue as healthy as possible, immediate and thorough cleansing of a rope burn is important. Vigorous scrubbing with moist gauze sponges and an antiseptic electrolyte solution removes devitalized tissue, blood clots, large particles of debris, and skin contaminants.

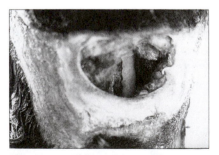 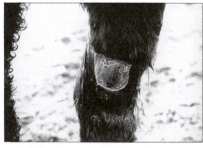

Fig. 16–12. This open wound was not sutured (left), but was bandaged. Bandaging allowed granulation tissue to form (right).

High pressure irrigation (flushing) with antiseptic solutions cleans the wound of deeper bacteria and debris. It may be necessary to debride discolored areas, because devitalized tissue contributes to the inflammatory response and provides nutrients for bacteria. A dark red or purple tissue color represents congestion and stagnant blood caused by bruising and crushing.

Heat damage interferes with a normal immune response within a wound, making it susceptible to infection. Use of Silvadene® Cream (a broad spectrum, over-the-

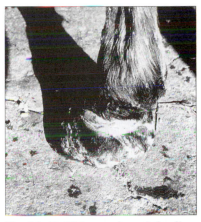

Fig. 16–13. This rope burn is healing well, but should stay bandaged.

counter human product), with or without aloe vera, protects tissue from drying. Silver ions in this preparation prevent the antibiotic from being inactivated by debris and discharge from the wound. The wound must be frequently cleaned, dressed, and bandaged to prevent infection.

Inflammation

An intense inflammatory response to thermal injury changes the way cells flow into the wound. White blood cells stick to vessel walls, and red blood cells mass together *(agglutinate)*. Toxins are released from dying cells, resulting in progressive tissue death. As blood vessels are blocked and constrict in response to injury, oxygen supply is reduced to the damaged area, leading to more cell injury and death—a vicious circle.

Corticosteroids and NSAIDs

Initially, a wound is isolated by the immune system and cleaned up by inflammatory cells. However, with excessive inflammation, edema and oxygen deficiency result. Corticosteroid or non-steroidal anti-inflammatory medications encourage dilation of the blood vessels, reduce cell adhesiveness, and enhance blood circulation, minimizing this process.

Aloe Vera

Aloe vera is useful in managing burns because it stabilizes blood vessels in damaged tissue, reducing leakage. Other reports find that aloe vera has an antibacterial effect, as well. *(Use only straight aloe vera extract, as mixtures containing aloe vera may be combined with potentially harmful chemicals.)*

Once a healthy granulation bed has developed over a rope burn, healing proceeds as it would for any other skin wound. With the presence of granulation tissue, the wound is as resistant to infection as is intact skin.

Eschar Formation

A coagulated crust of skin debris forms over the top of a rope burn. This crust is called an *eschar*. Not only does an eschar encourage harmful bacteria by providing nutrients, but it delays penetration of antibiotics to deeper tissues. An eschar that is brown-black in color is probably invaded by bacteria.

Oxygen is important to cellular metabolism, particularly the processes involving wound healing. Further, oxygen enhances the activity of white blood cells responsible for cleaning up dead tissue and bacteria. An eschar prevents atmospheric oxygen from reaching the underlying wound. As a wound heals, fragile, newly-formed skin cells compete with collagen-producing fibroblasts for oxygen.

An eschar should be removed from a wound as often as possible, to allow healing from the inside out. Its removal maintains a moist environment which aids the process of skin repair. Any remaining eschar usually separates from a wound as a granulation bed forms over a 2 – 4 week period.

Keloid Formation

A *keloid* may develop as a skin-like covering over proud flesh. This exaggerated scar protrudes above skin level. The wound surface resembles skin, but it remains fragile, dry, and crusty and lacks elasticity and strength derived from an underlying skin layer. Such wounds may require skin grafts to replenish a skin layer, or they are subject to chronic cracking and bleeding.

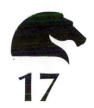

17

INJECTABLE
MEDICATIONS

Many pharmacological and biological products available for the horse come only in injectable form. As the number of available equine medicines increases with improved vaccines, antibiotics, and anti-inflammatory medications, more people are giving their horses injections.

When a veterinarian prescribes a course of therapy, the following factors are considered before any medication is given:

- Of primary consideration is the therapeutic goal: what specific disease process are we trying to alter, and what medication will do that?
- Is there an oral alternative that effectively side-steps the need for injections, or is more cost effective?
- What dosage is appropriate for the individual, and how often must the drug be given to maintain effective blood levels?
- How long must the therapy continue for therapeutic success?
- How can one evaluate a response to treatment?
- Will one drug interact adversely with another which is given at the same time?

- Does the horse suffer from a liver or kidney problem that might prevent normal excretion of the drug from the body?
- Is the horse pregnant or lactating, thereby precluding use of certain drugs?
- What adverse or allergic reactions might be anticipated from the medication?
- Can the horse be monitored for adverse reactions, and can rapid control of any allergic response be initiated?

Consideration of these factors for an entire course of therapy may best be left to a veterinarian's expertise. However, for the confident horse owner, administration of injectable products can save both time and money provided safe principles are followed.

Any time a substance is injected into a horse, be well-advised and educated about what the product is, what it will do, and why it is necessary. Good common sense about both purchase and storage of drugs can build a complete and safe equine emergency first aid kit.

Medicating with any drug should not be a haphazard "shot in the dark." Advice from a veterinarian can direct an owner or trainer to safe and effective formulations for an emergency. It is important to examine selection and storage of these drugs.

THE LABEL
Generic and Name Brands

Many products are available as both a generic or a proprietary name brand. In many instances, a generic product is pharmacologically identical to the more expensive name brand. However, in other instances, the carrier vehicle, preservatives, or suspension material of a generic form results in delayed or reduced absorption of the drug as compared to the name brand. Unless cost is prohibitive, it is better to purchase the proprietary name brand drug to ensure appropriate absorption and distribution of the active ingredient in the product.

Active Ingredient

It is equally important to carefully note the active ingredient of the drug or drugs. As an example of a confusing label, suppose the aim is to treat a horse with penicillin. For many years the familiar bottle of Pen-Strep® or Combiotic® was thought to serve this purpose. However, careful note of the label reveals that penicillin (at 200,000 units per ml) is combined with *dihydrostreptomycin*, another antibiotic which is a treatment of infections in cattle. Because of the way this combination antibiotic is formulated, a recommended dose of Combiotic® or Pen-Strep® provides plenty of dihydrostreptomycin for a horse, but *underdoses* the penicillin. If the injection's volume is increased to supply adequate penicillin, then dihydrostreptomycin is *overdosed* with possible side effects, including toxicity to the kidneys. Very few bacterial organisms contracted by a horse are susceptible to dihydrostreptomycin. It is therefore best to buy straight, uncomplicated procaine penicillin G (at 300,000 units per ml).

Refrigerated Medications

If products needing refrigeration, such as penicillin or vaccines, are shipped, they should arrive in an insulated container with cold packs that are still chilled. Many products, especially vitamins and vaccines, become unstable when exposed to heat, and are rendered inactive if they become warm for even a short period. It is best to deal with reputable sources like your local veterinary clinic. When dealing with mail-order or over-the-counter medications, check to ensure the company handles the drugs properly so there is no chance that the product is frozen or warmed during transport.

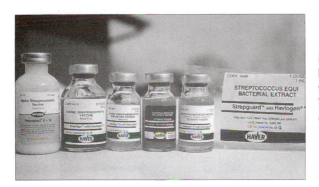

Fig. 17–1. Vaccines become unstable when exposed to heat. They should be kept cool during shipment.

Expiration Date

When purchasing injectable products, check the expiration date. Make sure there will be enough time for all the product to be used before that date. When buying through mail-order supply centers for veterinary products, the expiration date is difficult to evaluate until the product has been received. The dates indicate that if a drug is stored in the recommended manner, and if given at the recommended dose, the product will be effective until that date. It is best to throw away a drug that is past its expiration date, especially antibiotics.

Out-dated drugs do not often cause harmful reactions, but their reduced effectiveness can result in serious consequences, particularly with antibiotics for bacterial infections. Just as consistent underdosing of dewormers leads to resistant parasite strains, reduced effectiveness of antibiotics leads to antibiotic-resistant strains of bacteria, and consequently to severe infections. Therefore, out-dated products do little to improve the success of therapy.

Type of Drug

Intravenous drugs should not be injected into muscle, because they may cause irritating muscle reactions. As an example, there is currently no intramuscular preparation of phenylbutazone. Injection of the intravenous preparation into a muscle results in massive skin sloughing and pain. Then secondary bacterial infections of the skin develop. Myoglobin released from massive muscle breakdown travels to the kidneys and may obstruct their filtering systems, resulting in renal failure.

Moreover, injecting intramuscular medications, such as vaccines or penicillin, into a vein can cause an anaphylactic (severe allergic) reaction and death. Be sure to read all labels, and consult a veterinarian if there is any question about drug type.

SAFE STORAGE

Injectable drugs come in many forms:

- single-dose vials
- multiple-dose vials or bottles
- glass ampules
- prepackaged, single-dose, plastic syringes

Many drugs come in liquid form, already mixed with a saline solution. However, some drugs and vaccines are unstable in solution and are therefore freeze-dried (lyophilized). Then they are mixed with a saline solution or sterile water immediately before injection so the active ingredient is not degraded by storage.

If bottles of vaccine or other drugs sit for long periods, sediments may form in the bottom. Sediment particles may be important molecules of active ingredient that are no longer equally mixed in the solution. These substances should not be injected into muscle as sediments can create a noxious reaction at the injection site. If a drug has sedimented out, shake it. If it returns to normal and is not past its expiration date, it is still acceptable. If it does not mix together with shaking, or is past the expiration date, throw it away.

With lengthy storage, the tops of the vials may get dusty. It is best to clean the top of a bottle by swabbing it with alcohol before inserting a needle or withdrawing any medication. A dust-free cabinet or storage box reduces settling of grime and dust on the rubber stopper.

Storing injectable drugs in syringes for a lengthy time can result in injection of an inadequate dose, as some compounds are absorbed into the plastic walls of the syringe. When this happens, the horse does not receive the entire dose.

Any medication, whether in a bottle, vial, or syringe, should be carefully stored *out of reach of children or pets*, preferably in a locked cabinet or box. Needles accidentally discovered by children are a hazard to their safety. Accidental ingestion of many drugs can be poisonous to children or pets.

Environmental Stresses

Chemical incompatibilities within some drug preparations may result in premature precipitation of sediments, color changes, gas formation, or gelatinization (residue clinging to the sides of the bottle). Or, the drug may be inactivated without any visible change. These changes may occur due to interaction with preservatives or solvents in the drug, particularly if caused by pH changes, heat, or cold.

Injectable vitamin preparations are some of the products especially sensitive to environmental stresses. Most vitamin preparations are stable at acidic pH, from pH 2.0 – 6.5. The higher the pH, the less stable the preparation. In the presence of ultraviolet rays of sunlight, many vitamin preparations are inactivated. Heat greater than 75° F, or aeration by shaking, also contributes to vitamin instability. Contact with certain metals, especially in the presence of light, heat, or aeration, promotes rapid oxidation of vitamins. Trace elements of iron, copper, or cobalt will destroy the B-complex vitamins in a vitamin-mineral mix, therefore it is useless past the expiration date. Likewise, storing the mix in a metal container can also cause vitamins to become inactivated.

Vitamin Injection Storage

To effectively maintain the recommended shelf-life of vitamin injections, store them in a dark, cool place, free from any shaking. If the preparation is outdated, throw it away as it is probably ineffective.

Vaccine Storage

Heat stress is also dangerous to vaccines. They should be kept under

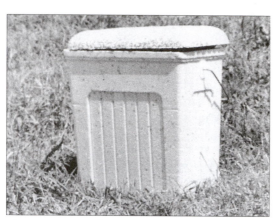

Fig. 17–2. Some drugs require refrigeration.

refrigeration, and not stored on the dashboard or seat of a truck for even a short time. When transporting vaccines, it is best to pack them in a small ice chest to keep them cool. A small amount of heat can make the product inactive. It is then better to throw a questionable product away, and purchase a fresh batch.

Contaminated Medications

Most injectable products have been heat sterilized, or filtered through Millipore® filter systems to reduce the risk of contaminating bacteria or foreign proteins. To limit the number of adverse reactions to injections, the products are ideally free of insoluble foreign particles or pyrogens, which are fever-producing substances.

If multiple-dose vials are used, as with flunixin meglumine (Banamine®), corticosteroids, certain hormones, tranquilizers or sedatives, or vaccines, beware of contamination of these bottles with dirt or used needles that can transfer blood or particles into the bottle. Any bottle suspected of such contamination should be discarded.

PRE-INJECTION PROCEDURES
Reading the Label

Before giving an injection, be sure the solution is well-mixed. Read the label several times to be certain it is the correct item. A wise practice is to read the label while picking up the bottle, read it again while withdrawing the medication, and once again while putting the bottle down prior to injection.

Using Clean Needles and Syringes

Whenever an injection is given to a horse, a brand new sterile syringe and needle should be used.

Needles should *never* be transferred from horse to horse because serious infections, such as Equine Infectious Anemia or protozoan blood parasites like *Piroplasmosis* can be transferred. Needles are inexpensive; there is no reason to save or salvage them.

Vials, syringes, and needles should be disposed of promptly so children or pets have no access to them. Burning these items after use is the preferred method of disposal, especially for biological products like vaccines.

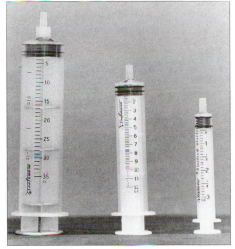

Fig. 17–3. The size of a syringe should be appropriate for the dosage to be given.

Cleaning the Site

Alcohol

Proper technique is essential to ensure a safe and clean injection. Many people still squirt alcohol (70% ethanol or isopropyl) on the area before needle insertion. However, studies have shown that even shaved or hairless skin must remain moistened in alcohol for *at least* 2 minutes before any antiseptic action is achieved. Moreover, not all microorganisms are susceptible to alcohol. A quick squirt of alcohol on top of fur and skin may remove some debris and dirt, but it accomplishes little more.

Effective Antiseptic Solutions

Combining 1.5% tamed iodine (Betadine®) or 0.5% chlorhexidine (Nolvasan®) with 70% alcohol greatly enhances its antiseptic action, although the solution still must contact every microscopic particle of hair and skin for 2 minutes.

Surgical scrubbing with tamed iodine solutions before injection is impractical but certainly provides a less contaminated injection site.

Remember that horses are quick to learn about painful procedures—the next time surgical soap is applied, the horse will be planning an exit from the situation, and the target will be a lot less stationary. Horses have long memories for painful experiences. It is no wonder that a horse responds to the sight of a syringe and needle in hand, or to the smell of alcohol applied to the skin just before the needle is inserted.

Handling the Horse

Always untie a horse before giving an injection, and have a restrainer hold the head if the injection is to be given in the rear end. The restrainer should stand on the same side as the person with the needle. The horse's head is pulled towards both people, and if it decides to kick, it automatically spins the hind end away.

If a horse is tied and violently reacts to needle insertion, it may lunge and throw itself against the rope. The horse's fright increases when it is unable to get free, and it can injure itself or a person in the struggle.

INTRAMUSCULAR INJECTIONS

Most of the time a horse suffers no ill consequences from an intramuscular (IM) injection given by a knowledgeable person, however, there are risks and adverse side effects that should be considered. It important to understand how to give intramuscular injections and what adverse reactions to watch for.

For a less experienced horse owner, some rules-of-thumb should be followed. The objective is to perform the procedure as quickly and painlessly as possible.

Injection Targets

Define the target for the injection ahead of time to avoid blind stabbing. The anatomy of the horse provides many major muscle groups which are safe for IM injection. Intramuscular injections can be given in the neck, rump, and thigh, and occasionally the pectoral muscles of the chest. Certain landmarks guide injection in each location.

Neck Injection

To avoid being kicked and hurt by a resentful horse, the neck and rump are the safest targets.

If the neck is used, note the triangular-shaped area of muscle bordered above by the nuchal ligament, below by the cervical spine, and

behind by the shoulder blade. If an injection is deposited within the ligament, it will not be appropriately ab-
sorbed. Be sure to stay away from the spine or the bony shoulder blade. Close to the spine is the *jugular furrow (groove)* which contains major blood vessels such as the carotid artery or jugular vein.

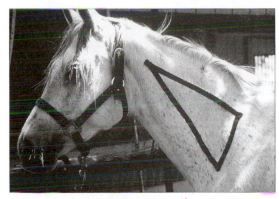

Fig. 17–4. The triangle indicates the area for IM injections in the neck.

If vaccine or medica-
tion that is not in-
tended for intravenous (IV) use is deposited in these vessels, serious and potentially fatal reactions can occur. Also, drugs injected around major nerve branches running along the jugular furrow may be harmful.

Rump Injection

The rump muscle is a large muscle mass located far from any vital structures. (At this location, it is also possible to avoid a kick that states an objection to the shot.)

On the large rump muscles (gluteals), the target site for injec-
tion is defined by drawing a line from the top of the croup to the point of the buttocks, and another line from the point of the hip to the dock. The intersection of these two lines is a safe muscle injection site.

There is a disadvantage in us-
ing the gluteal muscles, in that an abscess may form at the injection site. Because these muscle bundles are encased in a large, continuous sheet of connective

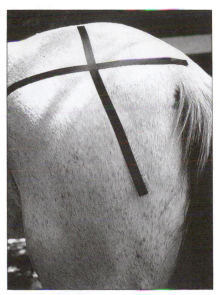

Fig. 17–5. Intersection of the two lines is the IM injection site on the rump.

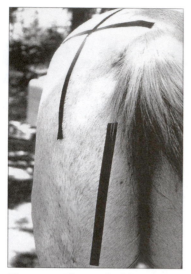

tissue *(fascia)*, an abscess can form under the tissue layers and spread up the loin and back. This spreading potentially leads to massive skin destruction and sloughing. Moreover, because the hip is located in an uppermost position, it is difficult to drain an infected injection site.

Thigh Injection

To avoid abscesses, inject into one of two large muscles that make up the thigh, along the back of the leg. These muscles are active in locomotion so exercise reduces soreness that may develop at the injection site. In the event of an abscess, infection in the thigh is constrained to a local area where it is easily lanced and drained.

Fig. 17–6. The vertical line indicates the IM injection site for the thigh.

Other Sites

Pectoral muscles are rarely used as they tend to become swollen and sore. They are used if multiple antibiotic injections are necessary for prolonged periods. These muscles are readily accessible and allow easy drainage.

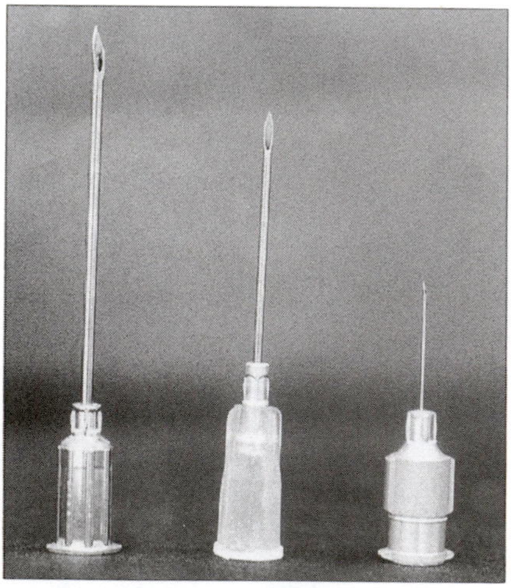

Size of the Needle

Equine muscle is thick and profusely laced with minute blood vessels. A needle should be long enough to penetrate deep into a muscle injection site to deposit the drug so the circulatory system can retrieve it from the muscle bed. A proper length of needle for most injections in the adult horse is 1H inches long, and 18 gauge or 20 gauge around. Foals require no more than a 20 gauge, 1-inch needle.

Fig. 17–7. There are different size needles available for every type of injection.

Inserting the Needle

The needle should be inserted decisively, with a quick thrust, perpendicular to the skin. Pinch a fold of neck skin to momentarily distract the horse, then thrust the needle in just to the side of the pinched skin. Punching the horse several times on the hindquarters before poking in the needle only alerts it to the fact that it is soon to be pricked. A quick thrust of the needle, with no warning to the horse other than a soothing voice and hand, is all that is required. Go for it, and do not hesitate.

Always insert the needle without the syringe attached. If a horse moves while a syringe is attached to the needle, its flopping further scares and irritates the horse. A moving needle lacerates surrounding blood vessels and muscle tissue. Once a needle is in place and the horse is standing quietly, attach the syringe.

Always pull back on the plunger before injecting the drug to be certain there is *no* blood in the hub of the needle. Accidental administration of vaccines or penicillin, as examples, into a blood vessel can result in an anaphylactic reaction (severe allergic reaction) and death. Always be sure no blood is leaking back through the needle. If a needle has penetrated a vessel or capillary and blood comes back, remove the needle, reinsert it, and start again.

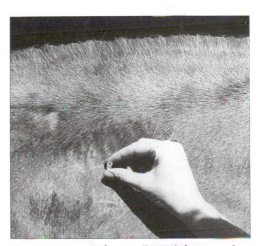

Fig. 17–8. Insert the needle and then attach the syringe.

If a needle is bent in a struggle, throw it away and start with a fresh one. Otherwise the needle may break and become embedded in deep muscle during the second insertion.

Adverse Reactions

With careful selection of the compounds a horse receives, and with clean injection technique, over 80% of adverse drug reactions can be avoided. A new era finds more horse owners assuming the responsibility of their horse's care by administering vaccines and medicines. This do-it-yourself approach to health management is commendable, but it must be backed up with comprehensive self-education. Knowing the risks and taking the necessary precautions ensures the horse's safety.

Abscess

Despite taking all precautions, some horses still experience adverse reactions to IM injections. A localized, firm, and tender swelling at the injection site may be a mild side effect, accompanied by muscle stiffness and soreness. However, if a swelling enlarges and softens, it may be developing into an abscess needing veterinary attention to lance, drain, and flush it. An abscess moves like a wave when touched, like a small water balloon, and is usually warm and sensitive to finger pressure.

Cellulitis

Whenever a needle penetrates skin, a horse receives a microscopic

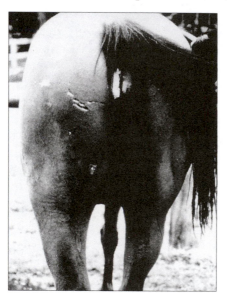

amount of bacteria. Normally, the local immune system surrounding this needle prick cleans up microorganisms that were introduced, and only a very small localized swelling may result, if anything.

However, if an infection persists and is left to simmer within the muscle, *cellulitis* can develop. Inflammation and obstruction of circulatory and lymphatic drainage systems causes the tissues around the injection site to become hot, painful, and swollen. Swelling compromises blood and oxygen supply to the affected tissues, worsening the swelling and infection.

Fig. 17–9. An infected injection site can rapidly swell to huge proportions.

Clostridial Bacteria

Localized cellulitis promotes *Clostridial* bacteria that prefer an anaerobic environment (without oxygen). These bacteria are rapidly lethal to a horse due to an overwhelming toxin production. Clostridial spores abound in manure, soil, and exist normally on a horse's skin. They enter the system as a horse eats, circulating harmlessly through the bloodstream. However, if Clostridial bacteria seed themselves in muscle tissue that is inflamed or dying, within 2 – 5 days, the site is overwhelmingly painful, far out of proportion to the actual amount of swelling. The area feels crackly like tissue paper *(crepitation)* due to gas bubbles trapped beneath the skin.

Careful monitoring of an injection site for several days reveals a problem before it becomes serious. Look for minute or excessive swelling, tenderness to finger pressure, lameness, or stiffness. More often than not, a mild reaction at the site of an injection resolves by itself within 3 – 4 days. Exercise, hot packs, massage, and DMSO hasten recovery. If swelling worsens, or seems abnormally enlarged or painful, contact a veterinarian immediately.

Fibrotic Myopathy

Whenever an infection occurs within a muscle mass, the inflamed tissue is ultimately replaced with scar tissue to varying degrees. If tissue within the thigh muscles scars to a large extent, it can result in a lameness syndrome called *fibrotic myopathy*. Forward extension of the hind leg is reduced due to mechanical constriction by fibrous scar tissue.

Fibrotic myopathy is commonly attributed to sudden sprint activities. A racehorse may tear muscle tissue as it bolts from the start gate. A cutting, roping, or gymkhana horse that abruptly slams on the "brakes," setting the hind legs far under it, can pull or tear a thigh muscle in the process. On rare occasions, however, this syndrome also develops from an infection after an IM injection.

Muscle Soreness

Remember that a horse has two sides to its body. If multiple injections are necessary, use as many different muscle groups as possible to limit soreness. A left-sided muscle group is used in the morning, and the right side at night. Remembering "right at night" avoids confusion.

Because a dressage horse depends on engagement of the hindquarters to collect and

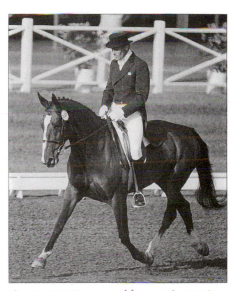

Fig. 17–10. Dressage riders prefer to give injections in the neck instead of the hind end.

perform symmetrical and rhythmic movements, most dressage riders prefer to give IM injections in the neck, away from the hind end. This method prevents loss of several days' training if a horse becomes stiff or sore from an injection.

Flu-like Symptoms

Sometimes a horse reacts adversely to an intramuscular vaccine by exhibiting flu-like symptoms, such as aching muscles, fever, depression, or lack of appetite. For horses known to be sensitive to vaccines, it is best to deposit vaccine in a hind end muscle group. Exercise improves circulation, reducing swelling and inflammation, and hastening resolution of the adverse reaction.

Sore Neck

Even more important, an injection into the neck can cause a horse to become so sore that it refuses to eat or drink—these efforts require stretching of a painful neck muscle. If a horse stops drinking, an impaction colic can develop, which is potentially life-threatening. A sore neck might discourage a foal from nursing, resulting in weakness and stress.

Fever

Anti-inflammatory drugs minimize fever and flu-like symptoms. It may be necessary, along with an inoculation, to administer a non-steroidal anti-inflammatory drug (NSAID), such as phenylbutazone, to a highly sensitive *adult* horse that consistently reacts negatively to vaccinations. (Horses less than 1 year old should never receive an NSAID without first consulting a veterinarian.)

Anaphylactic Shock

The worst complication arising from any injection is an allergic reaction *(anaphylactic shock)* which can abruptly kill a horse. Penicillin, some vitamin injections, and many of the non-steroidal anti-inflammatory drugs are implicated in these reactions, although any drug can cause anaphylaxis. The immune system of an individual that has previously been sensitized to a particular drug can react within seconds or minutes after the drug is deposited in a muscle. An overwhelming immune response suddenly assaults the body. The accompanying airway spasm and throat swelling rapidly lead to asphyxiation and shock. Without an immediate injection of *epinephrine*, the horse can lapse into cardiac arrest, and die. Epinephrine (adrenaline) opens the airways, allowing the horse to breathe. If a horse is experiencing an extreme anaphylactic allergic reaction, it may roll or convulse violently. Epinephrine can be injected anywhere by any injection method (IV, IM, SubQ, etc.) to achieve an instant result.

Warning Signs

Often a horse shows mild allergic symptoms before developing a full-blown anaphylactic reaction. Watch carefully for hives *(urticaria)* that may or may not itch and can be located anywhere on the body. Also, diffuse swelling of the limbs, head, or abdomen, an elevated respiratory rate, or behavioral changes, such as agitation or depression may signal an allergic response. Any combination of these problems may be warning signals that medication should be discontinued at once, and a veterinarian contacted. Profound hypersensitivity reactions can occur without warning; abrupt and fatal anaphylactic shock may be unavoidable.

Precautionary Measures

After administering a drug or medication to a horse, do not walk away immediately. Instead, stick around to watch for an adverse reaction which often peaks within 10 – 30 minutes.

To prevent adverse reactions from intramuscular injections:

- obtain a thorough drug history on each horse to identify previous allergic responses to certain medications
- affix a warning card on a horse's stall door to alert others of an allergy to specific drugs
- avoid mixing medications without first consulting a veterinarian
- properly dose a horse according to body weight and age to avoid excesses, and dose at appropriate time intervals
- read all labels to ensure that a drug is approved for IM administration
- throw away out-dated or improperly stored medicines

Above all, *avoid indiscriminate use of medications!* If a drug is not really necessary or is not recommended by a veterinarian, do not give it. Substitute oral preparations for intramuscular medicines whenever possible, particularly with vitamins or non-steroidal anti-inflammatory drugs. It takes longer for a drug to be absorbed from the intestine than it would through a muscle, yet it may ultimately be safer.

INTRAVENOUS INJECTIONS

Besides intramuscular injection, intravenous (IV) administration of medications is the most common means of injection in the horse. The horse's jugular vein is large and well-defined in the jugular furrow (groove) parallel to the underside of the neck. It swells as blood flow is briefly obstructed with finger pressure along the vein.

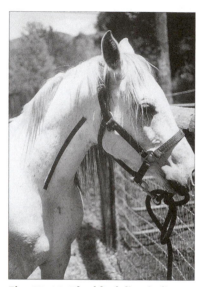

Fig. 17–11. The black line indicates the jugular furrow.

Not only is the jugular vein an opportune location for injecting medication, but it is the common site for collecting blood for Equine Infectious Anemia testing, complete blood counts, chemistry panels, blood typing, and drug testing. A blood tube with a vacuum in it permits rapid extraction of intravenous blood for these tests.

Many liquid medications are formulated for exclusive use as intravenous injections, such as phenylbutazone and potassium penicillin, but many substances can be given either intramuscularly or intravenously depending on how rapidly the effect is desired. Many sedatives and tranquilizers can be administered either way, but an immediate result is seen with IV injection. Any injection given intravenously should be a sterile preparation intended for IV use.

Administering IV Injections

If an injection is to be given IV, the needle can be inserted facing either toward the head or toward the heart, but remember that in the jugular vein, blood flows from the head to the heart. Once the needle is inserted into the vein, blood should only come back through the hub of the needle if the vein is compressed with finger pressure. If blood spurts vigorously from the needle without compressing the vessel, there is a strong possibility that it has been inserted into the carotid artery. *No medication should be administered in the carotid artery* because it would go directly to the brain and central nervous system, and could result in instant death.

If medication should be given directly into the blood vessel, but it leaks into surrounding tissue, serious skin irritation can lead to massive loss of skin in the area, and potentially to inflammation of the vein *(thrombophlebitis)*.

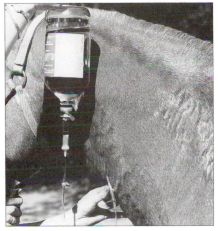

Phenylbutazone, sodium iodide, tetracycline, and guafenisin (a general anesthetic agent) cause this problem most often.

IV Catheter

If frequent IV medication must be given, or large volumes of electrolyte solutions are to be administered, an indwelling intravenous catheter is placed in the vein after clipping and scrubbing the insertion site. The catheter is a flexible plastic material that can safely remain in the jugular vein for up to 72

Fig. 17–12. An intravenous catheter for frequent IV administration.

hours if these sterilizing procedures are followed for its placement.

SUBCUTANEOUS INJECTIONS

Most medications are designed to be injected deeply into the horse's muscle tissue, or directly into the vein. However, sometimes a therapeutic medication is given subcutaneously, (subQ).

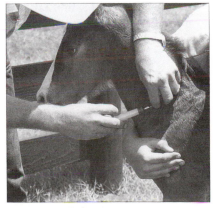

Injecting a horse subQ is difficult. This method of injection should not be attempted without advice and training from a veterinarian.

The loose skin behind the horse's elbow makes an ideal location for a subQ injection. The needle is placed just under the skin, but not into muscle, and the material is slowly injected. If the spot swells too much, the needle

Fig. 17–13. Subcutaneous injections are given just under the skin.

can be fanned in a semicircle to spread the medication out over a larger area. Medication or fluids given under a horse's skin are absorbed slowly, so there will be a lump at the injection site for several hours.

Local anesthetic is often placed subQ to numb an area for suturing or a scalpel incision. Fanning the anesthetic into the subcutaneous tissues increases the area of effect. Heparin is sometime administered for the prevention or treatment of laminitis, and it can also be given subQ.

INTRADERMAL INJECTIONS

An intradermal (ID) injection involves placing a needle inside the up-

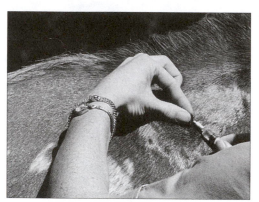

permost layer of the skin. This method is even more difficult than subQ injections. It should not be attempted without first being advised and trained by a veterinarian.

In some instances local anesthetic is injected intradermally. More commonly, the injection of a corticosteroid into nodular necrobiosis skin lesions involves an ID infusion. Also, use of Bacillus

Fig. 17–14. Intradermal injections are given inside the skin.

Calmette-Guerin *(See Chapter 15 for more information on BCG and sarcoids.)* to treat sarcoid tumors also requires intradermal injection for best results.

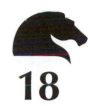

18

NON-STEROIDAL ANTI-INFLAMMATORY DRUGS

Equine athletic pursuits often result in sore muscles, swollen limbs, or mild lameness. It is not unusual for a horse owner or trainer to open the medical kit, and reach inside for a short-term anti-inflammatory solution to an ache or pain.

In theory, this practice seems sensible, and it is one we commonly apply to ourselves. Yet, our efforts to help a horse by numbing the problem with an anti-inflammatory drug may do more harm than good.

USE OF NSAIDS

The most overused and abused drugs available today are those belonging to the class of non-steroidal anti-inflammatory drugs (NSAIDs), particularly phenylbutazone ("bute") and flunixin meglumine (Banamine®). Bute and Banamine® are useful for a wide range of conditions. Aspirin is useful for very specific problems. Other, less common NSAIDs include dipyrone, Ketofen®, and naproxen.

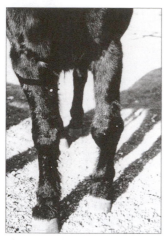

Fig. 18–1. NSAIDs can help a horse with chronic arthritis.

Benefits of NSAIDs

NSAIDs are powerful drugs, improving a horse's working capabilities. They are not stimulants. They simply allow a horse to perform up to normal capabilities, without lameness and pain. NSAIDs help control leg swelling, or reduce an out-of-control fever caused by infections. They can relieve spasms from muscle strain or a mild colic. They are helpful to the chronically arthritic horse to enhance its quality of life and the longevity of its performance career. Yet, NSAIDs should not be taken for granted and used indiscriminately.

Drawbacks of NSAIDs

Giving NSAIDs to a mildly lame horse while asking it for continued performance can aggravate an undiagnosed tendon or muscle injury. Or, if a horse with beginning signs of colic receives a dose of Banamine® or bute from a concerned owner, the pain seems to subside due to the anti-inflammatory effects of the drug. But the real problem goes unanswered. A horse only communicates via depression, lack of appetite, or pain, and the effect of the drug disguises these symptoms. Masking a serious colic condition, which may require surgery, permits the damage to intensify beyond repair.

Method of Action

When a horse is hurting from a wound, pulled muscle, colic, or arthritis, its body responds by producing substances called *prostaglandins*. Prostaglandins cause the cascade of events involved in the inflammatory process. Prostaglandins are short-lived molecules, and are only produced at or close to their site of action. They are produced upon demand and are not stored by the body. NSAIDs act as anti-inflammatory agents by inhibiting the normal production of prostaglandins.

At the site of action, prostaglandins stimulate contraction and permeability of the cells lining the blood vessels, causing leakage of fluids into surrounding soft tissues. This results in edema, and is seen as swelling.

At the same time, prostaglandins causes the smooth muscle of the blood vessel walls to relax, causing blood to pool in localized areas, which results in redness *(erythema)*.

Prostaglandins enhance the effects of other players in the inflammatory cycle, such as histamines and *bradykinin*. These chemicals attract white blood cells, and increase blood circulation to the inflammation site. Warmth is felt in the area due to increased blood flow and local blood pooling.

In addition to swelling, redness, and heat at a site of injury, prostaglandins make pain receptors super-sensitive, contributing to an exaggerated pain response.

Therefore, as anti-inflammatory agents, NSAIDs act as anti-prostaglandins. By inhibiting production of prostaglandins, NSAIDs reduce the spiraling events that result in inflammation and swelling; pain subsides as well.

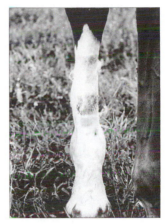

Fig. 18–2. Swelling of an injured site is caused by prostaglandins.

TYPES OF NSAIDS

Understanding the different pharmacological aspects of a drug is essential for its safe use. Manufacturer's labels and package inserts contain information about proper dosages and adverse side effects.

Different products within the NSAID drug class act better on some ailments than others. For example, bute is effective for musculoskeletal problems such as arthritis, a pulled muscle, or tendinitis. Flunixin meglumine is potent against gastrointestinal pain and endotoxemia.

Phenylbutazone

One of the least expensive and more potent examples of the NSAIDs is phenylbutazone, or bute. Once an intravenous dosage of bute is administered, it requires about ½ hour to begin blocking prostaglandin production. If given orally in paste, powder, or tablet form, it takes 2 – 3 hours to be absorbed from the gastrointestinal tract.

NSAIDs have no effect on the prostaglandins already produced. Therefore, once bute is administered, it does not take effect for 3 – 5 hours. This time lag is required for the body to break down enough of the previously manufactured prostaglandins. Total breakdown requires up to 12 hours. In the meantime, bute prevents additional prostaglandins from being produced.

If the blood level of bute is not maintained at a therapeutic level, prostaglandins begin to accumulate again, and the inflammatory cycle repeats itself. Depending on the ailment, bute protects against inflammation for 12 – 24 hours.

Flunixin Meglumine

Flunixin meglumine (Banamine®) is very useful for pain due to colic. It is also helpful against the effects of endotoxemia caused by a retained placenta, an overdose of rich feed, or a pituitary disorder. *(See Chapter 4 for more information on endotoxins.)* Banamine® is more potent than bute, and maintains its therapeutic effect for up to 30 hours.

Aspirin

Aspirin, which is rapidly excreted from the body, is only active for 6 – 8 hours.

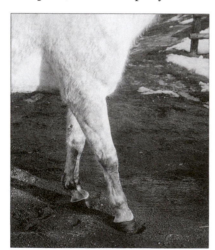

Fig. 18–3. Aspirin improves blood flow in horses with navicular disease.

Because of its short duration, aspirin is a poor anti-inflammatory drug for a musculoskeletal injury, or for anti-pyretic effects to reduce fever. Aspirin is a useful treatment for laminitis, navicular disease, colic due to obstruction of an intestinal blood vessel *(thromboembolic colic)*, or anterior uveitis.

Aspirin improves blood flow to limbs afflicted with laminitis or navicular disease. It helps manage thromboembolic colic, caused by the parasitic damage of *Strongylus vulgaris*. Aspirin also helps manage anterior uveitis cases by halting blood clotting in the eye. Pain, eye spasms, and the disease process abate.

Aspirin does these things because it alters the function of platelets. *Platelets* are a type of blood cell important to the blood clotting mechanism. Aspirin permanently alters platelet function, preventing blood clotting, for the life of that platelet.

The effect on platelets by a single dose of aspirin persists even after the bloodstream is cleared of the drug. This effect can last as long as 3 days.

Uses of NSAIDs	
Phenylbutazone	Effective against musculoskeletal injuries. Also effective against gastrointestinal pain.
Flunixin Meglumine	Effective against musculoskeletal injuries. Also effective against gastrointestinal pain and endotoxemia.
Aspirin	Effective to relieve laminitis, navicular disease, thromboembolic colic, or anterior uveitis.

Fig. 18–4.

NSAID TOXICITY
Stomach

While NSAIDs inhibit production of prostaglandins involved in the inflammatory process, they also interfere with production of prostaglandins necessary to normal physiologic function. Prostaglandin E2 protects the stomach lining by stimulating mucus production, and secretion of sodium bicarbonate by gastric cells to buffer the stomach's acid environment. Optimal blood flow to the stomach and intestinal tract is normally controlled by prostaglandin activity.

Without this protection, the stomach and intestines are prone to gastric ulcers. Ulcers are not only painful, but can be life-threatening.

Oral ulcers along the gums, palate, and tongue may accompany gastric ulcers. These ulcers are more common in horses receiving excessive NSAIDs orally, that is as paste, tablets, or powder. Mouth pain depresses appetite and performance suffers.

Kidneys

Prostaglandins also are responsible for maintaining normal blood flow, function, and water resorption abilities of the kidneys. In a dehydrated horse (due to lack of water, excessive sweating, bleeding, or severe colic) prostaglandins act as a protective device to dilate and enhance the blood supply to the kidney.

Irreversible, toxic effects may occur within 48 hours in dehydrated or blood volume-depleted horses that are given a single dose of a NSAID, particularly bute. The syndrome is known as *renal papillary necrosis,* and is fatal. Even if administered at recommended doses, bute can be a toxic product for a dehydrated horse.

Symptoms of NSAID Toxicity

Excessive amounts of NSAIDs damage the gastrointestinal lining with subsequent leakage and loss of proteins. Symptoms of NSAID-induced toxicosis and protein loss include diarrhea, edema of limbs and abdomen, blood loss in the feces, and weight loss. Some horses exhibit depression, loss of appetite, or abdominal pain due to gastric ulcers or edema of the intestinal lining.

A lower-than-recommended dose can cause toxicosis if given to a horse that is dehydrated, in pain, or stressed. Those horses respond to stress by producing internal corticosteroids. When internal corticosteroids are combined with a NSAID, steroid effects are amplified, resulting in toxicity.

Toxic effects occur with administration of excessive amounts of a NSAID over a short time (3 – 5 days), or by chronic dosing over months or years.

After more than a decade of use of many different non-steroidal anti-inflammatory drugs, equine practitioners have discovered that previously assumed safe doses in the horse can exert toxic effects if maintained at these levels too long. For example, 4 grams of bute a day for a 1,000-pound horse should not be administered more than 4 days in a row, assuming normal kidney and liver function. Once the drug has achieved therapeutic levels in the bloodstream, that level is safely maintained at 1 – 2 grams per day.

Allergic Reactions

Long-term use of NSAIDs (sporadic or consistent) can hypersensitize a horse to any drug in its class, and result in allergic reactions. These reactions range from a mild case of hives, or facial or limb edema, to a severe anaphylactic allergic reaction and death.

Some people may make a dangerous mistake—repetitive dosing with NSAIDs while applying a misguided theory that "if a little bit works, a lot must be better." A NSAID should never be repeated at less than 12-hour intervals unless specified by a veterinarian. Recommended dosing instructions per pound of body weight should never be increased.

Double Dosing

Another common mistake is to give an appropriate dose of one

NSAID, followed immediately by an appropriate dose of another NSAID. Toxic effects are additive, and this practice simulates a double dose of any single NSAID. Toxicosis results from combining NSAIDs.

If relief is not achieved from the initial drug treatment, there is no reason to believe relief will come from an additional product with a similar mechanism of action. There is a time lag of several hours until clinical relief is seen. The prostaglandin cycle is blocked immediately, but existing prostaglandins need to be metabolized and removed from the system. Adding more NSAIDs will not alter or speed up this process.

NSAIDs and Foals

Foals less than 6 – 8 months old are extremely susceptible to the toxic effects of NSAIDs. Under normal circumstances, newborn foals are never given NSAIDs. If it is a dire emergency, *a veterinarian* may decide to administer a NSAID.

The dangers of administration of NSAID medications to horses less than 1 year of age so far outweigh any possible benefits gained from anti-inflammatory or anti-pyretic effects, that a general rule-of-thumb should be followed: *never administer any NSAID to any horse under 1 year old.*

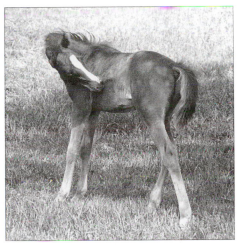

Fig. 18–5. Foals should not receive an NSAID except as recommended by a vet.

Professional Advice

Obtain professional veterinary advice before using NSAIDs. What "worked" for one horse may have no application to another. What seems to be a mild problem may be serious, requiring medical attention and expertise. It is easy to pick up the telephone and get professional advice, and has a less damaging toll on a horse's health than guesswork.

WITHDRAWAL FOR COMPETITION

There are legal responsibilities involved with the use of anti-inflammatory agents, as well. Drug levels are detectable in urine or blood up until 96 hours after administration. NSAIDs must be withdrawn from an endurance or competitive trail horse 3 – 4 days before the competition. Likewise, the American Quarter Horse Association forbids the use of any drug. The American Horse Shows Association's ruling states that a defined and limited amount of bute or Banamine® can be given. To comply with AHSA regulations, the maximum daily dose of bute should not exceed 2 grams per 1,000 pounds body weight. The recommended dose for Banamine® is 500 mg per 1,000 pounds body weight. Both drugs must be withdrawn 12 hours before competition, and should not be administered for more than 5 straight days without a day off the drug. One drug or the other is acceptable, but not both.

For racing, each state has its own rules and restrictions. Check with the State Racing Commission (of the state where the race will be held) to ensure the horse meets drug withdrawal requirements.

PREPURCHASE EXAMS

Be cautious during prepurchase examinations. An unethical seller who wants to mask a mild lameness problem may "improve" the examination results by using NSAIDs or other drugs.

ALTERNATIVES TO NSAIDS

Before grabbing a tube or tablets of a NSAID, examine other therapeutic alternatives such as rest, or hot or cold soakings. Rub a swelling with DMSO (dimethyl sulfoxide), or massage sore muscles. Examine shoeing practices that might have changed a limb's biomechanics enough to bring on lameness. Re-evaluate training methods, and the rate of increase in difficulty. Look to management, parasite control, and feeding changes to decrease the incidence of colic.

Remember, horses were designed to live on grasses, water, and salt. Anything else we put into their bodies must be evaluated for suitability and safety. The Federal Drug Administration (FDA) approves drugs at specified dosages and frequencies to comply with research studies in safety and efficacy. NSAIDs have a role in the horse world, provided they are used intelligently and in moderation.

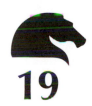

19

SAFE & EFFECTIVE RESTRAINT

Building a partnership that is based on trust is a goal that takes time, but is full of reward. Unfortunately, not all events in a horse's life are free from unpleasantness or pain. Some examples are wound doctoring, routine vaccinations, and administration of medications. Eventually the inevitable occurs, and the horse objects to a procedure.

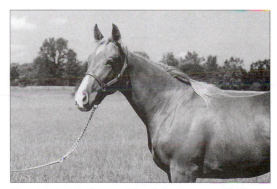

Fig. 19–1. A halter and lead rope are a mild form of restraint.

For some horses, administration of deworming pastes, use of electric clippers, or horseshoeing are traumatic experiences. Other horses object to benign grooming procedures like bathing, or pulling and braiding the mane.

The objectives of restraint are:
- to avoid getting hurt
- to prevent injury to the horse
- to get the job done effectively

Restraint of a half-ton animal obviously requires more than sheer human strength. A rearing horse can suspend a 200-pound man from the end of a twitch, and a horse recovering from general anesthetic can quickly flip two grown men off its neck. The brute strength of a horse should be addressed in a psychological arena, not in a physical showdown.

UNDERSTANDING HORSE BEHAVIOR
Natural Instincts

By using our human mind we can outwit a horse at its own game of resistance. To do so, we must understand the motivating influences behind the horse's contrary behavior. Horses evolved survival

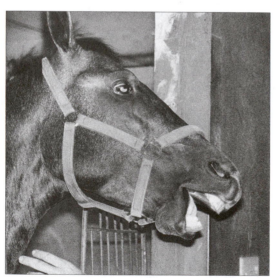

Fig. 19–2. Teeth can be used as a defensive weapon and also for aggression.

mechanisms to protect themselves from predators, such as the big cats. Their immediate response when threatened is to flee from the area. A flighty horse is only responding to natural instincts to run from a fearful situation. A response to a painful or scary event is to move away from the stimulus by backing up, lunging sideways, or rearing. If backed into a corner, or prevented from fleeing, a horse then reverts to using its built-in defense weapons—its teeth and hooves. This fear translates to biting, kicking, or striking, all of which are unacceptable behavior from a human point of view.

By understanding normal equine behavioral instincts, we can capitalize on them, and modify their behavior to the task at hand. Horses evolved in a herd hierarchy, and they accept a single dominant herd member as the leader. Because a horse is able to distinguish between dominant and submissive individuals, and respond accordingly, it is logical for humans to achieve dominance to successfully fulfill the objectives of restraint.

Learn to read a horse's behavioral cues, such as flattened ears, or bared teeth that indicate aggression, or a tightly clasped tail and hollow, tense back reflective of pain or fear. Other signals are more subtle, but perked ears, a relaxed posture, or droopy lip and eyes should be positively rewarded, because they are signs of cooperation.

CREATING CALMNESS

The temperament of an individual horse and its breed type are factors that may dictate a specific approach. However, certain fundamentals should be applied to restraint of any horse.

Environment

Make the situation appealing to the horse by working in a familiar environment that feels secure, and by using familiar equipment. Approach the horse quietly, and spend several minutes getting acquainted with its body language, and allowing it to become accustomed to the situation as well. Working off the near (left) side is comforting as most horses are accustomed to that. Talk to it in a quiet, calming tone of voice; a monotonous monologue can exert hypnotic effects upon the horse's psyche.

Reassurance

Take a few extra minutes to reassure the horse, and do not "mug" it. The horse will then begin to build confidence. More trust is gained by not overpressuring it, but proceeding when it is ready to accept the situation with some degree of reassurance. Reward any agreeable behavior with praise, and stroke its neck and face. Many horses like to be rubbed around the eye or over the withers.

Confidence and Patience

Looking a horse in the eye commands its attention. Act decisively, because hesitation promotes the horse's suspicion and enhances its anxiety and distrust. Humans easily transmit fear and nervousness to a horse. Slow and deliberate movements build confidence. Be firm with commands, and discipline appropriately.

Many horses are not necessarily fearful of a procedure, but may only be spoiled. These horses will respect a firm reprimand. Human efforts at psychological domination are a positive learning experience for the spoiled horse. Using sensitivity and patience teaches a horse about the necessity and benefits of submission to human will. Not only does this method make ground work more enjoyable for the horse and its handlers, but the horse's response to riding or driving training also improves. With respect comes obedience and cooperation.

An essential ingredient in any restraint conflict is to restrain our own fits of temper. Above all, stay cool and calm, and use the rational mind to command the situation. This advice sounds simple, but many of us know that self-restraint is not always easy during a battle of wills. It is always better to back off, count to ten (or fifty if necessary), and start over rather than to embark upon a counterproductive physical match with the horse.

Psychology

A horse should always be reacting to the people, rather than the people reacting to the horse. This goal is *not* accomplished by threatening the horse verbally or physically; instead, be mentally one jump ahead of the horse. Anticipate what it will do. Before it has even started to make that move, take steps to counter it, converting the move to something else. Unwanted behavior is diverted, and it also perplexes the horse, so now its attention is focused on the person. The horse looks to that person for a lead, accepting him or her as the dominant leader in the "herd."

This method of training requires empathy to individual equine personalities, and often is a gift with which one is born. Certain techniques can be learned by reading or attending seminars and clinics, but it is best to trust in common sense and sensitivity. Recipes for psychological modification should only be used as guidelines. Each person should find what works with an individual horse and stick to it.

Restraint of a fractious horse is not about physical force. Instead it depends on the mental approach and understanding of each horse's unique response to any given situation. Figure out what makes the horse tick, and take strides to mold this knowledge into a plan of human design, without reacting to the horse.

HANDLING PROCEDURES
Safe Area

When approaching a situation that will be disagreeable to a horse, work in an area free of entrapments such as machinery, vehicles, rakes, wheelbarrows, low overhangs, nails and latches, and electrical cords. Find level ground with enough space for safe movement. Children, bystanders, and pets (e.g. dogs and cats) should be asked to leave the working area. This practice ensures their safety, and prevents people from tripping over them while they work.

There should be at least two people involved in the procedure: the restrainer and the operator. The restrainer holds the horse while the operator performs the procedure. The restrainer should be a person who understands horses, and with whom it is easy to communicate.

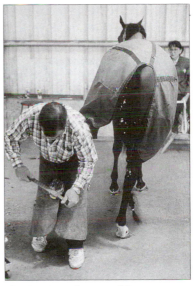

Fig. 19–3. A clear working area ensures the safety of the horse and handlers.

Dedicated Restraint

The restrainer must be confident and stay with the horse, not letting go at a jumpy reaction by the horse. If the restrainer lets go there is risk that the restrainer or operator could be hurt by a loose horse. Furthermore, letting go reinforces the adverse behavior and the horse now knows how to extract itself from the situation. Rather than submitting to the procedure, the horse intensifies its efforts to get away.

Safe Equipment

Check the safety of all equipment, using intact, well-fitting halters and stout lead ropes. Be sure all buckles and snaps are functional, and are likely to remain so if stressed.

Always keep hands and fingers out of the halter, and never wrap a lead line around the limbs or body. This practice prevents sprains, strains, or lost fingers if a hand is entangled in a rope as a horse reacts suddenly.

Standing Position

The best place to stand during any procedure is close to the horse, just behind the shoulder so it cannot strike out with a leg. An operator who is standing close to the horse when it suddenly throws its weight feels far less impact than if he or she stood a few feet away.

Never stand directly in front of any horse while performing a procedure. In this position, there are many ways for the horse to cause a problem, such as lunging, pawing, or rearing.

The restrainer usually stands on the same side as the operator, if possible. This position allows him or her to pull the horse's head towards the people, which automatically swings kicking hindquarters away.

METHODS OF RESTRAINT

Because a horse's instinct to flee is so intense, submissive behavior is induced by removing the ability to flee. Restraint of a horse's flight instinct is accomplished by either physical or chemical methods.

Application of any form of physical restraint depends on psychological wit to ensure success. Learn which physical restraint method works best for the horse and recognize when the desired effect has been achieved. Some horses may object so violently to certain restraining measures, such as stocks or a twitch, that more cooperation may be achieved by quietly asking the horse to submit to a procedure without any physical restraint. Experience teaches which horses respond best to a "least restraint" technique.

Physical restraint begins simply when we place a halter and lead rope on a horse. Assuming a horse knows how to lead, it will go where we go. Now that the horse is "in hand," more physical restraint can be applied as necessary.

Placing a horse in a safe stall limits its ability to plunge and flee across a paddock or pasture. A horse can be backed into a corner where it feels more under the control of the handler.

Stocks

Use of "stocks" confines a horse and severely limits its movements. Never be complacent about a horse in stocks because it is still able to kick or bite, or may attempt to jump out. A seat belt, snugly fit over the horse's withers, deters a tendency to leap upwards.

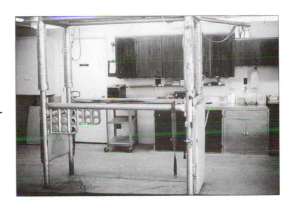

Fig. 19–4. Stocks with a restraining back strap made from a car seat belt.

Twitch

A *twitch* placed on the upper lip applies pressure to sensory nerves of the lip. It is uncomfortable enough to distract a horse's attention from other areas of the body. Evidence shows that endorphins are released by twitch application. Endorphins are narcotic-like substances produced in and released from the central nervous system, and they block referred pain from other parts of the body, causing the horse to relax.

An *easy twitch* is a piece of steel or aluminum clamped over a horse's nose sort of like a pair of pliers. A *chain twitch* is a device that winds a chain over the lip. A long handle is attached to the chain for increased leverage. If a horse throws its head and the twitch gets away from the restrainer, a chain twitch can become a flying "billy-club" capable of seriously injuring the restrainer, operator, or bystanders.

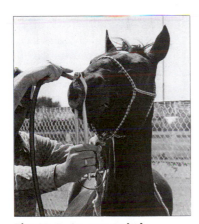

Fig. 19–5. An easy twitch.

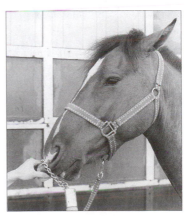

Fig. 19–6. A chain twitch.

An applied twitch should be held vertical to the ground, as twisting it sideways or upside-down is painful enough to elicit violent reactions from a horse. Do not pull on it or use it to lead a horse. For some horses, a twitch is a fearsome device; a normally tractable horse may strike out.

Lip Chain

The horse that fears and abhors twitches may respond positively to the use of a *lip chain*. A lip chain is placed over the upper gum just under the lip, and serves as a self-punishing device capable of train-

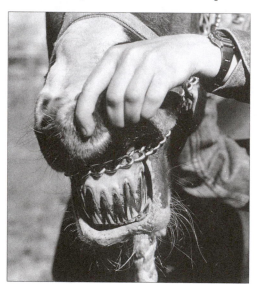

ing the horse. The lip chain is less intimidating than a twitch. Before applying the chain, running the fingers under the upper lip and along the gums provides a horse with a familiar taste of salt from the fingers and encourages confidence. Then the chain is quietly and smoothly slipped into place. If a horse exhibits undesirable behavior, the chain tightens over the gum and is painful, but as soon as the horse responds appropriately, it is instantly rewarded by release of pres-

Fig. 19–7. A lip chain is less intimidating than a twitch.

sure and pain. Rapid jerks on the chain by the restrainer are counterproductive and can result in rearing. A light, steady pressure is all that is necessary to keep the chain in place. The horse's response automatically tightens or loosens it.

Stud Chain

Instead of placing the chain under the lip, it can be applied over the nose as a *stud chain*. A firm jerk on a chain in this position causes pain to the nose, enforcing a verbal reprimand.

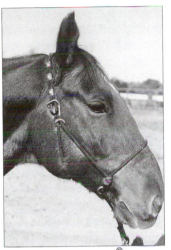

Fig. 19–8. A Be-Nice® halter.

Be-Nice® Halter

A Be-Nice® Halter works effectively on horses that react negatively by throwing their heads or rearing. The weight of the halter tightens the nose piece and pulls down on the poll section. If the "prongs" are placed downwards in contact with the poll, negative reinforcement is asserted when the horse raises its head. Dropping its head (and body) causes the pain to cease. A Be-Nice® halter can self-train by punishing and rewarding a horse instantly at the time of the behavior.

War-Bridle

Use of a "war-bridle" is overly threatening and painful to a horse if it is applied incorrectly or with anger. The rope passes over the poll and through the mouth as would a bit. This war-bridle places painful pressure on the poll and at the commissures of the mouth and the gums.

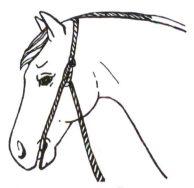

Fig. 19–9. A war-bridle.

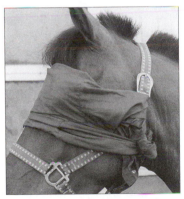

Fig. 19–10. A blindfold may be helpful when applying a twitch.

Blindfold

Blindfolding also prevents a horse from fleeing. It is now completely subservient to the restrainer because it has no idea of where to move. Occasionally, it is necessary to blindfold a horse to apply another physical restraint method such as a twitch.

Hobble

Another means of removing a horse's ability to escape is to tie one leg in a hobble. The leg is flexed at the knee, and a

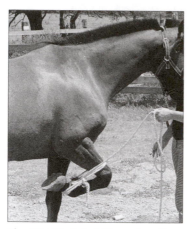

Fig. 19–11. A hobble makes the horse feel "crippled."

leather strap or soft cotton rope is placed around the forearm and pastern. If one leg is held off the ground, a horse feels "crippled." Its other limbs mildly fatigue. Many horses hop around in confusion as they try to free their leg. Occasionally, a horse overreacts by throwing itself to the ground. Others become subdued.

The goal is achieved when the horse recognizes the human as the "savior" who removes the hobble from the leg. Now the human is The Good Guy who presents the horse with the lesser of two evils: it can submit quietly with all four legs on the ground, or lose the use of one of its legs with a hobble.

Backing the Horse

Some horses prefer to back up to flee from an unpleasant situation. Unless there is a safe obstacle for them to back into, this flight behavior is incredibly frustrating. Forcing such a horse to rapidly back around and around a paddock may sufficiently fatigue its muscles so it willingly stops backing and allows the procedure. At the same time, the restrainer has achieved psychological domination over the horse.

Distracting Noises

Sometimes jiggling a halter distracts a horse's attention as it listens to the jingling buckles. Knocking on its forehead in a non-rhythmical pattern also diverts its attention to the feel and sound. Knock in a random pattern so it does not know when the next tap sequence is coming. The horse may temporarily tune in to this distraction, long enough to give an injection or apply a bandage.

Earing Down

Gently grabbing an ear and firmly pulling downward is another method of distraction. An ear should not be twisted or jerked as that can injure it. Downward traction is all that is required to achieve the necessary response. If performed properly, "earing" a horse rarely makes it head-shy afterwards, however, it is often difficult to grab hold of an ear on an already head-shy horse. A similar distracting method is to grab a fold of skin on the horse's neck and pinch it.

Cross-Ties

Cross-ties are a poor means of restraining a horse. Not only can a person be entangled in the cross-tie ropes, but a violently thrashing horse can rear up and flip itself over in the cross-ties, fatally injuring its head or neck. If cross-ties are the only available holding device, connect them with a quick-release buckle, and never leave a horse unattended in cross-ties.

Foal Restraint

Restraint of a foal requires a different technique than those used on grown horses. Foals often quiet down if the restrainer encircles the foal's chest with an arm, and runs the other arm around behind the buttocks. The tail can be pulled up gently, with no adverse effects, to stabilize the foal. Be sure the forward arm is not too high up on the neck so air flow through the trachea is not impeded. Pushing a foal against a safe wall, and placing a knee firmly into its flank while encircling it with the arms usually holds it steady so the operator can perform the necessary chore. Do not be fooled by a foal's size; the littlest newborn can crack someone's ribs or dent a head or shin.

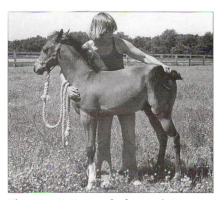

Fig. 19–12. Proper foal restraint.

Chemical Tranquilizers

For horses that do not comply with any form of physical restraint and threaten to injure a person or themselves, or for a horse that must be subjected to a painful procedure such as wound suturing, chemical restraint may be necessary. In this era of modern medicine it is no longer necessary to resort to the use of casting ropes that yank a horse off its feet and then submit it to being hog-tied. Chemical tranquilizers and sedatives diminish stress to both the horse and operator and prevent a horse from injuring itself.

Adverse Reactions

Tranquilizers and sedatives should be used under veterinary supervision, for although adverse reactions to these drugs are uncommon, they can occur. The horse's heart should be monitored with a stethoscope to check for any murmurs or arrhythmias. Sedatives or tranquilizers exert cardiovascular effects that can adversely affect a poor heart condition.

Many mortality insurance policies do not cover fatal accidents that occur from medication or drugs given without veterinary supervision.

Methods of Administration

Sedatives or tranquilizers can be administered either intravenously (IV) or intramuscularly (IM). If given into the vein, the effects are fairly immediate (within several minutes), but not as long-lasting as they are when given IM. An IM injection requires at least 10 minutes before the head drops and the horse's body relaxes.

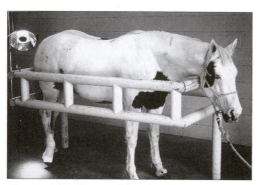

Fig. 19–13. A lowered head and relaxed body indicate sedation.

Different dose levels are calculated depending on whether the IV or IM route is used. Always discuss with a veterinarian how much and in what manner a drug should be given to avoid disastrous consequences. Learn about side effects for any drug given to a horse.

Excitement Prevents Tranquilizing

If a horse is excited and adrenaline is flowing before administration of a sedative or tranquilizer, the beneficial depressant effects of the drug may not be achieved. Adrenaline speeds up the heart rate and blood flow through the body, and results in flushing of the drug through the system too rapidly to affect the central nervous system.

Try to anticipate whether it would be advantageous to start with chemical restraint rather than getting the horse excited first. Once a horse is excited and a decision is made to try a chemical approach, it is best to wait 20 – 30 minutes for everyone to calm down before administering the drug. This method achieves an effective and less stressful result.

ALTERNATIVE SOLUTIONS

If a tactic is not working sufficiently, then stop and regroup. Think the situation over. Try to figure out what exactly is troubling the horse. Remember, the best approach is to use the *least* restraint necessary. Overpowering a horse mentally and physically elicits more of a fight. The objective is to convince a reluctant horse to *cooperate*. Cooperation does not mean that it willingly complies. Sometimes, just standing still is a sign of submission. Accept small winning steps, and reward cooperation. If necessary, seek professional help from a veterinarian.

Ideally, the goal is to train a horse to accept and tolerate a disagreeable event. Horses do not lie down, roll over, and just say, "Here, do what you will;" that will never happen. Be satisfied with incremental successes, and build on these. Maintain a bright, optimistic outlook, and this attitude will be transmitted to the horse.

Above all, stay rational and do not prematurely admit defeat. By drawing on reservoirs of psychological, physical, and chemical restraint, there is always a way to get the job done, both effectively and safely.

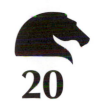

MANAGING THE CONFINED HORSE

Due to showing, racing, limited land resources, and for various other reasons, many horses are confined to paddocks, runs or stalls.

Stalls are a practical means of housing a large number of horses in a limited space, maximizing use of land and pasture resources. At horse shows and racetracks, a stall is usually the sole facility in which a horse is kept during its stay.

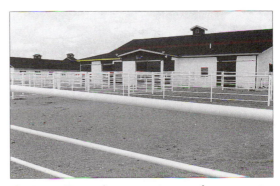

Fig. 20–1. For various reasons many horses must be confined to stalls or pens.

HERD INSTINCT

Studies reveal that under natural, free-ranging conditions, horses spend approximately 60% of their time grazing, preferably with the herd.

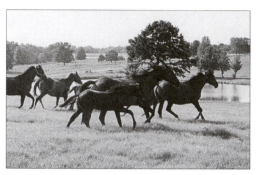

Fig. 20–2. Frolic and play are examples of social interactions within a herd.

Not only does frequent grazing satisfy a physiological need for roughage and a psychological need for chewing fiber, but grazing involves a fair amount of wandering and exercise during the course of a day.

As herd animals, horses enjoy the company of other horses. Grooming behavior, frolic, and play are just a few examples of social interactions between individuals within a herd. Horses like to touch, smell, and taste of each other. A pecking order, or social hierarchy, is established through social interplay as each horse assumes a comfortable and secure social position within the herd.

REASONS FOR CONFINEMENT

There are other circumstances, other than lack of acreage, which may cause an owner to prefer confining a horse indoors. Stalls provide shelter from wind and cold, rain or snow. Stalling a horse out of the sun also prevents sun bleach of a sleek and lustrous hair coat, giving a competitive advantage in the show ring.

If a horse suffers from a musculoskeletal injury requiring confinement for a lengthy period, a stall is instrumental in ensuring rest. A stall restricts movement, so bandages or limb casts stay clean and dry inside a well-bedded stall, hastening the healing process.

Some horses tend to self-destruct if left to run loose in a pasture or paddock. Nervous horses may unceasingly gallop a fence line, risking strain and exhaustion.

Mares in heat, or hormone-driven stallions may injure themselves or other horses during disputes across a pasture fence. Individuals that are too aggressive in the herd must be kept separate from other horses. For nervous or combative horses, housing within the quieting confines of a stall may prevent unnecessary mishaps. Dim indoor lighting and seclusion calms belligerent or nervous behavior.

Still other reasons induce us to stall our horses. A horse requiring a special diet can be fed appropriately without competition from a herd. Stalling a mare under lights during late winter or early spring hastens the onset of estrus so she can be bred earlier in the season. A mare due to foal is brought into a large foaling stall to provide a clean and sheltered environment that is easily monitored and safe from predators or dominant herd horses.

PSYCHOLOGICAL STRESS

What psychological stresses are imposed when we pull horses away from their social life, and isolate them? What happens when we remove access to grazing and movement by locking our horses inside a boxstall? They become dependent upon humans for feed, exercise, and companionship. Food may show up regularly two or more times a day, and in some cases free choice hay is available at all times. Yet, exercise and human companionship is only forthcoming for an hour or two a day.

For horses permanently stalled, 23 or 24 hours a day is a long time in which to do nothing, day after day. A lucky few have a door or window that opens to the outside, so they can stick their heads out the opening, and look at the world around them. Visual stimuli and sunlight are welcome diversions from overwhelming boredom. Horses provided with free choice hay have the luxury of fulfilling a ravishing need

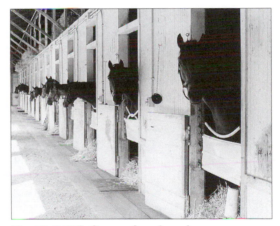

Fig. 20–3. Windows reduce boredom.

to chew fiber. But because a horse can only consume 2% – 3% of its body weight per day, it can only eat so much before becoming full of easily obtainable and highly nutritious hay. There is a lot of time left over for "hanging out" with no way to vent its pent-up energy.

Other stalled horses are fed a limited amount of hay twice a day, and may have no window or door through which to gaze upon the outside world. A belligerent horse or a stallion may be enclosed by metal bars or mesh fencing that prevents hanging a head out into the aisle of a barn.

Such horses experience no stimuli, no physical contact, and little or no exercise. Under such conditions, what do horses do?

Stall Vices

Not all horses fare well in the restrictive confinement of a stall. Removing a horse from a natural habitat (in which it could roam, graze, and interact within a herd) is an extreme form of stress. It is no wonder stall vices develop when a horse is confined.

A stall vice is a behavior developed as a result of stress. Once a behavioral pattern emerges, it is difficult to break the habit. If a problem is recognized in the beginning stages, measures can be taken immediately to alter the horse's environment. Initially, an unhappy horse may exhibit subtle behavioral changes while being saddled or ridden, or it may display uncharacteristic aggressive tendencies towards other horses or people. Ground manners may change, for example a horse may present a rear end as a person enters the stall, and lay its ears back in agitation. To a sensitive owner, such warning signals may be glaringly obvious, but the reason behind them can remain elusive.

Start by asking what has changed in a horse's routine, including:

- Has it been moved from a paddock to a stall?
- Is it stalled in a different location than before?
- Has a buddy horse left the premises, or a new arrival moved in next door?
- Have new employees assumed cleaning and feeding chores in the barn?
- Have feeding times been changed?
- Is the food quality different?
- Is it breeding season, a time that hormonally alters the behavior of mares and stallions?
- Have exercise levels changed?

If the horse could talk, it might say what is bugging it. In its own simple way, it is communicating distress by body language and mood. When people listen with all of their senses, they usually find the underlying cause.

Wood Chewing and Cribbing

Horses have a natural urge to chew. Wood chewers eat the insides of wooden stalls in an insatiable demand for fiber. It may also be due to boredom or lack of minerals. This behvior may result in splinters in the mouth. Swallowed splinters can lodge in the throat, or irritate or puncture an intestine, with serious consequences. Good quality pasture, and free-choice hay and salt will help prevent wood chewing.

Boredom may also spur a horse to latch its teeth onto an edge of the stall, a water container, or a feed bucket and swallow air. *Cribbing* is an incessant behavior pattern. It is speculated that cribbing activates narcotic receptors within the central nervous system, causing an addiction.

A horse that has been a cribber for very long can be identified by its teeth: the upper, front incisors are worn. They may also be hard keepers because they will turn away from food to nurture the habit. In addition, cribbers are predisposed to gaseous colic. *(See Chapter 13 for more information on colic.)* Cribbing can be controlled by feeding more often, providing more exercise and/or free time outside, or through the use of a neck brace, neck strap, or muzzle.

Abnormal Movement

Other stall vices are based on weird movement behavior, such as pacing, or weaving back and forth while standing in one place, remindful of the rocking motion used to calm an infant. Some horses dig holes of considerable depth in their stalls, while others kick at the walls with front or hind limbs, or both.

Stall Kicking

One of the more destructive stall vices is the habit of stall kicking. Not only does damage to a stall cost money to repair, but a horse can inflict serious damage upon itself. Splintered wooden walls and doors, bent metal components, and razor sharp edges result from damage to the structural integrity of the stall—and pose a serious hazard to a horse's vulnerable legs and face. If a door is kicked off its tracks or bent outward, a foot can get caught in a newly-made opening before the hazard is discovered.

The trauma on a horse's limbs as it kicks or paws at walls can strain or sprain ligaments, tendons, or muscles. Areas like the front of the knee *(carpus)*, fetlock, or back of the hock are particularly vulnerable to bruising and abrasion. Capped hocks or hygromas of the knee are caused by continuous trauma to bursal sacs underlying superficial

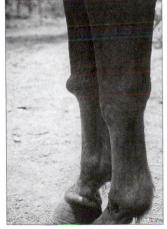

Fig. 20–4. A hygroma from constant stall kicking.

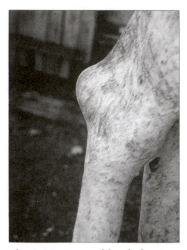

Fig. 20–5. Capped hock due to stall kicking.

tendons. Such blemishes are usually only of cosmetic significance, but if repeatedly aggravated, can develop into functional problems and impede performance.

Bruised muscle or connective tissue can develop serum or blood pockets, or an overwhelming inflammatory response known as *cellulitis*, which is accompanied by intense pain and swelling in the affected limb. Powerful impacts to the bottom of a foot as a horse kicks at a rigid wall can injure the coffin bone inside the hoof. The coffin bone can even fracture if an intense blow is sustained.

If a wooden structure is weakened by continual kicking, a solid impact can blow it apart, with a limb shooting through splintered wood. Serious lacerations can result.

Reasons for Stall Kicking

Anxiety and Frustration

What causes horses to kick or paw in a stall? Frustration at restriction of movement creates anxiety, leading to displacement activities like pawing and kicking. Transfer of pent-up energy also assumes the form of kicking or striking out at confining walls. If a horse sees other horses running at play, its frustration is intensified because it wants to join the frolicking herd.

Feeding Time

Some horses anticipate arrival of breakfast or dinner as soon as they spot the feeding person arrive at the barn. A horse displays an eager appetite by striking on a wall or door with its leg. What may start out as a small signal of impatience can escalate into an irrepressible habit.

Horses fed concentrated feed pellets finish their meal in less than an hour or two a day. Considering that in a range habitat, a horse intermittently grazes for about 16 hours a day, a stalled horse on a pelleted diet is remarkably bored. It may begin banging on the sides of its stall to get attention, or just to have something to do. This type of problem is readily resolved by feeding a grass hay diet to accommodate a need to chew roughage throughout the day.

Space and Relationships

Certain horses are extremely territorial about their space, and may be particular about a neighbor next door. Once pleasant relationships are established between horses, try to house them side-by-side. Keeping buddies in sight of each other reduces stress. Although they are unable to make physical contact, the visible presence of a buddy has a strong calming influence.

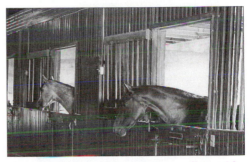

Fig. 20–6. Horses that get along well should be stalled next to each other.

Isolation Stress

Horses thrive with physical contact. A companionable horse who can not nuzzle and smell a neighbor by sticking its head out a door or over a partition may strike at the walls in frustration. Isolation for a normally social animal is a cause of anxiety. Individuals craving contact or companionship may relax with the introduction of a gentle goat or chicken, that lives in the stall with the horse. Herd relationships and bonding are established between a horse and any living creature. All it takes is a little imagination, and finding a suitable animal.

Loners

Certain horses prefer to be by themselves, perhaps because that is how they were raised and they are used to it. If a horse next door reaches toward the stall of a "loner," the loner horse may feel its space has been violated. In frustration and territorial intent, a loner horse kicks and strikes at an offending neighbor even if the friendly horse only glances its way.

New Surroundings

If a horse is moved to a new barn or is stabled at horse shows, not only are the surroundings new and different, but so are the other horses housed next to and across from it. Not all horse personalities get along in such enforced conditions, and the only separation may be a wooden partition with mesh fencing at the top. Feeling trapped and enclosed, a horse exhibits stress by striking at or kicking out at a neighbor. Walls of the stall take the brunt of the blows, but this activity may be the start of a terrible habit when a horse returns home.

Mares in heat, or stallions stalled next to stallions or cycling mares may pound on the walls from a breeding-related or physical dispute.

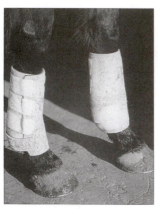

Fig. 20–7. Protective boots prevent injury.

Protection for Stall Kickers
Boots and Padding

Methods to protect a horse from wreaking physical damage to itself from stall kicking include armoring it with hock boots, fetlock boots, shin boots, or knee pads to protect these areas from trauma. Vinyl-covered foam padding on walls and doors reduces abrasions and trauma caused by striking a surface. Continual upkeep of padding is time-consuming and costly. Lining a stall with straw bales reduces the impact of hoof blows, but further limits the internal space within a stall, increasing a sense of claustrophobia and restriction of movement.

RELIEF FROM BOREDOM
Toys

Toys in a stall can relieve boredom and help prevent all types of stall vices. Hanging rubber or plastic balls give a horse something to bang or

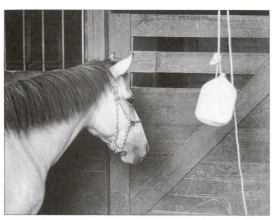

Fig. 20–8. A milk jug can be used as a stall toy.

chew on without risk of injury. Gallon water jugs can be hung from the rafters to create the same effect. Commercially available hanging plastic "apples" and "carrots" also serve as playthings for bored or restless horses.

Self-Exercise

When a horse is confined in a stall, it finds ways to wear off pent-up energy. Pacing, weaving, kicking, and pawing are all manifestations of a need to move. A horse that is stalled for most of the day should be allowed daily self-exercise in a large turn-out area or paddock. In this way it can vent its fire, buck and kick, and romp. If turn-out is not an option, then a stalled horse should be put on a "hot-walker" or hand walked for at least an hour per day. An occasional break in hand walking for a relaxing graze of fresh grass is also a benefit.

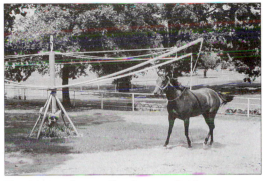

Fig. 20–9. A hot-walker is an outlet for energy.

Performance Exercise

Of course, the performance horse should be exercised properly for its particular event. However, calm easy riding occasionally in place of daily training helps to relieve stress. A horse should not feel that each time it is saddled it will be put under mental and/or physical pressure.

CHANGING THE ENVIRONMENT
Moving Outside

Along with exercise, perhaps the best cure for an anxious horse exhibiting stress behavior or a stall vice is to move it into the Great Outdoors. If possible, enlarge the spatial dimensions of an outdoor paddock relative to the previous size of its stall. Outside fence panels are used to restrict the area of movement if a horse is recuperating from an injury. Fresh air and sunshine, long distance views, and seeing other horses significantly calm a horse. Removing the restrictive walls of a

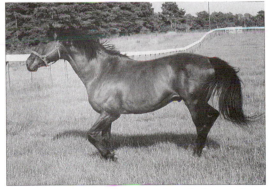

Fig. 20–10. Fresh air and sunshine help to calm a stressed horse.

stall also removes a rigid surface for a horse to kick.

Adjusting for Personality Conflicts

Recognizing personality conflicts between horses, and physically moving horses around until proper relationships are established reduces a horse's anxieties. It is also important to monitor how stable employees interact with a horse. An owner or trainer may find this interaction difficult to evaluate unless he or she arrives at the barn in time to watch reactions from the relationship. A horse may dislike a specific handler, groom, or helper. Anticipation at having to interact with a disliked person adds to a horse's stress level, with abnormal behaviors surfacing from underlying tension.

Changing Handlers or Location

If a once-happy horse starts stall vices or adverse behavioral patterns, it may be time to consider changing handlers or location. Possibly there is no specific reason for a horse's neurotic behavior other than a dislike of the surroundings or discomfort with a farm's routine. It may be worthwhile to move a distressed horse around on a property in an attempt to rule out certain neighboring animals, visual stimuli, noises, and physical locations before entirely moving a horse off the property.

Sometimes no matter where a horse is located on a particular farm, it remains stressed and unhappy. As soon as it is moved to a different facility, or to a new geographical location, it resumes a calm and quiet behavior by which the handlers have known it for years. Many of us can commiserate with specific geographical preferences. Most people at one time or another have personally encountered an uncomfortable situation. People exhibit spatial preferences; some people elect to sit on an aisle or in the back of a crowded auditorium, while others thrive in a crowd. In working environments, some people prefer a secluded cubby hole, and others want to be in the middle of the hubbub.

Horses are no different in seeking spatial arrangements to suit individual temperaments. Yet, their choices are limited by human arrangements of a limited land resource. By eliminating a natural, free-ranging habitat, people remove a horse's ability to seek its place in a geographical and social context. Placing walls around its restless spirit, and curbing its eating behavior to suit humans, reshape a horse's mental and physical state into something different from its natural predisposition.

Even within a restricted urban environment, people can listen to the message a horse conveys through its manners and actions. Fine tuning an environment and eliminating stresses channel a horse's energies into more useful applications than stall vices. Powers of concentration and learning abilities are improved in a happy horse, enabling it to give splendidly in athletic performance.

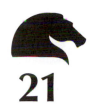
SAFE TRAVEL FOR THE EQUINE ATHLETE

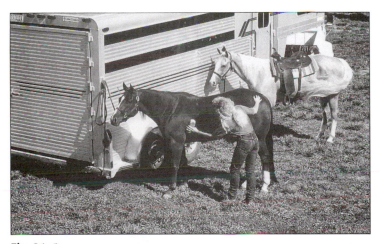

Fig. 21–1.

TRAVELING STRESS

For many people, traveling is stressful, upsetting the balance of every-day routine. Eating habits, sleeping patterns, and usual daily procedures are disturbed. When a horse's routine is disturbed, it may suffer from stress as well. However, the stresses on equine health can be minimized. Many studies provide useful information about how horses respond to long distance travel. Whether the horses are enclosed in a van, a trailer, or in a cargo hold on an airplane, they are a large animal confined within a small metal tube. Such confinement leads to both mental and physical stress. Even in this era of supertechnology, 6% of horses transported long distances become seriously ill. Records from the turn of the century reveal similar figures, indicating that in almost 100 years there has not been much reduction in life-threatening illness from transport stress.

Effects of Traveling Stress

Colic

Similar to people, horses are creatures of habit. They are happiest when familiar events occur each day on a consistent routine. It is known that feeding horses on a regular time schedule benefits intestinal health. When a horse expects a meal to appear, its stomach juices and saliva production increase. If the meal fails to arrive, the effects on a sensitive metabolism can cause gaseous colic because the body was geared up for an event that did not happen. Travelling stress can also cause intestinal upset and colic.

Monitoring the Long Distance Traveler

In one study of horses traveling by airplane half-way around the globe, specific health indicators such as heart rates were evaluated. Researchers hoped to find a way to monitor horses transported long distances. By using the information obtained from the airplane study, horse owners or trainers can minimize stress on traveling horses, and provide healthier conditions while a horse is in transit.

Increased Heart Rate

Fright is a form of stress and it can be evaluated by monitoring a horse's heart rate. On a long distance air flight of over 27 hours, horses' heart rates that averaged 52 beats per minute (bpm) before movement soared to 162 bpm at the first take-off. The average heart rate at the second take-off was 152 bpm, while the third resulted in heart rates averaging 130 bpm.

These results resemble the effect of conditioning—the horses gained experience and responded more favorably to each repetition of the experience. Conditioning horses to travel in a confined space, like a horse trailer, similarly diminishes stress from fear and anxiety.

Suppressed Immune System

Fear or stress increases the circulation of *cortisol* produced by the body. For a short trip, the cortisol response is minimal, but cortisol levels rise with longer transport, because the horse is under increased stress. Cortisol has an adverse impact on the immune system.

Transportation within a short distance causes no change in a horse's immune status. However, when horses travel long distances, the immune system is compromised. It cannot efficiently respond to challenge from microorganisms.

A study at Washington State University showed that horses traveling 700 miles over a 36-hour period had a depressed immune response. Not only is there a reduction in numbers of white blood cells to scavenge harmful microorganisms, but they are less effective at it. This suppression of the immune response predisposes a horse to infections.

Weight Loss

Another parameter that gives invaluable insight into transport stress of an individual horse is its body weight before and after transport. Within 12 hours, normal horses lose up to 33 pounds, or about 3% of body weight. Some of this weight loss is caused by varying degrees of dehydration. Horses that develop shipping fever lose about 51 pounds. The correlation of weight loss with development of infection is significant. Weighing horses before and after a long trip is useful for deciding if preventative care should be initiated.

Respiratory Disease

Environmental factors also have a profound effect on infection rates in horses. For example, as an airplane is in motion, air exchange occurs three times each minute. Air exchange greatly reduces the bacterial contamination of the environment, although continued environmental exposure to manure and urine eventually heightens bacterial counts. The number of colony forming units (cfu), both bacterial and fungal, number around 200 on a plane in flight. More than 5,000 cfu flourish when an airplane is stationary and loaded with horses.

Not only do the number of microorganisms increase when a plane is stationary, but temperature and relative humidity also are affected. In flight, temperature remains around 64° F. When a plane sits on the ground with long delays, the airline is only responsible for keeping the temperature between 45° – 85° F. Relative humidity escalates from an acceptable 47% while in flight to 90% when on the ground.

High temperature and humidity promote bacterial and fungal growth, increasing exposure of the lungs to microbes. Coupling these factors with a suppressed immune system due to stress develops a situation ripe for disease, particularly of the respiratory tract.

The greatest cause of loss in performance from illness or death is due to complications from respiratory disease, such as *pleuropneumonia* or *pleurisy*. Over 52% of "shipping fever" related illnesses occur *after* a horse arrives at its destination.

Elevated White Blood Cell Count

Before and after transit, blood samples are useful to evaluate impending infection. Cellular counts for horses that remain in good health have been compared to those that develop shipping fever. After transport, white blood cells do not elevate in normal horses, whereas within 2 days of arrival, horses developing shipping fever show an increase in total white blood cells.

Pre-Existing Respiratory Disease

Pre-existing respiratory disease predisposes a horse to serious respiratory disease from transit stress. In a horse with a pre-existing

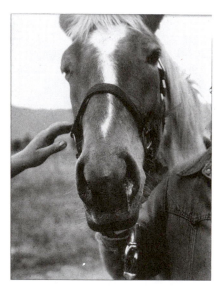

Fig. 21–2. Nasal discharge is a symptom of respiratory disease.

respiratory disease, the normal airway clearance mechanisms (such as coughing) are overwhelmed by increased temperature and humidity. A horse experiences more stress on its journey due to an overwhelming exposure to microorganisms, dehydration (correlated to weight loss), and delays in transit that prevent adequate air circulation and quality. These factors tip the scale of health and disease towards development of disease.

The best way to manage a traveling horse is to minimize stress. Common sense and humane practices during long distance transport of horses will improve the standards of health for equine travelers. Although a horse may not appear sick upon arrival to a far off destination, performance may suffer slightly, removing the winning edge in a competition. Careful monitoring of attitude, rectal temperature, body weight, and feed and water consumption can detect problems early on.

LONG DISTANCE TRAVEL PREPARATION

Although few horses are subjected to long distance air transport, similar principles can be applied to long distance travel between states. With competitions or breeding farms spaced thousands of miles away, multiple-day trailer trips are not uncommon. Certain steps can be taken to promote a more stress-free journey, and to control the continued health of the horses so they arrive in the best shape.

Physical Exam

A careful evaluation of each horse before shipment is of primary importance. Every state requires a health certificate for interstate transport. However, many states allow a 2 – 4 week lead-time during which a health certificate can be obtained. Health certificates are meant to screen out horses that are carrying a transmissible disease, such as lice, fungal dermatitis, *vesicular stomatitis* (caused by a virus), or viral respiratory illness, to name a few. Yet, a health certificate is also a safety precaution to identify a marginally or overtly sick horse that is about to be transported.

Not all illnesses are identified at the time of health inspection because there is an incubation period during which a horse is infected with disease, but has not developed clinical symptoms. Some horses will slip through even the most arduous screening process. However, careful examination of a horse just before transport improves the possibility of discovering a marginally ill horse.

With the additional stress of shipping, what may have normally developed into a mild upper respiratory viral infection can become sudden, severe pneumonia, leading to permanent respiratory damage or death. It is to a horse's advantage to be examined within several days of transport, rather than a protracted 2 – 4 weeks before. Even if a second veterinary visit is required so the necessary Coggins test (for Equine Infectious Anemia) paperwork is available in time for shipping, it is worth the extra trip.

Brand Inspection

Check with the state brand inspector to establish local laws pertaining to traveling away from home with a horse. Often a brand inspection is required for horses moving distances greater than 75 miles. A permanent brand inspection card can be issued that is legal for the horse's lifetime unless it is sold to a new owner. Each time a horse is purchased a new brand inspection must be obtained by providing proof of transfer of ownership.

Vaccinations

The vaccination status of a horse should be current and appropriate not only for the environment from which the horse originates, but for where it is going. To develop an adequate immune response to viral respiratory vaccines, boosters should be administered at least 2 weeks before travel. A veterinarian can administer vaccines at this time and obtain a blood sample for a Coggins test during the same visit. Then the next visit for a general physical exam and health certificate is scheduled for just a few days before a horse is expected to leave.

Unnecessary Antibiotics

Resist the impulse to start a horse on a preventative course of antibiotics before long distance travel. The problems that most commonly confront travelling horses stem from respiratory *viruses* for which there is no direct treatment; they must run their course. Yet once a viral infection is identified and diagnosed, a course of antibiotics may prevent bacterial infections that lead to pneumonia.

It used to be standard practice to give a horse a one-time injection of procaine penicillin just before shipping. This practice encourages development of bacterial resistance to antibiotics. A single injection does not instill a high blood level of antibiotic in the horse, nor does it persist long enough to effectively kill bacteria. There is no point in a single injection, and this practice should be discontinued.

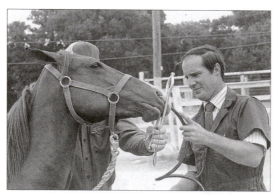

Fig. 21–3. Mineral oil minimizes gas build-up which can lead to colic or laminitis.

Mineral Oil

A horse that is a nervous traveler, and going a long distance, may benefit from a stomach tubing with a gallon of mineral oil just before departure. Mineral oil serves as a laxative to sustain intestinal motility, and it diminishes the build-up of gas within a nervous or stagnant bowel. Mineral oil also prevents absorption of endotoxin from the gut that can cause laminitis. Incidence of colic and associated laminitis are reduced by this practice, but only flighty individuals going long distances need mineral oil.

Maintain Air Quality

The environment in which a horse travels is of utmost importance to respiratory health. Good air quality and adequate ventilation are essential to keep temperature and relative humidity at safe levels. For horses hauled in trailers, exhaust pipes should be directed away from the intake air for the horses.

If a trailer or van stops moving for long periods, particularly in the summer, open the doors to allow circulation of fresh air through the horse stalls, or unload the horses and tie them outside. During stops, clean urine-soaked bedding and manure out of the trailer. Cleaning the area decreases bacterial and fungal contamination so numbers of microorganisms remain below an infective threshold.

Avoid long delays at international border crossings, ferry connections (found in parts of the United States and Canada), and at refueling stops. The longer horses are kept in a small, enclosed space with limited air circulation, the more the temperature and humidity rise, and the greater the exposure to microorganisms that challenge the respiratory tract.

Dust-Free Feeding

Always clean the mangers of stale hay and dust, and restock them with fresh, non-dusty hay. Fungal spores circulating in a trailer are decreased even more by providing vacuum-cleaned hay.

For respiratory tract clearance, horses should not be tied with their heads up high. If hay nets are tied low enough to encourage safe, head-down feeding, they allow small particles to fall down, away from a horse's airways. Nets should not be affixed so low that a horse can get a leg entangled in them.

Water and Electrolytes

Water should be offered at rest stops, at least every 4 hours. Electrolytes can be provided by oral paste or free choice to improve gastrointestinal function, and to stimulate natural thirst. Horses that do not drink strange water are at risk of serious dehydration. It is sometimes helpful to bring 5 – 10 gallons of water along from home.

Provide Companionship

To further minimize the stress of trailering, some horses settle into a better routine if accompanied by a calm equine companion experienced in such trips. The more times a horse undergoes an experience, provided it has not been alarmed or frightened, the more it is conditioned to traveling, and the less stress response it exhibits. Its immune system functions more efficiently, and is more capable of warding off the challenge of infection.

Traveling Backwards

Research at Texas A & M determined that the direction a horse faces is a more important factor than the distance traveled. Considerable muscular effort is required to retain balance while in motion. Horses that travel *facing the rear* of a trailer or transport vehicle are less affected by transit stress than are horses that are confined facing forward. In journeys farther than about 20 miles, analysis of blood samples shows an increase in muscle enzymes, reflecting the physical work that is required by a horse to maintain balance. A horse facing forward is unable to optimally use its hindquarters to diffuse the sway. By facing rearwards as a trailer, van, aircraft, or boat travels with jerky starts and hesitations, a horse easily shifts its weight to the haunches and maintains its balance with less effort.

PROTECTIVE BANDAGES

Whether or not to put leg wraps on a horse is a heated controversy, however from a veterinarian's point of view, horses wearing proper shipping bandages are rarely seen for trailer-inflicted injuries.

No matter how well a horse loads or rides, anything can happen. Suppose an adjacent horse with iron shoes loses its balance and steps on the horse's leg. Or, a horse can step on its own legs as it scrambles in the trailer due to sudden braking or a sharp curve.

Loading and unloading is the most dangerous time for legs. Trailer wraps provide a barrier between metal and flesh, and ground and flesh, particularly when loading or unloading a fractious, resistant horse. Moreover, if the flooring or ground is damp, a horse can slip and catch a leg on a ramp or on another limb, or a leg can slide underneath a step-up trailer.

Backing off a ramp is a shaky experience for a nervous or inexperienced horse. A leg can slip off the ramp, and with a convulsive jerk to regain footing, the horse can lacerate its leg on a sharp edge. If a foot wedges under the ramp, self-inflicted wounds or fractured limbs can result as a horse struggles to free its entrapped leg.

Some horses explode backwards when asked to load. If not armored with leg wraps, skidding across the pavement or gravel abrades and cuts thin skin.

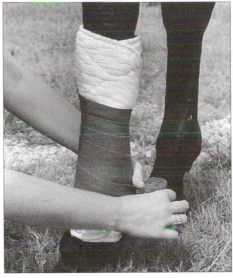

Fig. 21–4. Proper bandaging protects the legs from cuts and bruises.

Shipping Boots

There are many ways to apply shipping boots and bandages. It is important to cover the heel bulbs and pasterns as these areas are most likely to be injured. Wrapping the tendons and cannons is a good start, but if the bandages do not extend low enough, using bell boots will protect the heel bulbs. Then, a hind foot cannot lacerate a front limb.

Fleece-lined shipping boots with velcro closures take only moments to apply to all four legs although they are not as substantial as wrapping the legs with cotton quilting and "track bandages." Thick batting under the bandages pads the legs and is secured snugly into place, keeping the wraps from slipping.

For a short trip or in an emergency, use disposable diapers or cotton pads under an ace bandage. Be careful not to pull the ace bandage too tight or it will constrict the tendons.

Head Bumper and Tail Wrap

A head bumper protects the poll of a fractious horse in case it rears up and hits its head on the edge or top of the trailer.

A tail wrap prevents abrasion at the dock that can rub a horse's tail down to raw flesh. Commonly used are commercial neoprene tail bandages, or a track wrap or polo fleece. Be sure the tail wrap is not applied so tightly as to constrict blood flow through the tail, and not so loosely that it slips and falls off.

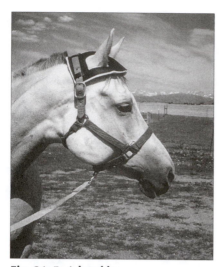

Fig. 21–5. A head bumper.

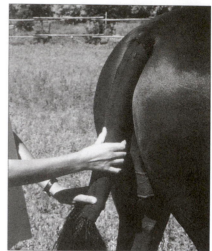

Fig. 21–6. A neoprene tail wrap.

Another way to protect the tail from rubbing on the door or butt bar is to fasten thick foam padding with duct tape over the butt chain. Also, place the horse's tail inside the trailer so it is not hanging loose and flying in the breeze. The tail can hook on a protrusion, frightening and seriously injuring the horse.

Bandaging the horse will probably take 20 minutes the first few times. With practice the whole exercise consumes no more than 5 minutes and may save the horse from a crippling injury. At the very least those few extra minutes may save on expenses for veterinary care, emotional hassle, and time nursing an injured horse.

SAFETY MEASURES
Training

A horse that is inexperienced in trailering can be conditioned to load and ride with a sense of confidence. Taking the time to accustom the horse to load and unload quietly minimizes injuries, and makes a more pleasureable experience for all. This conditioning can be accomplished by practicing loading and unloading with an experienced horse already in the trailer. Or, the novice horse can be fed in the trailer to give it a positive experience.

Once the horse confidently enters and backs out on command, take it on short rides to accustom it to the feel of movement. Again, a calm companion horse instills confidence into the learner. Longer trailer rides are introduced after the horse is conditioned to travel quietly. Each positive experience reinforces excellent trailering behavior.

Keep Doors Closed

Once a horse is loaded, a common mistake is to leave manger or escape doors open so the horse can look around while waiting to depart. This practice results in face and head lacerations and eye injuries. It only takes a spooky monster such as flying paper or a tractor driving by to cause a horse to jerk its head back through the open hatch. Occasionally a horse catches its head on a low door sill, which not only cuts the head, but panics it further.

The lesson here is simple. A horse spends most of its life with the freedom to look at the world around it. A few more minutes of gazing from the inside of a trailer is not worth the potential hazard. Close the manger and escape doors as soon as the horse is in the trailer.

Some horses are terrified of being in the trailer and an open manger or escape door is perceived as an escape route. For such individuals, these doors should be closed even before the horse is loaded in the trailer.

Tying the Horse in the Trailer

It is best to tie the head to the manger loop, or to an overhead tie loop. A horse with its head free in the trailer may try to turn around. The horse is then tightly wedged in a potentially life-threatening position.

A frightened horse without its head tied can also launch itself into the feeder. A poor traveler can inflict leg injuries to itself, and once it finds its front leg and head tightly wedged in the feeder, it is no longer a mildly reasonable animal.

When tying a horse's head, give it enough rope that it can comfortably move its head side-to-side, but cannot turn it backwards. The rope should not be so long that it can tangle in a leg or wrap around the head.

Commercially available "quick-release" snaps are the ideal way to tie a horse. The snap is easily released in an emergency with a quick snap of the special buckle, and it is difficult to snare fingers in the safety snap.

Always attach the butt bar or butt chain and close the door before tying a horse, and when unloading, always untie a horse before opening the trailer. A horse that is prone to bolting backwards can quickly pull on a lead rope, causing numerous problems.

A Butt Bar or Chain

A butt bar or butt chain adds a stop-gap for the unwelcome possibility that the back door of a trailer might fly open while it is moving. These

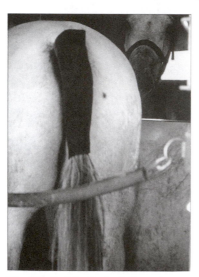

doors are known to fly open for a number of reasons, namely the loosening of bolts that hold down the door handles. Road vibration works nuts and bolts loose over time, so these areas should be inspected frequently. A horse kicking at the trailer door can kick it open with explosive force.

A butt bar or chain may keep the horse inside the trailer long enough for a flapping rear trailer door to be discovered. Also, it prevents a horse from leaning on the back door. A thousand pounds (or more) of weight pushing on the door weakens the hinges and door bolts over time, creating conditions for potential mishaps.

Fig. 21–7. A butt chain is an important safety device.

First Aid Kit

Whenever it is necessary to journey away from home with horses, take along a first aid kit expressly for them. The following list is a good starting place from which to build such a kit. A veterinarian may add to these supplies and provide information on how best to use them.

- Table salt and a clean container: mix 1 tablespoon salt per quart of water for saline rinse
- Tamed iodine antiseptic scrub
- Sterile gauze sponges
- Broad spectrum topical antibiotic ointment such as Silvadene® or Neosporin®
- Sterile Telfa® or Surgipad®
- Conforming roll gauze (Kling®)
- Elastikon® bandage (self-adhesive stretch tape)
- Bandage scissors
- Optional: broad spectrum oral antibiotic tablets
- Non-steroidal eye ointment for injury from branches, wind, dirt

- Easy Boot® in case a shoe is lost
- Thermometer

While on a long distance trip it is a good idea to stop every 3 – 4 hours to check on the state of affairs in the horse trailer, and to offer the horses fresh water. It is hard work for some horses to ride in a trailer, as they struggle to stay balanced through the twists and turns of the road, and the sway of the trailer. A half-hour rest stop allows horses to relax taut muscles while remaining tied in the trailer.

Recovery Time

Once a horse arrives at its destination after a long journey, monitor body temperature twice a day. A fever often develops 2 – 3 days after arrival in horses that have contracted an infection. With prompt diagnosis, aggressive therapy can dramatically alter the duration and severity of a disease. The faster a problem is recognized, the more quickly a horse responds to treatment, and the more likely that permanent effects will be prevented.

People expect their equine companions to understand where they are going, what is expected from them, and to immediately go to work upon demand. However, it is advantageous to plan a few extra days at the end of a journey to allow a horse to acclimate to a new environment, and to recover from the stress of transit.

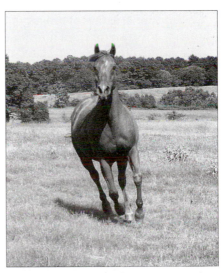

Fig. 21–8. Rest and relaxation is good for a horse after a long trip.

TRANSPORTING BROODMARES

Another performance horse besides the athlete is the broodmare that is transported to the breeding farm and back home again. After all the effort required to get a mare in foal, it is a shame to lose a fetus to the effects of transit stress. The greatest incidence of early embryonic death (EED) before 50 days of gestation occurs between days 15 – 20 and days 30 – 35.

A study at Colorado State University analyzed the effects of trailering on newly pregnant mares. During days 14 – 18, the mare's body must recognize the embryo for it to survive. Once it has passed this obstacle, at day 35 the embryo firmly implants in the uterus, and endometrial cups form to secrete progesterone hormones, which maintains the pregnancy.

There were 3 groups of mares studied. The 24 pregnant "control" mares remained at home between days 16 – 33 and had free access to food and water. A second group of 15 pregnant mares was trailered between days 16 – 22 of gestation for a 9-hour ride with no food or water. A third group of 15 pregnant mares experienced a similar 9-hour trailer journey between days 32 – 38 of gestation.

Hormonal assays of progesterone and cortisol were obtained on each mare. Progesterone is a hormone necessary to maintain pregnancy, and low levels are highly correlated to early embryonic death. Progesterone concentrations increased in the two groups of trailered mares as compared to the controls left at home, and progesterone levels in Groups 2 and 3 remained higher for a time upon return to the farm.

Of the 24 control mares, 3 lost their embryos. Another 3 of the 15 mares that were trailered between days 16 – 22 lost their embryos, and 1 of 15 mares trailered between days 32 – 38 lost her embryo. Therefore, there was no real statistical difference between any group of mares in this study. The mares that did abort started with lower progesterone levels, which may explain the loss of the embryo.

The study concluded that trailering mares during a critical time between days 16 – 33 has no influence on maintenance of pregnancy, and that transportation at that time poses a minimal risk for pregnant mares.

Endotoxin Study

Another study conducted at the University of California at Davis surveyed a different slant on early embryonic death. If a mare experiences any surge in endotoxin release before day 50 of gestation, endotoxin stimulates release of prostaglandin F_2-alpha. This particular prostaglandin interferes with function of the *corpus luteum* on the ovary that is responsible for progesterone secretion until about day 50 of gestation. By day 50, progesterone is secreted from other sources to maintain a high enough level for pregnancy to persist.

Endotoxin release accompanies stress-related syndromes such as colic, diarrhea, or other gastrointestinal disorders. It is of prime importance, then, that early term pregnant mares trailered for long distances receive ample food, water, and electrolytes while on their journey. This practice minimizes intestinal compromise that results in endotoxins.

Progesterone Supplements

To minimize the risk of early embryonic death from endotoxin in an early term pregnant mare during transport, the mare can be placed on a supplemental source of progesterone, such as Regumate®. This supplement is fed daily until day 50 or 60 of pregnancy. Oral Regumate® provides ample progesterone to maintain pregnancy even if the function of the corpus luteum is compromised by stress-induced endotoxin release.

BASIC TRAILERING TIPS

It is wise to have an RV mechanic do a complete check and maintenance on the trailer every year. Then, before every trip, running through the checklist and inspecting the mechanical features of electrical connections, brakes, tires, hitch, and bumper takes only a few minutes.

Always check the connections between the truck and trailer:

- ensure that the trailer ball is the right size
- make sure that locking pins are secure
- safety chains or cables should be strong enough to hold the trailer if the hitch comes off the ball
- check that the trailer ball is bolted on properly
- be sure the bumper is strong enough to pull the trailer, and that it is securely affixed to the truck frame with strong welds and/or stout bolts

Check the electrical connections, making sure the plug fits the socket and that the wiring is correct. When driving in the mountains, electric trailer brakes reduce wear-and-tear on the truck brakes and provide full braking power if needed.

Check the tire pressure of all tires (truck and trailer). Fully inflating tires to manufacturer's recommendations also reduces tire wear, and achieves the maximum gas mileage for the vehicle by reducing road friction. Take along spare tires (and a jack and lug wrench), for the truck and trailer.

When horse trailers are manufactured, often there is no safe place to affix a license plate. A common site for a license plate is just behind the back of a fender where it sticks out. In this position, the license plate can cut a horse on the lower leg if the horse paws or moves sideways. License plates are extremely sharp and easily cut through skin and tendons causing irreparable damage. Also, long lead lines can catch on the protrusion.

Mounting a license plate in a bracket with dull edges does not solve the problem. A horse still can catch a protruding edge, startling itself into injury to the face or legs. The problem is remedied by affixing the license plate on the back door of the trailer with or without a bracket. If fit flush with the door, no sharp projections offer any danger, while the license plate is still visible for legal purposes. As a temporary alternative, remove the license plate while the horse is tied to the trailer.

Clean out the trailer after every ride to remove manure and urine-soaked bedding and debris. Also pull out the trailer mats to allow the floor boards underneath to dry. Constant exposure to wet manure and urine inevitably rots the floor boards. Pulling up the mats and sweeping or hosing out the soiled bedding prolongs the life of the flooring and allows it to be inspected for weakness or rot.

The mangers should be swept clean after each trip. Otherwise, hay and grain will accumulate and mildew. Since most mangers are at nose level, mold spores and hay dust are inhaled into a horse's respiratory tract, possibly stimulating an allergic reaction and respiratory disease. Problems develop when a trailer is tightly enclosed without air exchange, or when a breeze stirs up dust from the manger.

Using a Trailer As a Hitching Post

It is often convenient to use the horse trailer as a hitching post. At a horse show, trailers may need to be parked on a treeless lot, leaving little choice where to tie a horse. At an endurance or competitive trail ride, horses are restrained next to a trailer off and on for several days during the course of a competition. While camping in many of the National Forests and National Parks, it is illegal to tie a horse to a tree or to permit the horse to graze on native forage. Because of such provisions or ecological laws, a trailer becomes the sole means of confinement. It is important for the trailer to have similar safety features as a stall, paddock, or pasture.

After parking and before opening the trailer doors, survey the area. It should be flat and free from dangerous obstacles all around. If the trailer is parked too close to an embankment the horse will be standing on an incline. Watch out for dangling overhead tree branches the horse might get tangled in.

If possible, analyze the direction the sun will travel through the sky, so the trailer will not receive too much sunlight during the day. Park so that horses are tied in the shade of a trailer to provide relief from direct sunlight.

Once the rig is parked, place some hefty rocks or wooden blocks in front and in back of a couple of tires as insurance that the trailer will not move.

Remember to untie the horse's head before releasing the butt bar or chain, so there will be no accidental bolting backwards while a horse is still tied. If more than one horse is along for the ride, it is always a good idea to unload a green horse first so it is not left behind as its companions are removed to the side of a trailer out of sight. If an inexperienced or nervous horse is left until last, it might work itself into a frenzy. It may paw vigorously to be let out, or strain on the butt bar, making it difficult to unload.

Unhitching the Trailer

When using a trailer as a hitching post, *never* disconnect a trailer from the truck. A frightened horse can easily pull an unhitched trailer which further panics the horse. Leaving a rig hooked up and placing rocks or wood blocks behind tires prevents these disasters. All doors and ramps should be closed before tying a horse to the trailer. An open manger, escape, or tack compartment door invites injury to a horse's face or legs. Usually these doors have sharp edges capable of lacerating the horse, so it is best to close them. Back doors or ramps should also be closed if a horse is tied near them. Some horses will try to load themselves, leading to a very tangled and frightened animal.

Safe Tying Methods

Tying two or more horses randomly to a trailer causes many problems. Only compatible horses should be tied side-by-side to prevent unruly behavior and potential injury. It is important to discourage conflicts between horses outside the trailer.

Lead ropes should be short enough so a horse will not entangle its leg or head, or its buckets in the line, but long enough that it can comfortably reach hay and water. A horse should have just enough lead to move side-to-side so it is not stuck in one spot. Excessively long lead lines can catch on the door of many trailers. Tie horses away from door handles to prevent a rope from getting caught. A tennis ball that has been cut open and placed over the door handle also prevents snagging of a lead rope.

To attach a lead rope onto the tie-in spot on a trailer, tie a quick-release safety knot that pulls loose with a swift tug on the dangling end in case of an emergency. Safety knots do not always pull free if a frightened horse heaves back on the line and tightens the knot. As an alternative, quick-release buckles, as used to tie a horse in the trailer, provide a safer way to fasten a halter buckle and a better guarantee of effective release.

Carry a sharp pocket knife at all times to cut a rope if a knot is too tight to release. A panicked and entangled horse does itself considerable damage if left to struggle for too long. A pocket knife quickly frees the horse from entrapment without endangering humans.

Caring for the Tied Horse

Feeding and Watering

Before attending to personal needs, set up hay nets and water buckets for each horse. Do not hang a hay bag or net too low or a horse can get tangled in it. Since a fair amount of hay generally falls out of a hay net onto the ground, be sure lead ropes are not so long that an unattended horse is tempted to rescue stray hay pieces off the ground. A long rope that is wound around a leg can cause serious physical damage. Too long a rope also allows a horse's head to lower where a halter can catch on a fender or other projection, resulting in fright and injury.

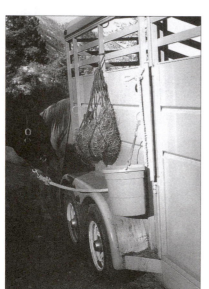

Fig. 21–9. A rope caught around a water bucket can create a problem.

Plastic or rubber water buckets are easily hung from a trailer using chains or nylon ropes with quick-release buckles. Buckets so suspended should be no lower than the horse's shoulder height so it has easy access to water or grain without snagging a rope around the bucket. A rope tangled with a bucket dumps out the contents and shortens a horse's line, possibly scaring it into an unpredictable reaction.

Water should be available at all times so a horse does not become dehydrated. Water is essential for muscular work and digestive processes. An average horse drinks 7 – 20 gallons each day, depending upon climate and exercise. Refills of fresh, clean water encourage adequate water intake to prevent colic, tying-up, or heat stress.

Some horses are finicky about strange water supplies, and subsequently do not drink well. Lightly treating water with cider vinegar or sugar disguises the strange taste, making the water more palatable. This trick is especially effective if a horse is conditioned to vinegar or sugar in the drinking water back home before the trip. Or, familiar water from home can be brought along for a finicky horse.

Electrolytes

It is difficult to provide free choice salt blocks to horses tied to a trailer. Supplementing with 1 – 2 tablespoons of a salt mixture in grain each day of the journey replaces essential electrolytes lost in sweat. This factor is particularly important if a horse is used for rigorous athletics or if subjected to high temperatures or humidity. A good mixture is produced by mixing one part potassium chloride (Lite® salt) with two parts sodium chloride (table salt). When supplementing a diet with salt in this manner, it is important that the horse is drinking well.

Blanketing

When horses are tied to a trailer for extended periods, they are unable to move about to warm muscles and maintain suppleness of tendons and ligaments. If night air is cold or breezy, it might be advantageous to blanket the horse, with either a sheet or heavier blanket appropriate for the weather. Blanketing keeps muscles warm, and provides a windbreak, if no shelter is provided by the trailer. If a horse has an ample hair coat and is used to the rigors of the environment, it may not be necessary to blanket. In the event of a driving rain or hail storm, horses can be loaded briefly into the trailer for respite from the elements. A horse that has exerted a tremendous athletic effort during an endurance or long distance competition may also benefit from a protective sheet or blanket to retain warmth in the muscles.

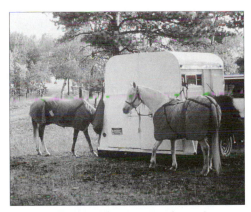

Fig. 21–10. A tied horse in cool weather should be blanketed to keep muscles warm.

Horses do not need to lie down in order to sleep. A unique anatomical arrangement called the *check apparatus* "locks up" the legs and keeps them from buckling as a horse sleeps. It is less dangerous to keep a horse tied so that it cannot lie down, than to lengthen its lead. If it has enough length of rope to lie down, it can also get entangled in it.

Hand Walking

It is more important than usual to adequately warm-up and cooldown any horse engaging in exercise after and before being tied to a trailer for a long period. Warm-up and cool-down time loosens kinked joints, tendons, ligaments, and muscles, providing circulation to adequately oxygenate tissues and remove toxic by-products. Suppleness improves as does performance, and tissue strain and fatigue is lessened.

A horse cannot move about at will when tied. Hand walk it at intervals after a day's athletics. Walking removes accumulated toxic by-products from muscle tissue, and improves circulation in the limbs so windpuffs do not develop overnight.

Alternatives to Tying

If it is unknown whether an inexperienced horse has been trained to tie for long periods, consider what it might do if startled. Depending on how they were trained, not all horses are excellent candidates for tying to anything. Some horses explosively fight such restraint when they discover they cannot get loose. Other horses have learned that if they pull hard enough, the rope or halter will break, freeing them completely.

If a flighty or devious horse lunges backwards with a violent tug on a lead line, considerable damage can be done. Not only will a horse endanger itself as it sits back on its haunches, threatening muscle strain from the effort, but stretching its head and neck can also result in injury. If a rope or halter breaks at this moment, a pulling horse can catapult backwards into another object or horse, or it can flip or fall down with impact. Serious injury to head or limbs may occur from such behavior.

Bring along a spare halter and lead rope in case they are damaged or broken. It is a serious inconvenience if this equipment is lacking.

Even a well-behaved horse is frightened if a stirrup iron, saddle, or other piece of tack snags on trailer fenders. Never leave a tacked horse unattended while tied next to a trailer. Dangling martingales, tie-downs, breast collars, stirrup leathers, and reins should be removed if someone cannot watch the horse.

When ill-behaved or frightened horses pull and fight being tied, other horses tied to the trailer are frightened as it rocks and vibrates.

Temporary Corral

There is a solution to the problem of confining a horse that has not been trained well and poses a danger to itself and others. Build a temporary corral out of fence panels, or PVC pipe. Fence panels, strapped to the side of the trailer for transport, are cumbersome, expensive, and time-consuming to assemble. Yet, they provide a safe solution to the problem. Rope can be used to fashion a "corral," however it is not as secure and can loosen or droop, inviting a horse to jump out.

If there is more than one trailer on a journey, a small holding corral can be fashioned by rigging panels, plastic pipe, or rope between the sides of the two trailers. A horse can move around freely, and lie down at will. Feed and water buckets are placed on the ground if desired or hung from the side of the trailer. Trailer fenders should be covered with chrome or rubber protector strips so the horse cannot cut itself. Remove the halter so the horse cannot snag it on anything.

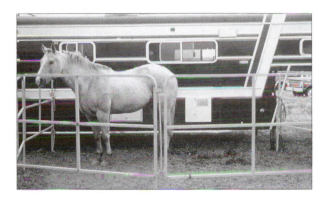

Fig. 21–11. Temporary corrals made of fence panels are a safe solution to confining horses while on the road.

If there are no other large vehicles or trailers to build a holding pen, another option is to purchase commercially available electric fence chargers that operate on solar power. These can create a temporary holding pen using fence stakes and electric wire. If remaining in one spot for a while, it may be necessary to build such an enclosure.

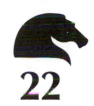

22

PREPURCHASE EVALUATION

SELECTION CRITERIA

Certain criteria should be considered when choosing a horse. Because demands on an athletic horse are so varied, some characteristics will be more important than others. Each horse must be judged according to its own merits.

Consult a trainer or reputable horseperson for an educated opinion about a horse's capabilities and level of training. A determined screening process weeds out candidates that, despite being fabulous horses, may not be athletic enough for the required tasks. A testing period also reveals horses that are soured to a specific athletic endeavor due to negative experiences.

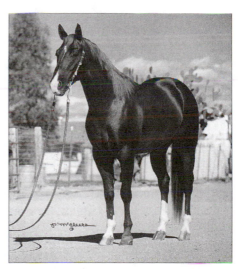

Fig. 22–1. Each horse should be judged on its own merits and the buyer's goals.

Age

An important consideration when purchasing a horse is its age. A young and green horse must be brought slowly through the ranks and schooled at the basics. Due to the rigorous demands of certain athletic pursuits and the differences in breed maturity, some horses should be allowed to mature to at least 5 years of age. This time allows for musculoskeletal maturity and development of mental concentration.

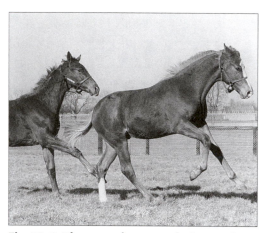

Fig. 22–2. The young horse needs time to develop musculoskeletal and mental agility.

There is always a beginning when every horse *and* rider is in the basic stages of learning. A novice rider should consider purchasing an experienced horse that can perform the intended task without compromising the safety of the rider.

An older horse, although initially lacking experience in a specific sport, usually is able to learn faster due to prior achievements. Physical maturity also provides the horse with the strength and stamina necessary for training and competing. A mature horse can be entered into a higher level of competition sooner than a youngster, provided it has mastered the basics of training. Of course if a horse is much older when beginning a performance sport, it may arrive at advanced levels too old to remain actively competitive.

Breed

Some breeds are genetically predisposed to excellence in certain athletic pursuits. The Arabian is bred for endurance and long distance competitive races. The Thoroughbred's speed makes it exceptional on the racetrack or as an event horse. The strong hindquarters of the Quarter Horse, Paint, or Appaloosa promotes their popularity in sprint sports like racing, cutting, barrel racing, and roping. The Standardbred displays exceptional speed at trotting and pacing. Warmbloods shine in dressage, jumping, eventing, and combined driving. Yet, there are horses with natural athletic talent which allows them to rise above breed prejudices and make their mark as versatile competitors.

Temperament

Brilliance in movement is not essential for athletic success. Scoring may depend on accuracy and obedience, flexibility and agility. The mind of the horse has as much to do with its performance as an inborn "way-of-going." Too often horses are purchased because of their beauty or athletic prowess. Without a sensible and accepting mind to "operate" these physical endowments, a gorgeous horse may be unsuitable for competition.

An excessively nervous horse may not hold up well under the stress of travel, training, and competition. It may also be prone to gastrointestinal disorders such as diarrhea or colic. A calm, observant attitude enables a horse to better cope with the bombardment of multiple stimuli as it campaigns. Also, observing a horse in the pasture or stable identifies serious vices such as cribbing, wood chewing, stall walking, weaving, or stall kicking.

Test Under Saddle

An essential criterion in assessing any horse is the potential for a partnership with the horse. Teamwork and trust are necessary elements to successful campaigning. A horse must be kind and forgiving. Judgement errors by a rider will occur on occasion, but the horse should continue to rely upon the rider for instruction. A temperamental and unpredictable character is dangerous, no matter how athletic the horse.

If possible, ride the horse being considered to determine the connection between horse and rider. Are its gaits enjoyable? Is it respectful and responsive? If the horse is experienced in a specific sport, ride it at its level of expertise or have a professional trainer or the owner do so. Note any quirks that may only show up under saddle.

Much information can be gained by trying out a prospect on more than one occasion. In this way, talent and temperament are more accurately assessed.

Intelligence and Attitude

A sport horse should be eager to learn, and intelligent so that it is able to learn. It should be able to think its way out of a crisis. This ability is often born as an innate cleverness, but also comes from experience and training. The horse should possess the inclination of "try" that encompasses courage, enthusiasm, and heart. Its attitude should be willing and bold, yet not reckless. The horse must accept discipline in all phases of training and competition.

So is this a description of the perfect horse? Individuals like this do exist, but as often happens, a horse can have all the desired characteristics in temperament, yet have an unsound limb, heart condition, or chronic respiratory disease, making it unfit for consistent performance.

Conformation

Conformational defects should be analyzed carefully to assess the possibilities of a physical breakdown. Such a breakdown can put a horse out of work, or worse, can pose a hazard to both horse and rider. Safety accompanies soundness. Ideal qualities include:

- big, solid, straight bones
- strong, uninjured tendons and ligaments
- flexible, pain-free joints
- strong, well-proportioned feet

Health Problems

When choosing a horse, consider the long-term effects if the horse has low-grade pain from foot soreness or mild arthritis. Will this pain interfere with stamina and willingness of the horse? Could the condition cause it to stumble and fall, or hesitate when asked to do something demanding? Will a currently mild problem progress to a crippling injury as greater athletic demands are placed on the horse?

A chronic respiratory problem may interfere with exercise tolerance at the desired level of training. The horse should be able to achieve rapid heart and respiratory recoveries after an exertion, so as not to compromise its metabolic status. Also, a known history of tying-up may preclude its purchase.

The rigors of athletic training place fantastic demands on the metabolic and musculoskeletal systems of a horse. If possible, start without any physical

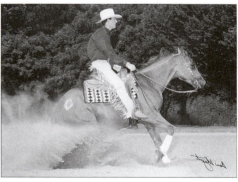

Fig. 22–3. A horse should be able to achieve rapid heart and respiratory recoveries after an exertion.

liability that may later interfere with active and safe participation in the chosen sport. Have a thorough prepurchase exam performed by a competent veterinarian who is well-versed in the athletic demands of the sport.

The Overview

It is helpful to make a list comparing the pros and cons of the horse. Put the price at the top of the list. Are the shortcomings on the "con" side acceptable when compared to the assets on the "pro" side? There will always be some less-than-perfect characteristics in the unproven individual that may work for one owner, but not for another.

Try not to set expectations too high, as it often leads to disappointment. View the purchase realistically, and be patient with the training process. Often it is impossible to fully appreciate how well a horse will respond to training until after purchase. If that individual does not respond well after a reasonable period, sell it and move on to another prospect rather than wasting time, emotional energy, and money on an unsuitable prospect.

PREPURCHASE EXAM

Regardless of whether a novice rider or a seasoned trainer is purchasing a horse, it is always prudent to ask a veterinarian to evaluate the horse before purchase. Even if monetary outlay for a horse is negligible, it is advisable to hire a skilled professional. Thorough assessment of a horse reveals disabilities that can halt an athletic career before it begins.

The cost of a thorough prepurchase exam should be factored into the initial purchase price. A veterinary prepurchase exam points out potential problems that one should be aware of before committing to an investment in a horse. Also, a veterinary exam is useful before leasing a horse to identify specific problems before assuming full responsibility and personal involvement with another person's horse.

During the hunting for a horse, a process of elimination finally reveals a suitable equine prospect. Try to maintain an objective distance until a prepurchase exam has been completed. If the decision is subconsciously made before a complete veterinary analysis, it is easy to ignore important facts that can spell disaster. It is difficult to divorce oneself from expectations and visions about the animal before a prepurchase exam. Then, if lameness or other unsound characteristics are discovered by a veterinarian, it is harder to walk

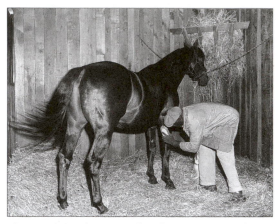

Fig. 22–4. Feed, care and maintenance must be remembered as part of the cost of a horse.

away from a purchase, especially if a deposit has already been made.

The danger in ignoring veterinary advice is that the buyer gets saddled with a horse that has a crippling disability. Expenses continue to mount, and it is difficult to resell the horse and regain the initial investment.

The Role of the Veterinarian

A veterinarian does *not* offer a "pass/fail" judgement on a horse. Normal procedure is for a veterinarian to carefully examine all visible features of a horse along with:

- a comprehensive motion evaluation
- flexion stress tests of the limbs
- analysis of respiratory and heart rate recovery with exercise
- diagnostic tests

Armed with complete information, a veterinarian describes for the buyer the good points and faults of an animal. A veterinarian describes the significance of the faults to the chosen sport. It is then the buyer's responsibility to decide if the imperfections or permanent injuries are acceptable. Some problems may only be cosmetic, while others may functionally impair athletic or breeding performance throughout a horse's lifetime.

Often, complaints arise that a prepurchase exam is non-committal on the part of the veterinarian. It is imperative that a buyer appreciate the role a veterinarian plays in the process. A veterinarian states facts discovered at the time of the prepurchase exam. It is a veterinarian's prerogative to speculate about future soundness and health of a horse, but there is no way one can really know. The buyer weighs pros and cons based on professional advice from a veterinarian and trainer. *The buyer assumes full responsibility for a decision to buy.* This determination is based on findings of not only a veterinary exam, but also the suitability of a horse for a buyer's personal goals as evaluated by the buyer.

Understanding the Prepurchase Exam

There are some points that should be clarified about what a prepurchase exam accomplishes, and how the buyer can help a veterinarian derive the most information from an exam.

Inherent in the purchase of any horse is a long-term commitment and responsibility to that animal. Such a decision should not be made on the spur of the moment. It is a mistake for a buyer to be pressured by a seller to quickly complete a deal. Schedule adequate time with a veterinarian to conduct a thorough exam. Enough pressure is placed on a veterinarian to present a buyer with a complete assessment without also encountering a urgency for immediate results.

Prepurchase exams require at least a couple of hours to complete. A buyer or agent for the buyer should be available during the entire exam, not only to handle the horse during examination procedures, but also to ride the horse, if necessary.

Ideally, all three parties (buyer, seller or agent, and veterinarian) should be present during the exam for full communication between all individuals, and to obtain information about the horse. This arrangement is not always feasible, especially in cases of out-of-state sales, but should be made whenever possible.

Avoiding a Conflict of Interest

It is important that all parties understand for whom the veterinarian is working. Usually, the person paying the veterinary fee is the buyer. That individual has, in fact, hired a veterinarian to act on his or her behalf. Therefore, the veterinarian is protecting the buyer's interests.

If a veterinarian usually works for both buyer and seller, hiring a different, impartial veterinarian to evaluate the horse eliminates a conflict of interest. This practice prevents accusations that a veterinarian has a vested interest in either the seller or the buyer that might prejudice the examination results. Hiring another veterinarian to do the prepurchase exam also avoids hard feelings.

If the buyer and seller both insist that their same, usual veterinarian perform the exam, no offense should be taken by a seller when problems with the horse are identified. At the same time, a buyer must trust that the veterinarian will be fair and maintain an objective viewpoint.

Medical Confidentiality

All reports of findings, diagnostic procedures, and radiographs belong as a legal medical record to the veterinarian. If a prepurchase exam has previously been performed on a horse, do not expect to call that veterinarian and obtain blanket information over the telephone. Under the ethics of medical confidentiality, none of this information can be released to another party without consent from the person who originally hired the veterinarian to perform the exam. A veterinarian must also contact the horse owner for consent to divulge medical history to a prospective buyer.

Disclosure Statement

Often at the time of a prepurchase exam a veterinarian or buyer will request a *disclosure statement* from a seller or agent to provide an historical background about the horse. The age of the horse, previous use, and current level of exercise or training give valuable information to a buyer and a veterinarian. If a horse has been retired to pasture for several months or years, a rest period may positively influence how "sound" an injured animal moves.

Information obtained from a disclosure statement includes a complete medical history, deworming and vaccination schedules, history of colic, prior surgeries, and disclosure of any medication or drugs a horse has previously or is currently receiving. This last item is a delicate issue as anti-inflammatory medications can mask problems of utmost concern to the animal's performance capabilities. A tranquilizer or sedative can alter a horse's disposition and behavior. All medications should be withheld at least 5 – 10 days before an examination.

Before the exam, it is also helpful for the veterinarian performing a prepurchase exam to receive a copy of the horse's medical record from the seller's veterinarian. Disclosure statements are not necessarily standard procedure, but are recommended to ensure fair representation of the horse by the seller.

Benefits of a Complete Exam

Some people are not interested in a complete prepurchase exam due to the cost involved. Requests such as "I just want you to look it over, Doc, and tell me if you see anything wrong" puts a veterinarian in an impossible situation. It is impractical to expect a veterinarian to perform a "partial exam" not only because very little information is obtained in an exam lacking thoroughness, but also due to legal implications involved in a prepurchase examination.

Compare buying a horse to purchasing a used automobile. If a person glances at a vehicle on a lot, or watches it drive into the driveway, all that can be said of that car is that it looks okay, and moves under power of its engine. On that basis, how can one tell if the brakes work, if the transmission is sound, or if the engine knocks and bangs? A cursory view does not determine if the frame or axles are bent, or if reconstructive body work has been done. Much the same can be said of an incomplete inspection of a potential equine athlete.

Detecting Problems

It is impossible to identify cardiac arrhythmias or murmurs without a stethoscope. Ophthalmic examination identifies corneal scars, cataracts, or vision problems. Use of hoof testers helps identify internal foot problems. Without placing a horse under a battery of tests which include manipulation of joints, tendons, ligaments, and muscles of the limbs, along with careful motion evaluation at all gaits, all a person can say about a horse standing at rest is that it looks okay. Perhaps a particular blemish or suspect musculoskeletal problem can be pointed out, but anything else about a horse's capabilities is pure speculation.

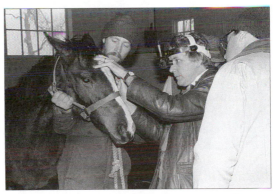

Fig. 22–5. An eye exam helps detect corneal scars, cataracts, and vision problems.

If possible, have the exam done at a location where there is access to both a hard-pack surface and a softer surface like grass or sand. A level surface enables a veterinarian to analyze foot placement and abnormal limb motion (winging, paddling) that may influence athletic soundness. An area with a slight incline is particularly helpful to identify a very subtle lameness.

The horse handler should be prepared to trot the horse in hand, and to longe the horse both directions. Ideally, the horse should not be exercised prior to the motion exam so as not to obscure problems that may improve as the horse warms up.

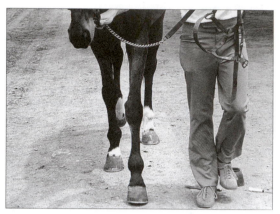

Fig. 22–6. A level surface can help detect poor foot placement.

Not all lameness problems are obvious until a horse is asked to perform the task for which its purchase is intended. Asking a jumping candidate to jump, a cutting prospect to cut, or a dressage horse to perform at its current level of training is desirable. While a horse is performing under the stress of these activities, subtle problems in the back, withers, or limbs may become visible to a skilled veterinarian.

Exercise may reveal other problems such as "roaring" (laryngeal hemiplegia), which is a serious impairment to airflow through the upper respiratory tract. In a mild case, the horse does not make a "roaring" noise, and the only way to identify paralysis of a cartilage in the throat is with an endoscopic exam.

For broodmares or breeding stallions, a fertility evaluation at the time of a prepurchase exam prevents disappointing surprises in the future.

Further Diagnostic Tests

Further diagnostic procedures include radiographic exam of specified areas of a limb, ultrasound exam of tendons, a complete blood count, blood chemistry tests, and drug tests.

A buyer and seller should expect a time lag for diagnostic tests upon which a sale may depend. Drug testing, blood work, and radiographic evaluation require a short period for results to be returned to and analyzed by the veterinarian. Some tests rely on outside laboratories which causes further delay.

Drug Testing

A drug screening test does not detect medication injected into a joint, nor does it identify all systemic medications that are available to suppress pain. To be completely certain that a horse has been off medication for at least several days prior to the scheduled exam, the horse can be moved to the buyer's boarding facility. Insurance policies can be purchased for a short time to cover accidental mishaps or illness while the horse remains in the prospective buyer's possession.

X-Ray Films

A single x-ray film of an area of concern on the leg does not provide complete information. To analyze a particular area on a limb, it is necessary to radiograph each joint separately, with four to five different directional views per joint.

A prepurchase exam identifies areas of concern that may require further evaluation with x-ray films, or in an unusual case, with diagnostic nerve blocks. A client should be prepared to spend as much money as is reasonably necessary to complete extra diagnostics. If not, a buyer is compelled to weigh a veterinarian's assessment without concrete radiographic evidence, possibly allowing an important defect to escape discovery. Clinical impressions are offered, but without x-ray films of suspect areas, it is difficult to determine if degenerative joint disease or osteochondrosis lesions are present in a joint. Permanent damage from previous infection or trauma in a bone is also difficult to identify without x-ray films. Radiographic examination of the foot often requires removal of the horse's shoes. The seller should be advised of this possibility and permission obtained ahead of time. Then the seller can make arrangements with the farrier to replace the shoes.

The Untrained Horse

If a horse has not yet been trained to the prospective desires of a buyer, it may be difficult to evaluate its ability for specific athletic pursuits. Yet, if trained under saddle, a horse should be ridden by the buyer, trainer, or seller during the examination.

It may be somewhat difficult to evaluate an untrained horse that is incapable of leading in hand, or unused to having its legs or body handled by humans. As a young horse jerks and fidgets, interpretation of results from limb manipulations or hoof testers may be confusing. Arrangements should be made to exercise a green horse freely in a confined arena. A buyer should be aware of limitations of a prepurchase exam under constraints where a veterinarian cannot perform a thorough, hands-on evaluation.

Looking Into the Future

Once obtained, results of diagnostic procedures are not always clear-cut. A predominant problem in the equine industry is use of x-ray films to determine if a horse suffers from a lameness that currently shows no physical symptoms. Commonly, veterinarians are asked to predict if a horse will continue to be "sound" and of athletic use in the *distant* future based on clinical findings and x-ray films taken on the day of an exam. Often the buyer also wants to know if a horse will retain its worth upon resale. It is expected that a veterinarian can clearly see into the future!

All a veterinarian can provide is an answer based on a clinical impression bolstered by past experience. As with any law of averages, some judgements can be wrong. Many issues cannot be factored into a professional opinion at the time of a sale. Some examples are:

- the type of work the horse will be asked to do
- how well a conditioning program develops the musculoskeletal system
- the terrain on which the horse will be exercised
- the expertise of the farrier
- age-related breakdowns

Navicular Radiographs

The deepest quagmire for prepurchase exams comes from radiographic evaluation of navicular films. At a recent convention of the American Association of Equine Practitioners, it was commented that 43% of legal problems over prepurchase exams stem from navicular x-ray films.

Navicular films alone are *not* a basis for diagnosing navicular disease. All information compiled from clinical history, clinical exam during exercise on different ground surfaces, hoof tester results, flexion tests, diagnostic nerve blocks, and navicular x-ray films must be gathered before arriving at a diagnosis.

Yet, great importance has been attached to the sole use of navicular films during a prepurchase exam. Buyers expect the films will predict the likelihood that a horse is currently afflicted with navicular disease or will develop it sometime in the future. Scientific evidence shows that navicular x-ray films do not completely correlate with clinical disease.

A horse may mimic navicular syndrome while simply suffering from bruised heels or imbalanced shoeing, although none of the navicular apparatus is abnormally affected. This horse may be incorrectly diagnosed as "navicular" without being given a chance to heal and show its true ability.

Not all horses with a true navicular disease syndrome have radiographic changes in their navicular bones. This lack of change may be because soreness comes from the soft tissue structures of the deep digital flexor tendon or the navicular bursa rather than from the bone itself. After a long lay-off and on a good day the horse may show no lameness and can slip through a lameness evaluation, complete with x-ray films, without identifying the problem.

On the other hand, many horses, especially athletes past 10 or 12 years, may show definite signs of wear-and-tear of the navicular apparatus on x-ray films without having any symptoms or history of lameness. Basing a judgement of navicular disease solely on radiographic findings is flawed and unjustified.

Liability for the Future

X-ray films of the feet need to be analyzed with utmost care, and not too much read into them. Veterinarians have been placed in a position where they are held liable for the future soundness of a horse while basing judgements and opinions on information gained over the course of a several hour exam. Such legal precariousness forces a veterinarian to be overly conservative and pessimistic in rendering an opinion.

Not only is this predicament an injustice to a veterinarian, but all too often a "pre-navicular" diagnosis is placed on a horse, condemning a horse and owner. For starters, a horse's value is diminished considerably, financially harming the seller. Secondly, it becomes increasingly difficult to find a buyer for that animal once word gets around. Thirdly, few insurance companies will insure a navicular horse for mortality.

Information for Assistance

In the old days people relied primarily on a philosophy of "buyer beware," but now with sophisticated instruments and a sophisticated level of education and expertise, veterinarians can help protect a buyer's interests. Arduous years of schooling and clinical experience develop trained eyes and skilled minds of equine doctors. These skills enable a veterinarian to identify problems during a prepurchase exam, but do *not* provide a crystal ball to see into the future.

The following points should be carefully considered:

- It is *the buyer's* decision to hire a veterinarian and to place trust in that person.
- Veterinarians are capable of human error.
- Through use and time, any horse may break down.
- There is no such thing as a guarantee on the health and soundness of any living being.
- No horse will be as perfect as those in our imaginations.
- The buyer makes the final decision on purchasing.

By knowing what to expect from a prepurchase exam, and by recognizing human limitations to make long-range predictions, a veterinary prepurchase exam enables a buyer to make an *informed decision* whether to purchase the horse.

For a horse that is basically sound in mind and body, a prepurchase exam is also a starting point from which a buyer can build a sound conditioning and feeding program. Noted weaknesses in conformation alert the buyer to areas that should be closely monitored during training. Problems with shoeing or imbalance of the feet are identified, and arrangements made to begin correction. This information gives a potential owner an intelligent foundation on which to develop an athletic prospect.

23

BREEDING THE PERFORMANCE HORSE

There may be times in the life of an equine athlete when it is unable to actively perform. During training or competition, a horse may sustain a musculoskeletal injury, requiring a lay-up of many months. If the idle horse is a mare, the down time may be used to advantage by breeding her.

Of all domestic farm animals bred in the United States, mares have the lowest reproductive efficiency; less than 60% of mares bred each year produce live foals. As with a performance athlete, sound management of the broodmare encourages her to perform to potential. Thoughtful planning and a prebreeding veterinary examination improve a mare's chances for conception and birth of a healthy foal.

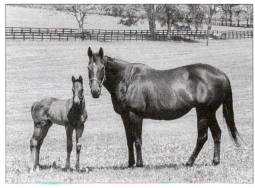

Fig. 23–1. Thoughtful planning leads to a healthy future athlete.

PREPARING FOR BREEDING

A mare cannot be pulled out of rigorous athletics and expected to im-

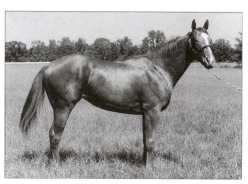

mediately conceive. If a mare is engaged in competitive athletics or on the show circuit, pull her out of work *at least 2 months* before breeding. This "let-down" period reduces her stress load and allows her reproductive pattern to settle into a regular cycling interval. Over several months her psychological state also adjusts to the relaxed environment.

Fig. 23–2. An athletic mare should stop work at least 2 months before breeding.

Likewise, the stress of competition reduces the fertility of a stallion. A let-down period of several days may be necessary for him, to improve the chance for conception on the first attempt.

Weight Problems

As an athletic mare is pulled out of performance, she may be too thin to encourage normal reproductive cycling. Once her athletic activity is minimized, she should begin to gain weight. Mares that are on a steady weight gain program *(flushing)* before the breeding period attain estrus 1 month sooner than mares that are not gaining weight. The fit breeding mare has a thin layer of flesh covering her ribs so they are not visible but can be felt as the hand is run lightly across the body.

A halter horse pulled from the show circuit may have the opposite problem from the athlete—it may be too fat. High energy rations should be removed immediately from the diet of a halter horse intended for breeding. It should be placed on a balanced maintenance diet with ample roughage and minimal grain. *(See Chapter 7 for more information.)*

THE MARE
Abnormal Estrous Cycles
Performance

Often, the stress of intense competition temporarily alters normal reproductive cycling. Some mares stop cycling altogether, or may display erratic heat cycles. A racetrack mare may have difficulty conceiving a foal during the first season after she has stopped racing.

Steroids

Anabolic steroids are sometimes used to "improve" a horse's body condition, growth, and muscling. Anabolic steroids have adverse effects on a mare's endocrine system. The mare that is influenced by the male sex hormone properties of these drugs has inconsistent or absent estrous cycles. If given repetitively, anabolic steroids can cause a mare to display stallion-like behavior. Once administration of the drug is stopped, the effects are reversible but may require several months for a mare to return to normal estrous cycles.

Pain

The performance horse that suffers from a serious injury that involves intense pain may have difficulty conceiving. Intense pain interferes with hormone production and may interrupt a normal estrous cycle.

The Mare's Reproductive Cycle

The mare is *seasonally polyestrus*, meaning that she cycles many times during the breeding season. Her optimal fertile period is between April and August (in the Northern Hemisphere), although many mares are bred earlier. Most mares stop cycling in the winter months *(anestrus)* between November and February. In February and March she enters a *transitional period*. Pituitary hormones controlling the reproductive cycle respond to longer daylight hours, stimulating the activity of the ovaries. The ovaries start producing follicles that eventually mature. Rupture of a mature follicle releases an egg for potential fertilization.

During the transitional period, estrous cycles are erratic, and may be prolonged without the production of an actual egg. Normally, during April through August, a mare cycles every 21 days, with visible signs of estrus (winking of the vulva, tail lifting, or frequent urinations) present for about 5 days.

Nature protects the survival of the species by maximizing fertility of both the mare and the stallion during the warmer times of the year. Then, a gestation period of 11 months allows a foal to be born into a welcoming and nutrient-rich environment for both mare and foal. By evaluating a mare's reproductive capabilities before the optimum breeding period, health problems can be addressed and resolved before the breeding season.

Each time a mare is bred, there is a risk of injury or uterine infection. If her fertility is coordinated with the proposed breeding date she will become pregnant with fewer breedings, avoiding these situations.

Hormonal Manipulation

Techniques to synchronize follicle maturation with the proposed breeding date include use of specific hormones or hormonal analogs, such as progesterone, prostaglandins, or human chorionic gonadotropin (HCG). However, hormonal manipulation of a mare is not practical until her ovaries are active and cycling.

If she is in the quiescent, winter anestrus, or just entering the transitional period around February or March, hormonal drug therapy may be ineffective in coordinating the timing for breeding. Only 20% – 30% of mares cycle and ovulate at regular intervals during February and March, whereas over 80% do so by April or May.

Artificial Lighting

To encourage mares to cycle earlier in the year, the erratic 2-month transitional period can be advanced by manipulating natural hormonal surges with artificial lighting. The photoreceptors of the eyes detect light, which sends a message to the *pineal gland* located behind the *hypothalamus* in the brain. The message mimics longer daylight hours of springtime, stimulating hormonal activity by the hypothalamus. As hormone secretions respond to the light, ovarian tissue is activated, and follicles form, mature, and ovulate. Each estrous cycle reoccurs approximately every 3 weeks to provide the breeder with many opportunities to get the mare in foal.

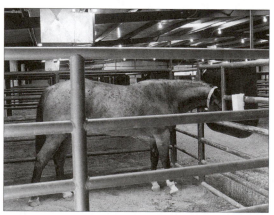

Fig. 23–3. Artificial lighting stimulates the mare's body to cycle earlier in the year.

Recommendations

For this method to work best, 16 hours of "daylight" is required. The type of light is not as important as the number of hours the mare is exposed to it. Incandescent, fluorescent, mercury vapor, and tungsten lights are all successful in stimulating a mare's reproductive activity. It is necessary to provide 2 months of lengthened daylight to enhance ovarian activity; a month later, follicles mature and ovulate. To maximize the use of artificial lighting, begin the program on December 1, with anticipated start of breeding to be March 1.

Lights should be turned on from 4:30 P.M. until 11 P.M. This schedule ensures a total of 16 hours of both natural and artificial light. A 200-watt incandescent bulb, or two 40-watt fluorescent bulbs are placed 10 feet above the mare in a 12 x 12 foot stall. There should be enough light to read a newspaper in the stall at eye-level with the mare. The mare should not be able to remove her head from the light source. If she does, the pineal gland is not stimulated by light.

As an energy-saving alternative, recent studies indicate that 1 – 2 hours of artificial light applied 8 – 10 hours after sunset may be sufficient to stimulate the pineal gland. Turning the lights on between 1 – 4 A.M. hastens the transitional period.

Blanketing and Food

A mare that is put under lights is also stimulated to shed out her winter coat. In a cold climate, premature shedding requires blanketing and shelter. The mare may require extra food to maintain good body condition. Remember, if an early breeding schedule is implemented in colder climates, indoor housing must be available to a mare foaling in January, February, or March to avoid climatic stress on the foal.

Preventative Medicine

A preventative medicine program, if not already in place, should be instituted before breeding. This program includes:

- deworming every 2 months with products approved for pregnant mares
- a rhinopneumonitis vaccine before breeding, and boosted at 5, 7, and 9 months of pregnancy to reduce the risk of viral abortion
- regular encephalitis, tetanus, and influenza boosters at appropriate intervals as determined by a veterinarian

The Mare's Prebreeding Exam

Ensuring the reproductive health of a mare from the onset avoids wasted time during the crucial breeding season, as well as unnecessary and repeated expenses that result in extreme frustration and financial loss. A veterinary prebreeding examination may detect external and internal abnormalities of a mare that can lead to reproductive failure.

General Physical Exam

To start, a general physical exam is performed to ensure the health of the heart and lungs, and the soundness of limbs and feet. Heart murmurs or arrhythmias reduce metabolic efficiency. Chronic lung disease interferes with the oxygen supply so important to placental and fetal health. A chronic cough from obstructive pulmonary disease (heaves) can cause enough straining to develop a "windsucking" vagina *(pneumovagina)* that pulls bacteria into itself, resulting in inflammation or infection.

Severe, chronic pain caused by arthritis, laminitis, or other limb problems can stress a horse enough to reduce her chances not only of conception but of carrying a foal to term. A mare with chronic laminitis poses an added reproductive risk. If the laminitic mare has difficulty with birthing or develops a uterine infection *(metritis)* after the birth, endotoxins may be absorbed into the bloodstream. Endotoxins may worsen an already crippling foot condition of laminitis.

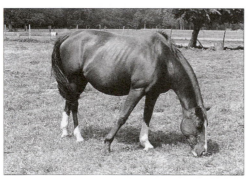

Fig. 23–4. This broodmare has a good body condition with her ribs barely showing.

Without good teeth, a mare is unable to meet nutritional needs important to maintaining pregnancy, fetal development, and lactation. Body condition is examined during the prebreeding exam so that appropriate nutritional adjustments can be discussed. Ideally, the mare's ribs should barely be visible. Therefore, a slow, controlled weight gain program can be implemented 1 – 2 months before the breeding season. Obesity is detrimental to conception and reproductive health, however, a malnourished horse is also at risk for infertility.

Examining the hair coat indicates the success of parasite control programs, and hormonal regularity. A rough coat may reflect internal health problems or an intestinal parasite load. A mare that is late in shedding her winter coat may also lack an appropriate hormonal response to the long daylight hours of breeding season.

Maturity

A mare should not be bred until she is sexually and skeletally mature to prevent additional stresses and demands on her own growing body.

The period of greatest fetal demand occurs in the last trimester (8 – 11 months) of pregnancy. A mare should not be bred any earlier than 3 years old. A mare bred as a 3-year-old approaches her fourth year before the foal taxes her system with rapid developmental growth and the subsequent energy demands of lactation.

External Exam of the Reproductive System

A common reason for failure to conceive, or for early embryonic death, is infection of the uterus (metritis). The unique anatomy of the *perineum*, which is the area around the anus and vulva, provides the first line of defense in protecting the uterus from bacterial invasion.

The Perineum

A normal mare has a vertical vulva with full *labia* (lips of the vulva) that are tightly aligned in a snug fit so that neither air nor feces can enter the vagina. In a normal mare, about 80% of the vulva is positioned below the pelvic brim, with the anus positioned very slightly behind or directly above the vulva so feces do not fall onto the labia.

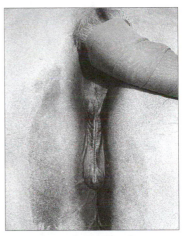

Tilted Vagina

In a mare with a tilted vagina, the labia sit high above the pelvic brim, the anus is pulled forward, and the vulva tilts horizontally. With the vagina tipped forward and the anus recessed inwards, feces fall directly onto the

Fig. 23–5. A normal perineum.

labia. The labia may gap, and then windsucking pulls air and feces into the reproductive tract. To check for windsucking, place the flat surface of the hands on each labial lip, and gently part them. In a windsucking mare, air is aspirated into the vulva as the labia are manually parted, resulting in a sucking sound. In many older mares, or in very thin horses, the position of anus and vulva is altered due to loss of muscle tone.

Vestibular Seal

The next barrier to uterine contamination is the *vestibular seal* created by the back portion of the vagina, the hymen if present, and the pelvic floor. If the vulva is tilted horizontally, constrictor muscles of the vulva and vestibule cannot prevent contamination of the reproductive tract.

Not only does a tipped vulva develop from age-related conformational changes or severe weight loss, but it can also be caused by an inherited defect from birth. Such fillies should be identified early so corrections can be made to enhance their future fertility. Keep in mind that conformation is heritable, and undesirable traits may be passed down from mare to foal. Normally, Mother Nature accounts for this problem by making poorly conformed mares unbreedable, but advances in scientific techniques encourage continued fertility and breeding of many of these mares.

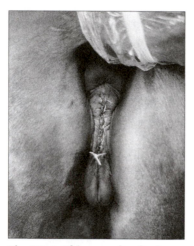

Fig. 23–6. This mare has had a Caslick's surgery.

Caslick's Surgery

Contamination to the reproductive tract may result in infertility from infection and subsequent scarring of the uterus. Once a mare with a forwardly tipped vagina has been bred and "settled," a *Caslick's* surgery *(episioplasty)*, performed by a veterinarian, closes the lips of the vulva to prevent contamination. Local anesthetic is placed along the borders of the vulva, tissue is trimmed away, and the two lips are sutured together to join as they heal. Several weeks before foaling, the Caslick's should be opened to allow normal birth of the foal without tearing.

Third Degree Perineal Laceration

Sometimes a foal is delivered with an improperly aligned leg, which tears the perineum. These mares should have the perineum reconstructed well ahead of the next breeding time to adequately clear a uterine infection from the system. In severe *third degree recto-vestibular lacerations*, as these are called, torn flesh between the rectum and the vagina allows feces to fall directly into the vagina. This condition requires three phases of surgical repair. Up to a year of healing time is necessary before breeding the mare again.

Udder Evaluation

In a prebreeding evaluation, the udder is examined for abnormalities in size or consistency, tumors or scar tissue, or evidence of previous or current *mastitis*. Mastitis is an inflammation of the udder. The thighs and underside of the tail are also examined for evidence of an abnormal vaginal discharge.

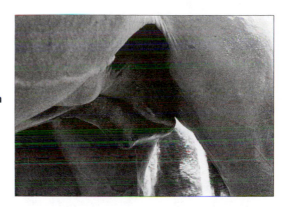

Fig. 23–7. A mare with mastitis.

Internal Exam of the Reproductive System

Rectal Exam

Once the mare's overall body health and external genitals have been thoroughly evaluated, examination of the internal reproductive tract can begin. Initially, a *rectal examination* is performed with the veterinarian inserting an arm covered by a lubricated, plastic sleeve into the rectum. The veterinarian then manually palpates the ovaries, uterus, and cervix to assess general health, activity, and abnormalities. Size of the ovaries is determined, while the amount of follicular activity present on each ovary ascertains if the mare is currently cycling. The tone and size of the uterus and cervix establish if fluid, tumors or abscesses, adhesions, or scar tissue are present. A flaccid and doughy feeling uterus may signal infection within or abnormal endocrine function.

A *maiden mare* that has never been bred should be examined rectally to determine if all appropriate reproductive "equipment" is present; that is, two ovaries, a cervix, and a normal shaped and positioned uterus. On rare occasions, abnormalities such as lack of an ovary, tumor of an ovary, or a split cervix may be felt.

Vaginal Exam

After thoroughly washing the perineum and wrapping the tail to prevent pulling debris inwards, the next step is a *vaginal speculum exam* to visually inspect the vagina for:

- inflammation
- congestion
- vaginal cysts
- abnormal discharge
- vaginal or vulvar tearing from prior births
- cervical lacerations or adhesions

The *cervix* is the third barrier to uterine contamination, and its integrity is important to reproductive health. In a maiden mare, a *hymen* may be present, and can be broken down at this time. Blood is spermicidal and interferes with semen fertility, therefore, it is best to open the hymen before breeding.

The color and moistness of mucous membranes within the vagina reflect vaginal health and endocrine function. Air bubbles may indicate chronic windsucking, while a collection of fluid on the vaginal floor warns of other serious problems.

Urine Pooling

An important cause of infertility in some mares is a syndrome known as urine pooling *(vesiculo-vaginal reflux,* or VVR) on the floor of the vagina. Urine is not only spermicidal, but it is an irritant which can cause inflammation of the vagina *(vaginitis),* inflammation of the cervix *(cervicitis),* and inflammation of the uterus with subsequent infertility. If urine is not entirely voided clear of the reproductive tract, small, residual amounts drain forward to collect on the vaginal floor. The veterinarian can see the urine (when the speculum is in place) with a flashlight. Suspect fluid can be analyzed biochemically to confirm that it is urine.

A mare with a tipped vulva is particularly susceptible to urine pooling. In a normal vulva, entry into the vagina requires an upward path, ensuring that urine is drained down and out. A tipped vulva directs the entry downward, therefore, urine tends to flow into the vagina. It occurs very slightly during estrus when the reproductive tract relaxes, or if a Caslick's surgery is improperly sewn.

Surgery

To correct urine pooling, *urethral extension surgery* "builds" a urethral tunnel from pre-existing shelves of tissue within the vagina. Urine travels outward through the tunnel, and cannot collect within the vaginal cavern. In one study, this surgery resulted in a conception rate of 92% of mares with previous urine pooling, and 65% carried foals to term.

Maiden Mare

A maiden mare is a mare of any age who has never been exposed to semen. Once she has been "bred," whether she conceives or not, she is no longer a maiden. The untouched uterus is a sterile environment. In a maiden mare, the reproductive exam often stops after rectal palpation and a vaginal exam. There is no reason to assume any possible uterine infection unless conformation of the vulva appears suspect, or if vaginal inflammation or urine pooling has been confirmed.

For a mare that has been bred, with or without conception, or for a poorly conformed maiden mare, the prebreeding exam continues.

Bacterial Culture of the Uterus

A bacterial culture is obtained directly from the uterus to determine whether there is an infection of the uterine lining. A very long cotton swab is passed through the cervix, guarded in a plastic sheath. A protective cap on the end of the sheath is pushed open once in the uterus, and uterine secretions soak into the swab for 30 seconds. The swab is pulled back into the sterile protective sheath and removed from the reproductive tract. The sample is sent to the lab to be checked for bacterial growth over the next 48 hours. If bacterial growth does occur, the lab can determine the antibiotic to which the bacteria is susceptible.

Effectiveness of Bacterial Culture

By itself, bacterial culture of the uterus has a poor correlation with the presence of actual disease. As many as 61% of mares with infection of the uterus do not show significant bacterial growth when a culture is taken. Other mares may have non-harmful bacteria resident in the uterus, with no accompanying disease. Bacteria are detected in the uterine linings of 80% of mares up to 3 days after breeding, and up to 30 days after foaling. A normal mare's immune system quickly clears them from the reproductive system.

However, bacterial culture and antibiotic sensitivity testing of the superficial uterine lining is helpful in confirming other diagnostic findings, such as:

- an abnormal-feeling uterus
- presence of fluid or urine pooling
- continued infertility
- results from uterine biopsies and cellular evaluation *(cytology)*

Specific bacteria, such a beta-hemolytic Streptococci, *Klebsiella, Pseudomonas, E. coli,* and yeasts, are significant if found on the culture. An infected uterus needs to be treated with local antibiotics and/or antibiotic injections before breeding.

Cellular Evaluation of the Uterine Lining

The swab used to gather secretions from the uterus also collects cells from the uterine lining. In the lab, the swab is rolled onto a glass slide, stained, and examined under a microscope for inflammatory cells, debris, or bacteria. The presence of specific inflammatory cells provides warning signals about the duration and severity of an infection.

Uterine Biopsy

The most informative diagnostic tool for analyzing the viability, health, and structure of the equine uterus is the *uterine biopsy.* A special instrument is inserted through the cervix into the uterus, and its movable jaws are closed to tear off a deep tag of tissue. The uterine lining *(endometrium)* of the mare, unlike humans, has no nerve endings, therefore a horse does not feel the tug or tearing of tissue as the biopsy is taken. The tissue sample is prepared at the laboratory by slicing it microscopically thin for examination under a microscope. A random sample provides adequate information about overall uterine health.

Infertility Due to Uterine Infections

Often, infertility is caused by uterine infections in the deep tissue layers. These can only be inspected by biopsy of the tissue. Microscopic evaluation identifies infection, inflammation, or scarring *(fibrosis)* of the glands that support uterine nutrition. There is a direct correlation of biopsy findings with fertility, which makes this procedure an invaluable diagnostic tool. A Kenney classification system categorizes the degree of uterine *pathology*, or disease, and predicts the mare's chance of success.

Kenney Classification System

Grade I Uterus

A Grade I uterus has at least an 80% chance of conception, with minimal or no pathological changes (infection, inflammation, or gland scarring) present in the endometrium.

Grade II Uterus

A Grade II describes moderately severe inflammation and gland scarring that interfere with the ability of the endometrium to adequately support a foal to term. A Grade IIA uterus is associated with a 50% – 80% chance of success of maintaining a pregnancy. A mare with this classification has a reasonably good possibility for return to Grade I status with appropriate treatment. A Grade IIB uterus has more widespread abnormalities in the endometrium, and will have limited success (10% – 50%) of carrying a foal to term.

Grade III Uterus

A Grade III classification is the most severe, with irreversible, widespread inflammatory changes and periglandular scarring, providing less than a 10% chance of conception and carrying a foal to term. Widespread scarring in the uterus decreases uterine motility during a critical period when normal motility is essential for continued pregnancy.

With diminished uterine motility, an embryo may not migrate throughout the uterus during days 5 – 15 after conception. Embryonic migration stimulates chemical signals which block the release of prostaglandins from the uterus. Without embryonic migration, prostaglandins are released. Prostaglandins cause a premature reduction of the hormone, progesterone, which is necessary for maintaining early pregnancy. The fetus is then lost. Extensive scarring of the uterus, and particularly of the glandular areas, also reduces nutrient supplies essential to support a developing embryo.

Kenney Classification System		
GRADE	**CHANCE OF CONCEPTION**	**PATHOLOGY**
Grade I Uterus	**at least 80%**	**minimal or none**
Grade II Uterus **Grade IIA** **Grade IIB**	**50% – 80%** **10% – 50%**	**moderately severe: may reverse with treatment**
Grade III Uterus	**less than 10%**	**irreversible, widespread damage**

Fig. 23–8.

Breeding For Excellence
Scientific Interference

The days of spontaneously breeding a mare in a whimsical moment have pretty much vanished, as quality stallions and mares must schedule time for propagation of the species. With human interference and manipulation of reproductively less efficient animals, we may, in fact, perpetuate the necessity of scientific manipulation. Mother Nature no longer selects for reproductively sound horses that breed and foal without human assistance. Many other variables arise as we breed for athletic performance and beauty, and remove the natural selection process for reproductive efficiency. A poorly conformed, slanting vagina, urine pooling, or an infected uterus often are medically or surgically repaired. These problems are genetically passed to the foal, allowing continued propagation of problems that would never have remained under normal circumstances.

Promoting Genetic Improvement

Only with conscious recognition of undesirable traits, and a concerted effort to eradicate these characteristics will a breeder promote continued improvement of horses. Discuss suspected flaws with a veterinarian and other breeders. Be hypercritical of a mare.

Before breeding, carefully assess the contribution the mare can make to the horse population. Breeding a mare that is crippled due to conformational defects does little to improve the equine world at large, and may produce a foal with similar problems.

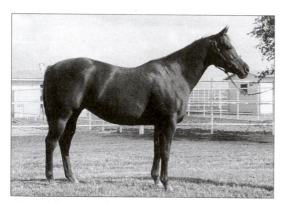

Fig. 23–9. Carefully assess the contribution a mare can make if she is bred.

Breeding an excellent mare to a poor stallion, or vice versa, is a huge mistake. Do not cut corners by diluting good stock. The initial cost of breeding the mare is only a small part of raising a foal to performance age, therefore, put money into the initial investment by selecting an excellent quality mare *and* stallion. Selecting an excellent stallion ensures improvement of the genetic pool. Analyze the performance of the sire and his offspring, and the compatibility of conformational aspects between the stallion and mare.

THE STALLION

A breeding stallion has a unique place in the performance world. Not only is it possible to ride him as a performance horse, but his genetic characteristics will be passed on to future generations. Because of this lasting influence, a stringent selection process should be applied to the stallion by both the potential stallion owner and the broodmare owner looking for the perfect complement to the mare.

The stallion's disposition and temperament are vital to the enjoyment of the stallion and his progeny. A bad-tempered stallion is hazardous to his handlers, to farm personnel, and to broodmares. A bad disposition is potentially passed to the foal. It is wise to geld a dangerous stallion rather than risk passing this genetic tendency on to future offspring.

Before investing in a breeding stallion, evaluate the stallion's performance results. If he has progeny old enough to compete, track their performance results, both successes and failures. Examine the offspring to see if the desired characteristics are passed to succeeding generations. Pedigree may suggest potential, but recent generations of offspring prove or disprove the athletic value of a specific genetic line.

When considering a stallion, match him to a mare with a complementary body type and strength. Find a stallion with similar desirable characteristics to reinforce them in the foal, and with characteristics that improve or correct the weak components of the mare. If the mare has too many faults, consider breeding a different mare rather than risking passing her conformational defects to the foal. A mare or stallion that has been retired due to lameness caused by conformational problems should not be considered as a breeder. There is no sense in breeding the mare or stallion only to create a foal with a similar unsoundness.

Breeding Performance

Not only do good looks, strong conformation, and an impressive athletic record make a stallion excellent for propagating these desirable traits, but he must be able to perform his duties as a breeding horse.

To adequately evaluate a stallion's reproductive capacity, his semen should be collected and analyzed. In the process of collecting semen, information is also gained regarding the stallion's libido and breeding behavior. Some stallions are intimidated by the breeding process due to bad experiences. It is valuable to discover if the stallion is aggressive and difficult to handle when presented with a mare in heat, or if he has trouble attaining and holding an erection, mounting the mare or dummy, or achieving ejaculation. However, it is premature to make too many assumptions about the performance of an inexperienced stallion in his first attempts.

The breeding stallion must be able to rise on his hind legs to mount a mare or a phantom breeding dummy. Some breeding sheds in Kentucky have created special facilities to place a mare in a low point on the ground to allow an arthritic stallion easier access to her. Such management considerations by the breeding farm are as important as the overall health of the stallion because they ensure the success of live coverage.

A thorough exam evaluates the soundness of the stallion's breeding capabilities. A breeding exam starts with a thorough history and general physical examination of the stallion's overall health. Deworming and vaccination schedules are reviewed, and prior experience or problems associated with breeding are discussed. A complete history of medical or surgical events should be disclosed at this time to determine if a past problem is injurious to a stallion's career as a breeding horse.

General Physical Exam

The breeding stallion should be in good flesh, neither too fat nor too thin. His teeth should be fully checked for problems that can interfere with his continuing good condition. His heart and lungs should be examined at rest and with exercise to detect abnormalities. A broodmare owner with the intent of using a stallion at stud also should carefully critique the stallion's straightness of limbs, size and health of feet, and general body proportions to determine if the stallion will complement the mare. Remember that the stallion contributes half the genetic information, therefore, his defects can be passed on to the offspring.

Heritable Abnormalities

It is important to identify the existence of undesirable, heritable traits such as a retained testicle (cryptorchidism), a scrotal or umbilical hernia, parrot mouth, combined immunodeficiency disease (CID), or eye cataracts. These abnormalities are all passed down in a genetic link, and the presence of one or more of such heritable traits renders a stallion as unfavorable for breeding.

Other syndromes that are not entirely linked to genetics but may have a heritable tendency are developmental abnormalities like angular limb deformities, osteochondrosis, or cervical spinal malformation which can lead to *wobbler syndrome*. Ascertain if the stallion has a history of such problems in his lineage or in his get.

Investigate soundness problems that have developed in the stallion or his offspring. Identify conformational abnormalities that interfere with continual soundness, like angular limb deformities, too long a pastern slope, or post-legged hindquarters. The mare contributes half of the genetic information to the foal, therefore, not all problems can be traced exclusively to the stallion.

Reproductive Exam

Examination of both the internal and external genital structures is an important part of a stallion's breeding exam. The prepuce is checked for injuries, scars, or tumors. Both testicles are measured with calipers across the widest part of the scrotum, and their consistency is determined by manual palpation.

The Testicles

The testicles should feel firm, whereas a soft, mushy, or hard consistency may indicate degeneration or disease. A rectal exam or internal ultrasound exam evaluates the health of the internal genital glands.

Testicular size is highly correlated to the amount of sperm output, which determines fertility. Although a young colt may begin producing viable semen by 13 months of age, most stallions are not purposely put to stud until they are 2 – 3 years old. A 2 or 3-year-old stallion should have testicles that each measure 5 centimeters or more. Size of the testicles depends on the age of a stallion, with maximum size attained by age 6. Testicular size is heritable; if a stallion has undersized testicles, not only is he potentially a poor sperm producer, but small testicles could be passed on as an undesirable trait.

The size of the testicles does decrease with a horse in training, the stress of competition (especially racing), and with medication such as anabolic steroids.

The Penis

After the stallion is lightly teased, his penis is examined for skin lesions consistent with melanomas, squames, sarcoids, warts, or summer sores. Evidence of inflammation around the urethra may signal a mild infection or a venereal disease.

Venereal Disease Testing

EIA and EVA

As part of a general physical exam, the stallion should be blood tested for Equine Infectious Anemia (EIA) and Equine Viral Arteritis (EVA). Both viral diseases are potentially passed venereally to the mare. EVA can be passed to other mares by the respiratory route. Not all stallions shed EVA virus in their semen but the semen should be evaluated as this virus can cause abortion. Any mare to be bred to a stallion that has tested positive for EVA should be vaccinated before breeding.

Another venereal disease is caused by yet another virus, equine herpes virus-3 or *equine coital exanthma.* Stallions or mares may be asymptomatic carriers, but horses with active herpes lesions should not be bred by live coverage, although the virus does not interfere with conception rates.

CEM

A stallion that is imported into the United States from Europe must be quarantined for *contagious equine metritis* (CEM), a bacterial infection caused by *Taylorella equigenitalis.* The stallion only carries the bacteria as a surface contaminant on his penis, whereas infection of a mare persists in her reproductive tract. A stallion's immune system does not respond to the disease by building antibodies that circulate in the blood.

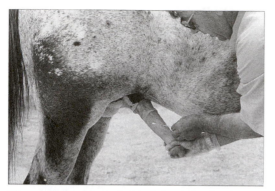

Therefore, blood testing a stallion for exposure to the bacteria does not identify a carrier stallion. The only way to determine CEM infection is by taking repeated bacterial cultures swabbed directly from the penis.

Fig. 23–10. Taking a bacterial culture for CEM.

Bacterial Culture

Both before and after ejaculation, a bacterial culture is taken by gently inserting a cotton swab into the urethra. Then the swab is taken to a lab which can determine the presence of other bacterial organisms that can be transferred from the stallion to the mare through the semen. Some bacteria can cause a serious enough infection in the mare that it will prevent conception or induce spontaneous abortion.

Semen Evaluation

The semen is evaluated for its quality by collecting samples on successive days until the semen quality has stabilized. Evaluating the semen in this manner gives a realistic picture of how much sperm a stallion can produce, its color and structure, and how vital the sperm is.

Color

The color of the semen is examined for blood *(hemospermia)* or urine; both substances damage fertility by killing sperm cells.

Motility

One of the most important aspects of semen fertility is the *motility* of the sperm, which is the ability of the sperm to move. The activity of the sperm and its propensity to swim in a forward direction is called *progressive motility*. A drop of semen is placed on a warm slide and examined under a microscope immediately after collection to determine the percent of sperm that are motile compared to those that are inactive. An ideal sample would be one with over 80% of sperm showing active progressive motility, but over 50% motility is considered acceptable. Raw semen of fertile stallions retains over 10% motility for 6 hours. If semen motility is diminished to less than 10% in under 2 hours, conception rates are poor.

Structure

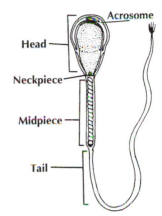

The structure *(morphology)* of individual sperm cells is important to their effective motility. Sperm with defective tails are unable to swim forward, and may travel in circles or in reverse. The head of the sperm must be perfect for the *acrosome* of the head eventually penetrates the waiting egg. Even if a sperm is able to swim to its destination, a defective acrosome would prevent it from fertilizing the egg. Ideally, more than 60% of the sperm cells should be normal with less than 10% major structural defects.

Fig. 23–11. Structure of a sperm.

Concentration

The *concentration* of sperm is important to a stallion's fertility. This figure is obtained by a spectrophotometer that counts the total number of sperm cells in a measured sample. The minimum concentration necessary to ensure conception of a mare is estimated at 5×10^8 (500 million) sperm cells per inseminated dose.

Other Factors Affecting Fertility

Stress Level

The stress of competition reduces the fertility of a stallion and has a marked effect on his breeding performance. This fact should be considered if a mare is booked to a stallion that is actively campaigning between breeding dates. Semen that had ample potency on collection may be infertile at insemination 12 or more hours later. This is particularly significant if semen is to be transported long distances.

Semen Extenders

Semen extenders that provide the sperm with adequate energy and nutrients are a vital aspect of the longevity of shipped semen. An extender must be matched for compatibility with each stallion's semen. An ideal semen extender will increase the conception rates of mares receiving transported semen.

Season

The season the stallion is bred also affects his fertility. April through August is the normal breeding season in the Northern Hemisphere. These summer months offer the optimum fertile period for breeding, not only for the stallion, but also for the mare.

Siring Records

The potency of a stallion with a past breeding history can be put to the test by examining his siring records. This is particularly helpful when selecting a stallion for transported semen, as the costs of semen collection, air transport, and insemination can escalate with each estrous cycle if the mare does not conceive. If a stallion has a history of standing to stud, it is possible to categorize him as a satisfactory, questionable, or unsatisfactory breeder.

Satisfactory Breeder

The satisfactory breeder achieves at least a 75% conception rate during a single breeding season. A satisfactory breeder can potentially accommodate a large booking for the season if the season is extended from mid February to mid August, and the mares are presented to him at staggered cycles. It is possible for a fertile stallion to be booked to as many as 45 mares for natural cover, or to 125 mares for artificial insemination if his semen quality is consistent throughout the breeding months.

Questionable Breeder

A stallion would fall into the questionable category if he has problems with libido, effective ejaculation, or if his semen quality is marginal.

Unsatisfactory Breeder

The unsatisfactory breeder is the stallion that has poor semen quality leading to low fertility. A stallion with heritable defects or venereal disease is excluded as breeding stock, and by definition is unsatisfactory.

Maintaining a Stallion's Health

The breeding stallion is a performance horse that can continue in his duties well into his twenties if he is properly cared for and condi-

tioned. An idle stallion becomes obese and un-
healthy, and is prone to
laminitis, colic, and heart
failure. A stallion's body
condition score should be
carefully monitored to ensure the quality of his diet.
A stallion that is exercised
on a regular program has
greater longevity in the
breeding sheds. Turning
the stallion into a paddock
or pasture each day is primarily good for his mental
state, but forced exercise
for 30 – 60 minutes a day is
required to keep him fit
and in prime metabolic
condition.

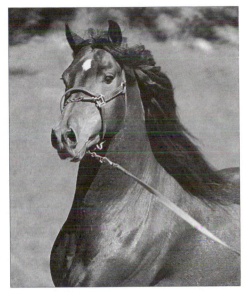

Fig. 23–12. Exercise and nutrition ensure a stallion's health and reproductive longevity.

ARTIFICIAL INSEMINATION

This era of advanced supertechnology has enhanced the options on how to have a mare bred, and to whom. If alternative methods of breeding such as artificial insemination (AI), (shipped cooled or frozen semen), or embryo transfer are employed, carefully research the stallion. Major, unrecoverable expenses can be incurred in collecting a stallion and shipping semen that has low fertility or viability. For long distance breeding methods or for embryo transfer, plan ahead to work out problems such as airline schedules, show schedules, or synchronizing ovulation for embryo transfer candidates. Check with the breed registry if methods other than live cover *are allowed* so the foal can be registered.

Artificial insemination may be used on mares at the breeding farm, or for mares living long distances from a stallion. Costs incurred by using artificial insemination include semen collection, transport of cooled or frozen semen to the mare at home, along with veterinary fees to collect the stallion and to inseminate the mare.

Advantages of AI

Artificial insemination is beneficial not just to the mare owner, but also to the stallion owner. Because one collection of semen can be divided into multiple inseminations, more mares can be bred than with natural cover.

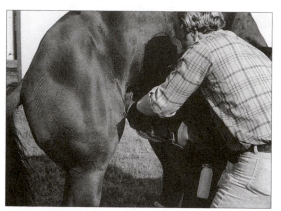

Fig. 23–13. Collecting semen for AI.

Breeding Several Mares at Once

It is common practice to collect semen from a stallion on the premises, and having synchronized several mares to the same estrous cycle, all the mares can be bred at the same time. Not only does the stallion have to perform as stud fewer times to breed all the mares, but this facilitates management 11 months later when it is time to monitor the mares for foaling.

Reduced Risk of Injury

There is less risk of physical injury to both the mare and stallion if the stallion does not have to approach or mount a mare to breed her. AI reduces the chance of infecting a mare with a hidden bacterial venereal disease, especially if antibiotics are added to a semen extender used for shipping semen to a distant location.

Breeding Mares With Foals

If a mare has a foal by her side it is often easier and safer to use AI. The mare accepts the breeding without having to protect her foal, and the mare and foal need not be shipped to the stud farm.

Breed Registries and AI Regulations

Not all breed registries approve artificial insemination. It is wise to check with the registry before embarking on that route, and to have all the appropriate paperwork in hand and registry fees paid before breeding expenses begin to add up. The registry may require blood typing to ensure that the foal is truly the offspring of the stated mare and stallion.

Where AI Is Forbidden

The Jockey Club of America does not permit any form of AI for Thoroughbred horses, nor do the American Miniature Horse Association or the Standard Jack and Jennet Registry of America.

Where AI Is Allowed

In contrast, the Arabian Horse Registry of America (AHRA) for purebred Arabians, the International Arabian Horse Association (IAHA) for part-bred Arabians, and the American Morgan Horse Association (AMHA) permit any form of artificial insemination, using liquid or frozen transported semen. Many Warmblood associations, like the American Hanoverian Society, Inc., the American Holsteiner Horse Association, and the Swedish and Dutch Warmblood registries approve AI for their mares.

Other registries with liberal policies for the use of transported semen include the Pinto Horse Association of America, the American Saddlebred Horse Association, the American Hackney Horse Society, the Peruvian Paso Horse registries, and some draft horse registries.

Where AI Is Conditional

The American Quarter Horse Association (AQHA) does not approve use of transported or preserved semen. AI is allowed only if both the stallion and mare are on the same premises and the mare is bred immediately after semen collection. The American Paint Horse Association (APHA) and the Appaloosa Horse Club, Inc. (ApHC) permit the use of AI with similar stipulations as for the AQHA, but the semen can be preserved for up to 24 hours.

The United States Trotting Association has variable regulations on the use of transported semen, so it is best to check the registry in the state.

BREEDING MANAGEMENT

Whether breeding is accomplished by natural mating at a breeding farm, by artificial insemination, or by cooled or frozen, shipped semen, expenses can run quite high before a mare is declared "in foal."

First, there is a stud fee. Then, there is the cost of daily "mare care" while a mare remains at the breeding farm. The cost of transportation to deliver her to the breeding farm, and home again, must also be considered.

Breeding Contract

Usually, a written contract is executed between stallion breeder and mare owner. Read the contract thoroughly; make sure all wording is understandable. Discussion of mare care and liability for veterinary services while the mare is at the breeding farm should be included in the contract to avoid misunderstandings.

Find out if the stud fee includes semen collection charges if transported semen is to be used. If not, veterinary expenses can add up if the stallion must be repeatedly collected for a mare that fails to conceive on the first cycle she is bred.

Many stud farms require a uterine biopsy and bacterial culture of the mare's uterus before entering into a breeding contract. The costs of a prebreeding evaluation for the mare must be further considered when determining the financial feasibility of breeding a mare.

Most stud fees include a *live foal guarantee* (LFG), meaning that if the mare fails to conceive, aborts, or gives birth to a dead foal, the mare owner is not liable to pay the stud fee or is promised a breeding the following season at no charge. Review the contract for a clause stating a live foal guarantee, or the stud fee and related expenses may be lost.

Teasing Programs

It is essential to find a reputable breeding facility that manages a competent breeding operation. Valuable time is lost without proper teasing techniques, teasing frequency, and record-keeping.

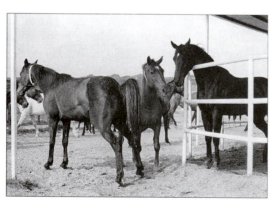

Fig. 23–14. Valuable time is lost without proper teasing techniques.

Interview the stallion manager about the farm's record-keeping and a consistent daily teasing program to detect when a mare is in heat. One of the largest causes of "infertility" is management's failure to identify if a mare is in estrus and ready for breeding. An excellent teasing program is a key to success so a breeder can identify when a mare is in heat. This identification may be difficult for mares with "silent" heats who refuse to show to any stallion, or who show to only one particular stallion. In these cases, daily rectal palpation or ultrasound may be necessary to identify breeding time if not using natural coverage.

Careful attention to teasing records also minimizes the number of times a stallion is required to inseminate a mare. The fewer times he must breed her or be collected reduces the chances for injury and infection, and increases the number of mares he can breed in a season.

Booking to a Stallion

Long before it is time to breed a mare, arrangements should be made with the stallion manager to "book" the mare in time for the breeding season ahead. A stallion can only breed so many mares each season, especially if he is involved in a show or performance schedule. To avoid profound disappointment at finding a stallion's bookings filled, plan as much as a year in advance. *(Editor's Note: For a complete and very detailed book on all subjects of equine breeding, read **Breeding Management & Foal Development** published by Equine Research, Inc.)*

APPENDIX

Parts of the Horse

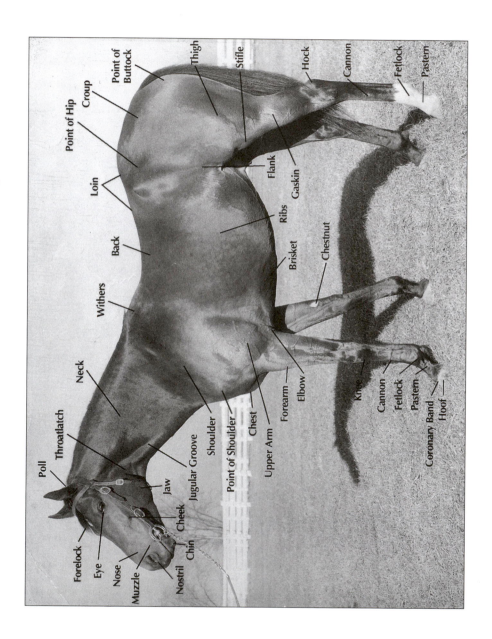

Bones of the Horse

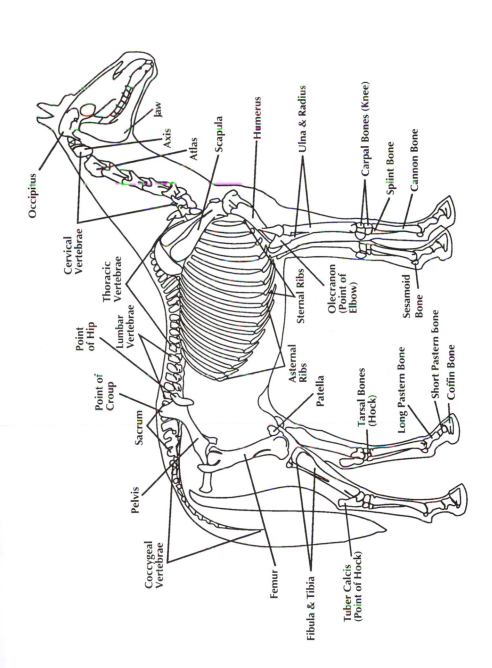

Muscles of the Horse

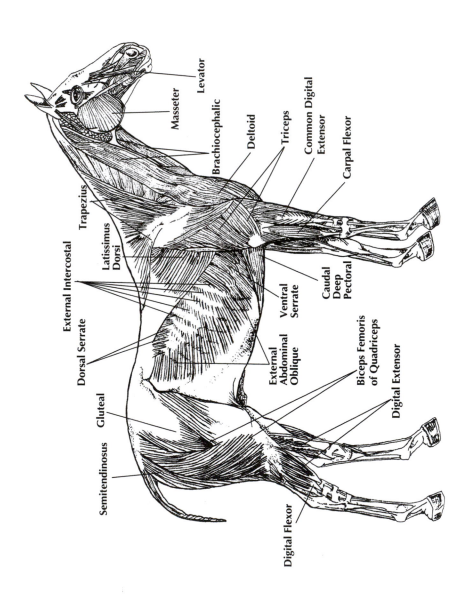

Bibliography

Adams, O.R. *Lameness in Horses.* Third Edition. Lea and Febiger, Philadelphia, 1979.

Alsup, E.M. "Dimethyl Sulfoxide." *Journal of the American Veterinary Medical Association,* Vol. 185, No. 9 (November 1984), pp. 1011 – 1014.

Antikatzides, T.G. "Soft Laser Treatment of Musculoskeletal and Other Disorders in the Equine Athlete." *Equine Practice,* Vol. 8, No. 2 (February 1986), pp. 24 – 29.

Asquith, R.L., E.L. Johnson, J. Kivepelto, and C. Depew. "Erroneous Weight Estimation of Horses." *Proceedings of the American Association of Equine Practitioners* (1990), pp. 599 – 607.

Austin, S.M., J.A. DiPietro, J.H. Foreman, G.J. Baker, and K.S. Todd. "Parascaris Equorum Infections in Horses." *Compendium on Continuing Education,* Vol. 12, No. 8 (August 1990), pp. 1110 – 1118.

Baker, D.J. "Rationale for the Use of Influenza Vaccines in Horses and the Importance of Antigenic Drift." *Equine Veterinary Journal,* Vol. 18, No. 2 (1986), pp. 93 – 96.

Balch, O.K., M.H. Ratzlaff, M.L. Hyde, and K.K. White. "Locomotor Effects of Hoof Angle and Mediolateral Balance of Horses Exercising on a High-Speed Treadmill: Preliminary Results." *Proceedings of the American Association of Equine Practitioners* (1991), pp. 687 – 705.

Banks, William J. *Applied Veterinary Histology.* Williams and Wilkins, Baltimore, 1981, pp. 245 – 261.

Barber, S.M. "Second Intention Wound Healing in the Horse: The Effect of Bandages and Topical Corticosteroids." *Proceedings of the American Association of Equine Practitioners* (1989), pp. 107 – 116.

Baucus, K.L., S.L. Ralston, et al. "The Effect of Copper and Zinc Supplementation on Mineral Content of Mare's Milk." *Equine Veterinary Science,* Vol. 9, No. 4 (1989), pp. 206 – 209.

Baucus, K.L., E.L. Squires, S.L. Ralston, and A.O. McKinnon. "The Effect of Transportation Stress on Early Embryonic Death in Mares." *Proceedings of the Equine Nutrition and Physiology Symposium* (1987), pp. 657 – 662.

Baxter, G.M. "Equine Laminitis." *Equine Practice,* Vol. 14, No. 4 (April 1992), pp. 13 – 22.

Baxter, G.M. "Wound Healing and Delayed Wound Closure in the Lower Limb of the Horse." *Equine Practice,* Vol. 10, No. 1 (January 1988), pp. 23 – 31.

Bayly, W.M., H.D. Liggitt, L.J. Huston, and W.W. Laegreid. "Stress and Its Effect on Equine Pulmonary Mucosal Defenses." *Proceedings of the American Association of Equine Practitioners* (1986), pp. 253 – 262.

Beeman, M. "Conformation: The Relationship of Form to Function." *Quarter Horse Journal* Reprint.

Bennett, D. "Principles of Conformation Analysis." Selected Articles from *Equus* 117 – 177.

Bertone, J.J., J.L. Traub-Dargatz, R.W. Wrigley, D.G. Bennett, and R.J. Williams. "Diarrhea Associated With Sand in the Gastrointestinal Tract of Horses." *Journal of the American Veterinary Medical Association* (December 1988), Vol. 193, No. 11, pp. 1409 – 1412.

Blagburn, B.L., D.S. Lindsay, C.M. Hendrix, and J. Schumacher. "Pathogenesis, Treatment, and Control of Gastric Parasites in Horses." *Compendium on Continuing Education*, Vol. 13, No. 5 (May 1991), pp. 850 – 857.

Booth, N.H. and L.E. McDonald, eds. *Veterinary Pharmacology and Therapeutics*. Fifth Edition. Iowa State University Press, Ames, 1982.

Bradley, R.E., T.J. Lane, R.F. Jochen, B.P. Seibert, and K.M. Newcomb, "Distribution and Frequency of Benzimidazole Resistance in Equine Small Strongyles." *Equine Practice*, Vol. 8, No. 2 (February 1986), pp. 7 – 11.

Bramlage, L. and Editorial Staff. "Surgical Repair of Bowed Tendons." *Thoroughbred Times* (February 1992), pp. 22 – 24.

Bramlage, L.R., N.W. Rantanen, R.L. Genovese, and L.E. Page. "Long-term Effects of Surgical Treatment of Superficial Flexor Tendinitis by Superior Check Desmototomy." *Proceedings of the American Association of Equine Practitioners* (1988), pp. 655.

Bridges, C.H. and E.D. Harris. "Experimentally Induced Cartilaginous Fractures (Osteochondritis Dissecans) in Foals Fed Low-Copper Diets." *Journal of American Veterinary Medical Association*, Vol. 193, No. 2 (July 1988), pp. 215 – 221.

Bryans, J.T. "Control of Equine Influenza." *Proceedings of the American Association of Equine Practitioners* (1980), pp. 279 – 285.

Buffa, E.A., et al. "Effect of Dietary Biotin Supplement on Equine Hoof Horn Growth Rate and Hardness." *Equine Veterinary Journal*, Vol. 24, No. 6 (1992), pp. 472 – 474.

Burch, G.E. "Transcutaneous Electrical Stimulation." *Equine Practice*, Vol. 7, No. 9 (October 1985), pp. 6 – 11.

Carleton, C.L. "Basic Techniques for Evaluating the Subfertile Mare." *Veterinary Medicine* (December 1988), pp. 1253 – 1261.

Carlson, G.P. "Medical Problems Associated With Protracted Heat and Work Stress in Horses." *Compendium on Continuing Education*, Vol. 7, No. 10 (October 1985), pp. 542 – 550.

Clabough, D. "Streptococcus Equi Infection in the Horse: A Review of Clinical and Immunological Considerations." *Equine Veterinary Science, Vol. 7*, No. 5 (1987), pp. 279 – 283.

Clarke, A.F., T.M. Madelin, and R.G. Allpress. "The Relationship of Air Hygiene in Stables to Lower Airway Disease and Pharyngeal Lymphoid Hyperplasia in Two Groups of Thoroughbred Horses." *Equine Veterinary Journal*, Vol. 19, No. 6 (1987), pp. 524 – 530.

Clayton, H.M. "Comparison of the Stride of Trotting Horses Trimmed With a Normal and a Broken-Back Hoof Axis." *Proceedings of the American Association of Equine Practitioners* (1988), pp. 289 – 298.

Clayton, H.M. "Time-Motion Analysis in Equestrian Sports: The Grand Prix Dressage Test." *Proceedings of the American Association of Equine Practitioners* (1989), pp. 367 – 373.

Clayton, H.M. *Conditioning Sport Horses*. Sport Horse Publications, Saskatoon, Saskatchewan, Canada, 1991.

Coffman, J.R. "Muscle Fibers: Coupling and Contraction and Energy Metabolism." *Equine Sportsmedicine*, Vol. 3, No. 2 (1984), pp. 1 – 3.

Coffman, J.R. "Stress and the Racehorse." *Equine Sportmedicine*, Vol. 3, No. 4 (1984), pp. 1, 7 – 8.

Colles, C.M. "A Technique for Assessing Hoof Function in the Horse." *Equine Veterinary Journal*, Vol. 21, No. 1 (1989), pp. 17 – 22.

Colles, C.M. "The Relationship of Frog Pressure to Heel Expansion." *Equine Veterinary Journal*, Vol. 21, No. 1 (1989), pp. 13 – 16.

Collier, M., et al. "Electrostimulation of Bone Production in the Horse." *Proceedings of the American Association of Equine Practitioners* (1981), pp. 71 – 89.

Collins, L.G., and D.E. Tyler. "Phenylbutazone Toxicosis in the Horse: A Clinical Study." *Journal of the American Veterinary Medical Association*, Vol. 184, No. 6 (March 1984), pp. 699 – 703.

Colquhoun, K.M., et al. "Control of Breeding in the Mare." *Equine Veterinary Journal*, Vol. 19, No. 2 (1987), pp. 138 – 142.

Cook, W.R. "Diagnosis and Grading of Hereditary Recurrent Laryngeal Neuropathy in the Horse." *Equine Veterinary Science*, Vol. 8, No. 6 (1988), pp. 431 – 455.

Cook, W.R. "Recent Observations on Recurrent Laryngeal Neuropathy in the Horse: Applications to Practice." *Proceedings of the American Association of Equine Practitioners* (1988), pp. 427 – 478.

Cook, W.R. "Some Observations on Form and Function of the Equine Upper Airway in Health and Disease: 1. The Pharynx." *Proceedings of the American Association of Equine Practitioners* (1981), pp. 355 – 391.

Cook, W.R. "Some Observations on Form and Function of the Equine Upper Airway in Health and Disease: 2. The Larynx." *Proceedings of the American Association of Equine Practitioners* (1981), pp. 393 – 451.

Cook, W.R. *Specifications for Speed in the Racehorse: The Airflow Factors.* The Russell Meerdink Company, Ltd., 1993.

Cook, W.R., et al. "Upper Airway Obstruction (Possible Asphyxia) as the Possible Cause of Exercise-Induced Pulmonary Hemorrhage in the Horse: An Hypothesis." *Equine Veterinary Science*, Vol. 8, No. 1 (1988), pp. 11 – 26.

Cox, J.H. and R.M. DeBowes. "Colic-like Discomfort Associated With Ovulation in Two Mares." *Journal of the American Veterinary Medical Association*, Vol. 191, No. 11 (December 1987), pp. 1451 – 1452.

Cox, J.H. and R.M. DeBowes. "Episodic Weakness Caused by Hyperkalemic Periodic Paralysis in Horses." *Compendium on Continuing Education*, Vol. 12, No. 1 (January 1990), pp. 83 – 88.

Crawford, W.H., R. Vanderby, Jr., et al. "The Energy Absorption Capacity of Equine Support Bandages." *V.C.O.T.*, Vol. 1 (1990), pp. 2 – 9.

Crowell-Davis, S., W. Crowell-Davis, and A. Caudle. "Preventing Trailering Problems: Part II." *Equine Practice*, Vol. 9, No. 1 (January 1987), pp. 32 – 33.

Currey, J.D. "The Mechanical Consequences of Variations in the Mineral Content of Bone." *Journal of Biomechanics*, Vol. 2 (1969A), pp. 2 – 11.

Currey, J.D. "The Relationship Between Stiffness and the Mineral Content of Bone." *Journal of Biomechanics*, Vol. 2 (1969B), pp. 477 – 480.

Custalow, B. "Protein Requirements During Exercise in the Horse." *Equine Veterinary Science*, Vol. 11, No. 1 (1991), pp. 65 – 66.

Cymbaluk, N. "Water Balance of Horses Fed Various Diets." *Equine Practice*, Vol. 11, No. 1 (1989), pp. 19 – 24.

Derksen, F.J., et al. "Chronic Obstructive Pulmonary Disease Roundtable Discussion." *Equine Practice*, Vol. 13, No. 5 (May 1991), pp. 25 – 28. *Equine Practice*, Vol. 13, No. 7 (July/August 1991), pp. 15 – 19.

Derksen, F.J. "Physiology of Airflow in the Athletic Horse." *Proceedings of the American Association of Equine Practitioners* (1988), pp. 149 – 158.

DiPietro, J.A. and K.S. Todd. "Anthelmintics Used in Treatment of Parasitic

Infections of Horses." *Equine Practice,* Vol. 11, No. 4 (April 1989), pp. 5 – 15.

DiPietro, J.A., T.R. Klei, and D.D. French. "Contemporary Topics in Equine Parasitology." *Compendium on Continuing Education,* Vol. 12, No. 5 (May 1990), pp. 713 – 720.

Divers, T.J. and D. Dreyfuss. "Evaluating the Horse With a Poor Racing Performance." *Veterinary Medicine* (May 1990), pp. 522, 529.

Drudge, J.H. and E.T. Lyons. *Internal Parasites of Equids With Emphasis on Treatment and Control.* Hoechst-Roussel Agri-Vet Company, 1986.

Drudge, J.H. and E.T. Lyons. *Internal Parasites of Equids With Emphasis on Treatment and Control, Revised 1989.* Hoechst-Roussel Agri-Vet Company.

Drudge, J.H., E.T. Lyons, and S.C. Tolliver. "Strongyles—An Update." *Equine Practice,* Vol. 11, No. 4 (April 1989), pp. 43 – 49.

Duren, S., C. Wood, and S. Jackson. "Dietary Fat and the Racehorse." *Equine Veterinary Science,* Vol. 7, No. 6 (1987), pp. 396 – 397.

Dwyer, Roberta M. "The Practical Diagnosis and Treatment of Metabolic Conditions in Endurance Horses." *Equine Practice,* Vol. 8, No. 8 (September 1986), pp. 21 – 33.

Dyer, Robert M. "The Bovine Respiratory Disease Complex: A Complex Interaction of Host, Environmental, and Infectious Factors." *Compendium on Continuing Education,* Vol. 4, No. 7 (July 1982), pp. 296 – 307.

Editorial Staff. *Dynamics of Equine Athletic Performance. Proceedings of the Association of Equine Sports Medicine* (1985), Veterinary Learning Systems Co., Inc.

Editorial Staff. "Conformation." *Practical Horseman* (May 1992), pp. 54 – 60, 90 – 91.

Editorial Staff. "Round Table on Interval Training." *Thoroughbred Times* (February 1992), pp. 14 – 21.

Editorial Staff. *Proceedings of a Roundtable on Equine Influenza* (December 1987), Coopers Animal Health, Inc.

Editorial Staff. "Hyperkalemic Periodic Paralysis Presents Medical and Ethical Challenge." *Journal of the American Veterinary Medical Association,* Vol. 202, No. 8 (April 1993), pp. 1203 – 1209.

Edwards, Gladys Brown. *Anatomy and Conformation of the Horse.* Dreenan Press, Ltd., Croton-on-Hudson, New York, 1980.

England, J.J. "Veterinary Virology, Part II: Pathogenesis of Viral Infections." *Compendium on Continuing Education,* Vol. 6, No. 2 (February 1984), pp. 145 – 154.

Equine Respiratory Medicine and Surgery. *Equine Veterinary Journal,* Vol. 19 (September/October 1987), No. 5.

Erickson, B.K., Erickson, H.H., and Coffman, J.R. "Exercise-Induced Pulmonary Hemorrhage During High Intensity Exercise: Potential Causes and the Role of Furosemide." *Proceedings of the American Association of Equine Practitioners* (1989), pp. 375 – 379.

Essen-Gustavsson, B., D. McMiken, et al. "Muscular Adaptation of Horses During Intensive Training and Detraining." *Equine Veterinary Journal,* Vol. 21, No. 1 (1989), pp. 27 – 33.

Ewert, K.M., J.A. DiPietro, J.H. Foreman, and K.S. Todd. "Control Programs for Endoparasites in Horses." *Compendium on Continuing Education,* Vol. 13, No. 6 (June 1991), pp. 1012 – 1018.

Fadok, V.A. and P.C. Mullowney. "Dermatologic Diseases of Horses, Part 1: Parasitic Dermatoses of the Horse." *Compendium on Continuing Educa-*

tion, Vol. 5, No. 11 (November 1983), pp. 615 – 622.

Foil, L.D. and C.S. Foil. "Arthropod Pests of Horses." *Compendium on Continuing Education*, Vol. 12, No. 5 (May 1990), pp. 723 – 730.

Foil, L.D. and C.S. Foil. "Dipteran Parasites of Horses." *Equine Practice*, Vol. 10, No. 4 (April 1988), pp. 21 – 38.

Foil, L.D., et al. "The Role of Horn Fly Feeding and the Management of Seasonal Equine Ventral Midline Dermatitis." *Equine Practice*, Vol. 12, No. 5 (May 1990), pp. 6 – 14.

Fox, S.F. "Management of Thermal Burns—Part 1." *Compendium on Continuing Education*, Vol. 7, No. 8 (August 1985), pp. 631 – 639.

Fox, S.F. "Management of Thermal Burns—Part 2." *Compendium on Continuing Education*, Vol. 8, No. 7 (July 1986), pp. 439 – 444.

Frape, D.L. "Dietary Requirements and Athletic Performance of Horses." *Equine Veterinary Journal*, Vol. 20, No. 3 (1988), pp. 163 – 172.

Frazier, C. "Cardiac Recovery Index." *AERC Endurance News* (September 1992), pp. 4 – 6.

Frazier, D. "Equine Dietary Adaptation: Cardiac Recovery Index." *AERC Endurance News* (November 1992), pp. 10 – 15.

Fredriksson, G., H. Kindahl, and G. Stabenfeldt. "Endotoxin-Induced and Prostaglandin-Mediated Effects on Corpus Luteum Function in the Mare." *Theriogenology*, Vol. 25 (1986), pp. 309 – 316.

Freestone, J.F. and G.P. Carlson. "Muscle Disorders in the Horse: A Retrospective Study." *Equine Veterinary Journal*, Vol. 23, No. 2 (1991), pp. 86 – 90.

French, D.D. and M.R. Chapman. "Tapeworms of the Equine Gastrointestinal Tract." *Compendium on Continuing Education*, Vol. 14, No. 5 (May 1992), pp. 655 – 661.

French, D.D., T.R. Klei, and G.E. Hackett. "Equine Parasites: Dollars and Sense." *Equine Practice*, Vol. 10, No. 5 (May 1988), pp. 8 – 14.

Fricker C., W. Riek, and J. Hugelshofter. "A Model for Pathogenesis of Navicular Disease." *Equine Veterinary Journal*, Vol. 14 (1982), pp. 203 – 207.

Gach, J. "Trailer Studies Reveal Fewer Harmful Effects Than Expected." *Equus* 120 (1987), pp. 12 – 16.

Genetzky, R.M. "Chronic Obstructive Pulmonary Disease In Horses — Part 1." *Compendium on Continuing Education*, Vol. 7, No. 7 (July 1985), pp. 407 – 414.

Gerring, E.L. "All Wind and Water: Some Progress in the Study of Equine Gut Motility." *Equine Veterinary Journal*, Vol. 23, No. 2 (1991), pp. 81 – 85.

Getty, Robert, ed. *Sisson and Grossman's The Anatomy of the Domestic Animals*. Volume 1. WB Saunders Company, 1975.

Gillespie, J.R. and N.E. Robinson, eds. *Equine Exercise Physiology 2*. ICEEP Publications, Davis, California, 1987.

Gillis, C. and D. Meagher. "Tendon Response to Training." *The Equine Athlete*, Vol. 4, No. 5 (September/October 1991), pp. 26 – 27.

Ginther, O.J. *Reproductive Biology of the Mare*. McNaughton and Gunn, Inc., Ann Arbor, Michigan, 1979.

Glade, M.J. "Feeding Innovations for the Performance Horse." *Equine Veterinary Science*, Vol. 4, No. 4, pp. 165 – 166.

Goetz, T.E., C.H. Boulton, and G.K. Ogilvie. "Clinical Management of Progressive Multifocal Benign and Malignant Melanomas of Horses With Oral Cimetidine." *Proceedings of the American Association of Equine Practitio-*

ners (1989), pp. 431 – 438.

Goetz, T.E., G.K. Ogilvie, et al. "Cimetidine for Treatment of Melanomas in Three Horses." *Journal of the American Veterinary Medical Association*, Vol. 196, No. 3 (February 1990), pp. 449 – 452.

Goodman, N., et al. "An Equine Roundtable Discussion on Lameness." *Equine Practice*, Vol. 12, No. 8 (September 1990), pp. 28 – 33.

Gorham, S. and M. Robl. "Melanoma in the Gray Horse: The Darker Side of Equine Aging." *Veterinary Medicine* (May 1986), pp. 446 – 448.

Grant, B.D., L.J. Smith, et al. "Hill Training for High-Speed Performance Horses." *The Equine Athlete*, Vol. 1, No. 1 (December 1988), pp. 6 – 7, 15 – 16.

Green, E., et al. "Endotoxemia Roundtable Discussion." *Equine Practice*, Vol. 14, No. 9 (October 1992), pp. 7 – 12. *Equine Practice*, Vol. 14, No. 10 (November/December 1992), pp. 13 – 18. *Equine Practice*, Vol. 15, No. 1 (January 1993), pp. 7 – 14.

Griffiths, I.R. "The Pathogenesis of Equine Laryngeal Hemiplegia." *Equine Veterinary Journal*, Vol. 23, No. 2 (1991), pp. 75 – 76.

Hackett, G.E., C. Uhlinger, R. Mitchell, F.B. McCashin, and S. Conboy. "Continuous Deworming Programs: Roundtable Discussion." *Equine Practice*, Vol. 14, No. 7 (July/August 1992), pp. 13 – 18. *Equine Practice*, Vol. 14, No. 8 (September 1992), pp. 27 – 33.

Halldordsottir, S. and H.J. Larsen. "An Epidemiological Study of Summer Eczema in Icelandic Horses in Norway." *Equine Veterinary Journal*, Vol. 23, No. 4 (1991), pp. 296 – 299.

Hamm, D. and E.W. Jones. "Intra-Articular and Intramuscular Treatment of Noninfectious Equine Arthritis (DJD) With Polysulfated Glycosaminoglycan (PSGAG)." *Equine Veterinary Science*, Vol. 8, No. 6 (1988), pp. 456 – 459.

Harkins, J.D. and S.G. Kamerling. "A Comparative Study of Interval and Conventional Training Methods in Thoroughbred Racehorses." *Equine Veterinary Science* (January /February 1990), pp. 45 – 51.

Harkins, J.D. and S.G. Kamerling. "Effects of Induced Alkalosis on Performance in Thoroughbreds During a 1600 Meter Race." *Equine Veterinary Journal*, Vol. 24, No. 2 (1992), pp. 94 – 98.

Harman, J. "Acupuncture for Horses." *AERC Endurance News* (August 1991), pp. 8 – 9.

Harper, Frederick. "Control of the Broodmare's Reproductive Cycle." *Equine Veterinary Science*, Vol. 9, No. 2 (1989), pp. 112 – 115.

Harris, P. and D.H. Snow. "Plasma Potassium and Lactate Concentrations in Thoroughbred Horses During Exercise of Varying Intensity." *Equine Veterinary Journal*, Vol. 23, No. 3 (1992), pp. 220 – 225.

Hart, C. "Equine Conformation of the Top Endurance Athlete." *AERC Endurance News* (August 1990), pp. 10 – 11.

Hayes, Horace M. *Points of the Horse.* Arco Publishing Company, Inc., New York, 1969.

Haynes, Peter. "Obstructive Disease of the Upper Respiratory Tract: Current Thoughts on Diagnosis and Surgical Management." *Proceedings of the American Association of Equine Practitioners* (1986), pp. 283 – 290.

Henneke, D.R. "A Condition Score System for Horses." *Equine Practice*, Vol. 7, No. 8 (September 1985), pp. 13 – 15.

Herd, R.P. "Epidemiology and Control of Equine Strongylosis at Newmarket." *Equine Veterinary Journal*, Vol. 18, No. 6 (1986), pp. 447 – 452.

Herd, R.P. and A.A. Gabel. "Reduced Efficacy of Anthelmintics in Young

Compared With Adult Horses." *Equine Veterinary Journal*, Vol. 22, No. 3 (1990), pp. 164 – 169.

Hickman, J. "Navicular Disease—What Are We Talking About?" *Equine Veterinary Journal*, Vol. 21, No. 6 (1989), pp. 395 – 398.

Hintz, H.F. "Factors Which Influence Developmental Orthopedic Disease." *Proceedings of the American Association of Equine Practitioners* (1988), pp. 159 – 162.

Hintz, H.F., et al. "Effects of Protein Levels on Endurance Horses." *Journal of Animal Science*, Vol. 51 (1980), p. 202.

Hintz, H.F. "Biotin." *Equine Practice*, Vol. 9, No. 9 (October 1987), pp. 4 – 5.

Hintz, H.F. "Effect of Diet on Copper Content of Milk." *Equine Practice*, Vol. 9, No. 8 (1987), pp. 6 – 7.

Hintz, H.F. "Protein Needs of the Equine Athlete." *Equine Practice*, Vol. 8, No. 6 (1988), pp. 5 – 6.

Hintz, H.F. "Some Myths About Equine Nutrition." *Compendium on Continuing Education*, Vol. 12, No. 1 (1990), pp. 78 – 81.

Hintz, H.F. "The 1989 NRC Estimates of Protein Requirements." *Equine Practice*, Vol. 11, No. 10 (1989), pp. 5 – 6.

Hintz, H.F. "Weighing Horses." *Equine Practice*, Vol. 10, No. 8 (1988), pp. 10 – 11.

Hodgson, D.R. "Exertional Rhabdomyolysis." *Current Veterinary Therapy 2*, WB Saunders Co., Philadelphia, 1987, pp. 487 – 490.

Hodgson, D.R. "Myopathies in the Athletic Horse." *Compendium on Continuing Education*, Vol. 7, No. 10 (October 1985), pp. 551 – 556.

Honnas, C.M., J. Schumacher, and P.W. Dean. "Laryngeal Hemiplegia in Horses: Diagnosis and Surgical Management." *Veterinary Medicine* (October 1985), pp. 752 – 763.

Houpt, K.A. "Thirst in Horses: The Physiological and Psychological Causes." *Equine Practice*, Vol. 9, No. 6 (June 1987), pp. 28 – 30.

Houston, C.S. *Going Higher: The Story of Man and Altitude.* Little, Brown, and Company, Boston, 1987.

Huddleston, A.L., P. Rockwell, D.N. Kulund, and R.B. Harrison. "Bone Mass in Life-Time Tennis Athletes." *Journal of the American Medical Association*, Vol. 244 (1980), pp. 1107 – 1109.

Hurtig, M.B., S.L. Green, H. Dobson, and J. Burton. "Defective Bone and Cartilage in Foals Fed a Low Copper Diet." *Proceedings of the American Association of Equine Practitioners* (1990), pp. 637 – 643.

Hustead, D. "Vaccines: What's Ahead?" *Large Animal Veterinarian* (March/April 1990), pp. 8 – 11, 36 – 37.

Ivers, T. "Osteochondrosis: Undernutrition or Overnutrition?" *Equine Practice*, Vol. 8, No. 8 (September 1986), pp. 15 – 19.

Ivers, T. "Cryotherapy: An In-Depth Study." *Equine Practice*, Vol. 9, No. 2 (February 1987), pp. 17 – 19.

Jeffcott, L.B. "Osteochondrosis in the Horse—Searching for the Key to Pathogenesis." *Equine Veterinary Journal* (1991), Vol. 23, No. 5, pp. 331 – 338.

Jennings, S., T.N. Meacham, and A.N. Huff. "Management of the Brood Mare." *Equine Practice*, Vol. 9, No. 1 (January 1987), pp. 28 – 31.

Jones, W.E. "Muscular Causes of Exercise Intolerance." *Equine Veterinary Science* (1987), Vol. 7, No. 5, pp. 312 – 316.

Jones, W.E. *Equine Sports Medicine.* Lea and Febiger, Philadelphia, 1989.

Jones, W.E. *Sports Medicine for the Racehorse.* Second Edition. Veterinary Data, Wildomar, California, 1992.

Jones, W.E., ed. *Nutrition for the Equine Athlete.* Equine Sportsmedicine News, Wildomar, California, 1989.

Kiley-Worthington, M. "The Behavior of Horses in Relation to Management and Training—Towards Ethologically Sound Environments." *Equine Veterinary Science,* Vol. 10, No. 1 (1990), pp. 62 – 71.

King, J.N. and E.L. Gerring. "The Action of Low Dose Endotoxin on Equine Bowel Motility." *Equine Veterinary Journal,* Vol. 23, No. 1 (1991), pp. 11 – 17.

Knight, D.A., A.A. Gabel, et al. "Correlation of Dietary Mineral to Incidence and Severity of Metabolic Bone Disease in Ohio and Kentucky." *Proceedings of the American Association of Equine Practitioners* (1985), pp. 445 – 461.

Knight, D.A., A.A. Gabel, et al. "The Effects of Copper Supplementation on the Prevalence of Cartilage Lesions in Foals." *Equine Veterinary Journal,* Vol. 22, No. 6 (1990), pp. 426 – 432.

Knight, D.A., S.E. Weisbrode, L.M. Schmall, and A.A. Gabel. "Copper Supplementation and Cartilage Lesions in Foals." *Proceedings of the American Association of Equine Practitioners* (1988), pp. 191 – 194.

Kohnke, J. "Liquid Vitamin Supplements." *Equine Practice,* Vol. 8, No. 10 (1986), pp. 7 – 9.

Kopp, K. "Do Horses Bend?" *Equus* 115, pp. 31 – 38, 110.

Koterba, A. and G.P. Carlson. "Acid-Base and Electrolyte Alterations in Horses With Exertional Rhabdomyolysis." *Journal of the American Veterinary Medical Association,* Vol. 180, No. 3 (February 1982), pp. 303 – 306.

Kronfeld, D.S. "Symposium Sheds New Light on Equine Ventilatory Adaptations, Muscle Glycogen." *DVM Magazine* (September 1989), pp. 12, 14.

Kronfeld, D.S. and S. Donoghue. "Metabolic Convergence in Developmental Orthopedic Disease." *Proceedings of the American Association of Equine Practitioners* (1988), pp. 195 – 202.

Kurcz, E.V., L.M. Lawrence, K.W. Kelley, and P.A. Miller. "The Effect of Intense Exercise on the Cell-Mediated Immune Response of Horses." *Equine Veterinary Science,* Vol. 8, No. 3 (1988), pp. 237 – 239.

Laegreid, W.W., L.J. Huston, R.J. Basaraba, and M.V. Crisman. "The Effects of Stress on Alveolar Macrophage Function in the Horse: An Overview." *Equine Practice,* Vol. 10, No. 9 (1988), pp. 9 – 16.

Landeau, L.J., D.J. Barrett, and S.C. Batterman. "Mechanical Properties of Equine Hooves." *American Journal of Veterinary Research,* 44 (January 1983), p. 100.

Lawrence, L.M., K.D. Bump, and D.G. McLaren. "Aerial Ammonia Levels in Horse Stalls." *Equine Practice,* Vol. 10, No. 10 (November/December 1988), pp. 20 – 23.

Leadon, D.P., C. Frank, and W. Backhouse. "A Preliminary Report on Studies on Equine Transit Stress." *Equine Veterinary Science,* Vol. 9, No. 4 (1989), pp. 200 – 201.

Leadon, D.P. "A Summary of a Preliminary Report of an Investigation of Transit Stress in the Horse." *AESM Quarterly,* Vol. 3, No. 2 (1988), pp. 19 – 20.

Leadon, D.P., et al. "Environmental, Hematological and Blood Biochemical

Changes in Equine Transit Stress." *Proceedings of the American Association of Equine Practitioners* (1990), pp. 485 – 490.

Lee, A.H., S.F. Swaim. "Granulation Tissue: How to Take Advantage of It in Management of Open Wounds." *Compendium on Continuing Education*, Vol. 10, No. 2 (February 1988), pp. 163 – 170.

Lee, A.H., S.F. Swaim, et al. "Effects of Nonadherent Dressing Materials on the Healing of Open Wounds in Dogs." *Journal of the American Veterinary Medical Association*, Vol. 190, No. 4 (February 1987), pp. 416 – 422.

Lee, S. and C.L. Davidson. "The Role of Collagen in the Elastic Properties of Calcified Tissues." *Journal of Biomechanics*, Vol. 10 (1977), pp. 473 – 486.

Lees, M.J., P.B. Fretz, and K.A. Jacobs. "Factors Influencing Wound Healing: Lessons From Military Wound Management." *Compendium on Continuing Education*, Vol. 11, No. 7 (July 1989), pp. 850 – 855.

Lees, M.J., P.B. Fretz, J.V. Bailey, and K.A. Jacobs. "Second Intention Wound Healing." *Compendium on Continuing Education*, Vol. 11, No. 7 (July 1989), pp. 857 – 864.

Liu, I.K.M. "Update on Respiratory Vaccines in the Horse." *Proceedings of the American Association of Equine Practitioners* (1986), pp. 277 – 282.

Lopez-Rivero, J.L., et al. "Comparative Study of Muscle Fiber Type Composition in the Middle Gluteal Muscle of Andalusian, Thoroughbred, and Arabian Horses." *Equine Sportsmedicine* (November/December 1989), pp. 337 – 340.

Lopez-Rivero, J.L., A.M. Diz, E. Aguera, and A.L. Serrano. "Endurance Training in Andalusian and Arabian Horses." *Equine Practice*, Vol. 15, No. 4 (April 1993), pp. 13 – 19.

Lopez-Rivero, J.L., et al. "Muscle Fiber Size in Horses." *The Equine Athlete*, Vol. 3, No. 2 (March/April 1990), pp. 1 – 11.

Lopez-Rivero, J.L., et al. "Muscle Fiber Type Composition in Untrained and Endurance-Trained Andalusian and Arab Horses." *Equine Veterinary Journal*, Vol. 23, No. 2 (1991), pp. 91 – 93.

MacFadden, K.E. and L.W. Pace. "Clinical Manifestations of Squamous Cell Carcinoma in Horses." *Compendium on Continuing Education*, Vol. 13, No. 4 (April 1991), pp. 669 – 676.

MacNamara, B., S. Bauer, and J. Lafe. "Endoscopic Evaluation of Exercise-Induced Pulmonary Hemorrhage and Chronic Obstructive Pulmonary Disease in Association With Poor Performance in Racing Standardbreds." *Journal of the American Veterinary Medical Association*, Vol. 196, No. 3 (February 1990), pp. 443 – 445.

Mal, M.E., T.H. Friend, D.C. Lay, S.G. Vogelsang, and O.C. Jenkins. "Physiological Responses of Mares to Short Term Confinement and Social Isolation." *Equine Veterinary Science*, Vol. 11, No. 2 (1991), pp. 96 – 102.

Manning, T. and C. Sweeney. "Immune-Mediated Equine Skin Diseases." *Compendium on Continuing Education*, Vol. 8, No. 12 (December 1986), pp. 979 – 986.

Martin, R.K., J.P. Albright, W.R. Clarke, and J.A. Niffenegger. "Load Carrying Effects on the Adult Beagle Tibia." *Medicine and Science in Sports and Exercise*, Vol. 13 (1981), pp. 343 – 349.

McCarthy, R.N. "The Effects of Exercise and Training on Bone." *Trail Blazer Magazine* (August/September 1991), pp. 16 – 17.

McIlwraith, C.W., ed. *AQHA Developmental Orthopedic Disease Symposium* (1986), Amarillo, Texas.

McMiken, D. "Muscle Fiber Types and Horse Performance." *Equine Practice*, Vol. 8, No. 3 (March 1986), pp. 6 – 14.

Melick, R.A. and D.R. Miller. "Variations of Tensile Strength in Human Cortical Bone With Age." *Clinical Science*, Vol. 30 (1966), pp. 243 – 248.

Meschter, C.L., et al. "The Effects of Phenylbutazone on the Intestinal Mucosa of the Horse: A Morphological, Ultrastructural, and Biochemical Study." *Equine Veterinary Journal*, Vol. 22, No. 4 (1990), pp. 255 – 263.

Meyers, M.C., G.D. Potter, et al. "Physiologic and Metabolic Response of Exercising Horses to Added Dietary Fat." *Equine Veterinary Science*, Vol. 9, No. 4 (1989), pp. 218 – 223.

Moore, J.N. and D.D. Morris. "Endotoxemia and Septicemia in Horses: Experimental and Clinical Correlates." *Journal of the American Veterinary Medical Association*, Vol. 200, No. 12 (June 1992), pp. 1903 – 1914.

Morris, E.A. and H.J. Seeherman. "Clinical Evaluation of Poor Performance in the Racehorse: The Results of 275 Evaluations." *Equine Veterinary Journal*, Vol. 23, No. 3 (1991), pp. 169 – 174.

Morris, E.A., et al. "Scintigraphic Identification of Skeletal Muscle Damage in Horses 24 Hours After Strenuous Exercise." *Equine Veterinary Journal*, Vol. 23, No. 5 (1991), pp. 347 – 352.

Morris, E.A. and H.J. Seeherman. "Equisport: A Comprehensive Program for Clinical Evaluation of Poor Racing Performance." *Proceedings of the American Association of Equine Practitioners* (1989), pp. 385 – 397.

Morris, E.A. and H.J. Seeherman. "Evaluation of Upper Respiratory Tract Function During Strenuous Exercise in Racehorses." *Journal of the American Veterinary Medical Association*, Vol. 196, No. 3 (February 1990), pp. 431 – 438.

Morris, E.A. and H.J. Seeherman. "The Dynamic Evaluation of Upper Respiratory Function in the Exercising Horse." *Proceedings of the American Association of Equine Practitioners* (1988), pp. 159 – 165.

Mullowney, P.C. "Dermatologic Diseases of Horses, Part IV: Environmental, Congenital, and Neoplastic Diseases." *Compendium on Continuing Education*, Vol. 7, No. 1 (January 1985), pp. 22 – 32.

Mullowney, P.C. "Dermatologic Diseases of Horses, Part V: Allergic, Immune-Mediated, and Miscellaneous Skin Diseases." *Compendium on Continuing Education*, Vol. 7, No. 4 (April 1985), pp. 217 – 228.

Munroe, G.A. "Cryosurgery in the Horse." *Equine Veterinary Journal*, Vol. 18, No. 1 (1986), pp. 14 – 17.

Murray, M.J. "Phenylbutazone Toxicity in a Horse." *Compendium on Continuing Education*, Vol. 7, No. 7 (July 1985), pp. 389 – 394.

Naylor, J.M., et al. "Familial Incidence of Hyperkalemic Periodic Paralysis in Quarter Horses." *Journal of the American Veterinary Medical Association*, Vol. 200, No. 3 (February 1992), pp. 340 – 343.

Neely, D.P., I.K.M. Liu, and R.B. Hillman. *Equine Reproduction*. Hoffman-La Roche, Inc., 1983.

Nilsson, B.E. and N.E. Westlin. "Bone Density in Athletes." *Clinical Orthopedics*, Vol. 77 (1971), pp. 179 – 182.

Oldham, S.L., G.D. Potter, et al. "Storage and Mobilization of Muscle Glycogen in Exercising Horses Fed a Fat-Supplemented Diet." *Equine Veterinary Science*, Vol. 10, No. 5 (1990), pp. 353 – 359.

Pascoe, J.R. "Exercise-Induced Pulmonary Hemorrhage." *Equine Veterinary Science*, Vol. 9, No. 4 (1989), pp. 198 – 200.

Peyton, L.C. "Wound Healing in the Horse Part 2: Approach to the Treatment of Traumatic Wounds." *Compendium on Continuing Education*, Vol. 9, No. 2 (February 1987), pp. 191 – 200.

Peyton, L.C. "Wound Healing: The Management of Wounds and Blemishes in the Horse—Part 1." *Compendium on Continuing Education*, Vol. 6, No. 2 (February 1984), pp. 111 – 117.

Piotrowski, G., M. Sullivan, and P.T. Colahan. "Geometric Properties of Equine Metacarpi." *Journal of Biomechanics*, Vol. 16 (1983), pp. 129 – 139.

Pollit, C. "Monitoring the Heart Rate of Endurance Horses." *Trail Blazer Magazine* (May 1992), pp. 16 – 17.

Pollit, C. "Monitoring the Heart Rate of Endurance Horses, Part 2." *Trail Blazer Magazine* (July/August 1992), pp. 8 – 11.

Pollit, C. "The Role of Arteriovenous Anastomoses in the Pathophysiology of Equine Laminitis." *Proceedings of the American Association of Equine Practitioners* (1991), pp. 711 – 719.

Pool, R.R. "Adaptations of Bones, Joints, and Attachments of the Limbs of the Horse in Response to Developmental and Infectious Diseases and to Biomechanical Forces Encountered in Athletic Performance." *Proceedings from the Denver Area Veterinary Medical Association Seminar* (January 1991).

Pool, R.R. "Developmental Orthopedic Disease in the Horse: Normal and Abnormal Bone Formation." *Proceedings of the American Association of Equine Practitioners* (1988), pp. 143 – 158.

Pool, R.R. "Pathophysiology of Athletic Injuries of the Horse: Bones, Joints, and Tendons." *AESM Quarterly*, Vol. 3, No. 2 (1988), pp. 23 – 29.

Pool, R.R. "Pathogenesis of Navicular Disease." *Proceedings of the American Association of Equine Practitioners* (1991), p. 709.

Porter, Mimi. "Physical Therapy for Equine Athletes." *AESM Quarterly*, Vol. 3, No. 3 (1988), pp. 40 – 43.

Porter, Mimi. "Techniques of Treatment." *Equine Veterinary Science* (March/April 1991), pp. 191 – 194.

Porter, Mimi. "Therapeutic Electricity." *Equine Veterinary Science* (January / February 1991), pp. 59 – 64.

Porter, Mimi. "Therapeutic Electricity: Physiological Effects." *Equine Veterinary Science* (March/April 1991), pp. 133 – 140.

Porter, Mimi. "Therapeutic Ultrasound." *Equine Veterinary Science* (July/August 1991), pp. 243 – 245.

Porter, Mimi. "Therapeutic Ultrasound." *Equine Veterinary Science* (September/October 1991), pp. 294 – 299.

Poulos, P.W., and M.F. Smith. "The Nature of Enlarged 'Vascular Channels' in the Navicular Bone of the Horse." *Veterinary Radiology* (1988), Vol. 29, pp. 60 – 64.

Powell, D., et al. "Rhinopneumonitis Roundtable Discussion." *Equine Practice*, Vol. 14, No. 4 (April 1992), pp. 8 – 12. *Equine Practice*, Vol. 14, No. 5 (May 1992), pp. 30 – 36. *Equine Practice*, Vol. 14, No. 6 (June 1992), pp. 17 – 20.

Pratt, G.W. "An In Vivo Method of Ultrasonically Evaluating Bone Strength." *Proceedings of the American Association of Equine Practitioners* (1980), pp. 295 – 306.

Pratt, G.W. "The Response of Highly Stressed Bone in the Race Horse." *Proceedings of the American Association of Equine Practitioners* (1982), pp.

31 – 37.

Pugh, D.G. and J.T. Thompson. "Impaction Colics Attributed to Decreased Water Intake and Feeding Coastal Bermuda Grass Hay in a Boarding Stable." *Equine Practice*, Vol. 14, No. 1 (January 1992), pp. 9 – 14.

Rabin, D.S., N.W. Rantanen, et al. "The Clinical Use of Bone Strength Assessment in the Thoroughbred Race Horse." *Proceedings of the American Association of Equine Practitioners* (1983), pp. 343 – 351.

Ralston, S.L. and K. Larson. "The Effect of Oral Electrolyte Supplementation During a 96 Kilometer Endurance Race for Horses." *Equine Veterinary Science*, Vol. 9, No. 1, pp. 13 – 19.

Ralston, S.L. "Common Behavioral Problems of Horses." *Compendium on Continuing Education*, Vol. 4, No. 4 (April 1982), pp. 152 – 159.

Ralston, S.L. "Nutritional Management of Horses Competing in 160 Kilometer Races." *Cornell Vet*, Vol. 78, No. 1 (1988), pp. 53 – 61.

Ralston, S.L. "Patterns and Control of Food Intake in Domestic Animals." *Compendium on Continuing Education*, Vol. 6, No. 11 (1984), pp. 628 – 634.

Reef, V.B., B.B. Martin, and A. Elser. "Types of Tendon and Ligament Injuries Detected With Diagnostic Ultrasound: Description and Follow-up." *Proceedings of the American Association of Equine Practitioners* (1988), pp. 245 – 248.

Reef, V.B., B.B. Martin, and K. Stebbins. "Comparison of Ultrasonographic, Gross, and Histologic Appearance of Tendon Injuries in Performance Horses." *Proceedings of the American Association of Equine Practitioners* (1989), p. 279.

Reilly, D.T. and A.H. Burstein. "The Mechanical Properties of Cortical Bone." *Journal of Bone and Joint Surgery*, Vol. 56A (1974), pp. 1001 – 1022.

Reinemeyer, C.R. "Anthelmintic Resistance in Horses." *Equine Veterinary Science*, Vol. 7, No. 6, pp. 390 – 391.

Reinemeyer, C.R., S.A. Smith, A.A. Gabel, and R.P. Herd. "Observations on the Population Dynamics of Five Cyathostome Nematode Species of Horses in Northern USA." *Equine Veterinary Journal*, Vol. 18, No. 2 (1986), pp. 121 – 124.

Reinemeyer, C.R. and J.E. Henton. "Observations on Equine Strongyle Control in Southern Temperate USA." *Equine Veterinary Journal*, Vol. 19, No. 6 (1987), pp. 505 – 508.

Richardson, D.W. "Pathophysiology of Degenerative Joint Disease." *Equine Veterinary Science*, Vol. 11, No. 3 (1990), pp. 156 – 157.

Ridgway, K.J. "Cardiac Recovery Index: Avoiding Inappropriate Utilization." *AERC Endurance News* (October 1991), pp. 5 – 7.

Ridgway, K.J. "Respiration as an Evaluation Parameter for Distance Riding." *AERC Endurance News* (October 1990), pp. 4 – 5.

Ridgway, K.J. "Exertional Myopathies." *Proceedings of the American Association of Equine Practitioners* (1991), pp. 839 – 843.

Robb, E.J. and D.S. Kronfeld. "Dietary Sodium Bicarbonate as a Treatment for Exertional Rhabdomyolysis in a Horse." *Journal of the American Veterinary Medical Association*, Vol. 188, No. 6 (March 1986), pp. 602 – 607.

Robinson, N.E. *Current Therapy in Equine Medicine 2*, WB Saunders Company, 1987.

Robinson, N.E. and R. Wilson. "Airway Obstruction in the Horse." *Equine Veterinary Science*, Vol. 9, No. 3 (1989), pp. 155 – 160.

Robinson, N.E., et al. "Physiology of the Equine Respiratory Tract and

Changes in Disease: The Role of Granulocytes." *Proceedings of the American Association of Equine Practitioners* (1984), pp. 253 – 261.

Roche, J.F., L. Keenan, and D. Forde. "Some Factors Affecting Fertility of the Mare." *Equine Practice*, Vol. 9, No. 1 (January 1987), pp. 8 – 13.

Romeiser, K. "Tying-Up: Old Problem, New Twist." *Equus* 126, pp. 60 – 64, 128 – 129.

Rooney, J. "Passive Function of the Extensor Tendons of the Fore and Rear Limbs of the Horse." *Equine Veterinary Science*, Vol. 7, No. 1 (1987), pp. 29 – 30.

Rose, R.J. and D.R. Lloyd. "Sodium Bicarbonate: More Than Just a 'Milkshake'?" *Equine Veterinary Journal*, Vol. 24, No. 2 (1992), pp. 75 – 76.

Rubin, S.I. "Non-Steroidal Anti-Inflammatory Drugs, Prostaglandins, and the Kidney." *Journal of the American Veterinary Medical Association*, Vol. 188, No. 9 (May 1986), pp. 1065 – 1068.

Rude, T.A. "Vaccines, Bacterins, Toxoids Can Cause Allergic Reactions." *DVM Magazine* (May 1989), pp. 42 – 44.

Ruff, C.B. and W.C. Hayes. "Bone Mineral Content in the Lower Limb." *Journal of Bone and Joint Surgery*, Vol. 66A (1984), pp. 1024 – 1031.

Ruggles, A.J. and M.W. Ross. "Medical and Surgical Management of Small-Colon Impaction in Horses: 28 Cases (1984 – 1989)." *Journal of the American Veterinary Medical Association*, Vol. 199, No. 12 (December 1991), pp. 1762 – 1766.

Ruth, D.T. and B.J. Swites. "Comparison of the Effectiveness of Intra-Articular Hyaluronic Acid and Conventional Therapy for the Treatment of Naturally Occurring Arthritic Conditions in Horses." *Equine Practice*, Vol. 7, No. 9 (October 1985), pp. 25 – 29.

Schott II, H.C., D.R. Hodgson, J.R. Naylor, and W.M. Bayly. "Thermoregulation and Heat Exhaustion in the Exercising Horse." *Proceedings of the American Association of Equine Practitioners* (1990), pp. 505 – 513.

Schott II, H.C. "Aspects of Heat Production, Dissipation, and Exhaustion in the Exercising Horse." *AERC Endurance News* (November 1991), pp. 5 – 6.

Scott, B.D., G.D. Potter, et al. "Growth and Feed Utilization by Yearling Horses Fed Added Dietary Fat." *Equine Veterinary Science*, Vol. 9, No. 4 (1989), pp. 210 – 214.

Scraba, S.T. and O.J. Ginther. "Effects of Lighting Programs on Onset of the Ovulatory Season in Mares." *Theriogenology*, Vol. 24 (1985), pp. 667 – 679.

Shabpareh, V., E.L. Squires, V.M. Cook, and R. Cole. "An Alternative Artificial Lighting Regime to Hasten Onset of the Breeding Season in Mares." *Equine Practice*, Vol. 14, No. 2 (February 1992), pp. 24 – 27.

Shaw, K., et al. *Strongid® C: A Roundtable Discussion.* Pfizer, Inc., 1990.

Shively, M.J. "Equine-English Dictionary: Part 1—Standing Conformation." *Equine Practice*, Vol. 4, No. 5 (May 1982), pp. 10 – 20, 25 – 27.

Smith, C.A. "Electrolyte Imbalances and Metabolic Disturbances in Endurance Horses." *Compendium on Continuing Education*, Vol. 7, No. 10 (October 1985), pp. 575 – 584.

Smith, J.D., et al. "Exercise-Induced Pulmonary Hemorrhage Findings, A Workshop." *Equine Practice*, Vol. 14, No. 1 (January 1992), pp. 19 – 25. *Equine Practice*, Vol. 14, No. 2 (February 1992), pp. 9 – 15. *Equine Practice*, Vol. 14, No. 3 (March 1992), pp. 28 – 32.

Smith, M.J. "Electrical Stimulation for Relief of Musculoskeletal Pain." *The Physician and Sportsmedicine*, Vol. 11, No. 5 (May 1983), pp. 47 – 55.

Snow, D.H. "Sweating and Anhidrosis." *Equine Sportmedicine*, Vol. 5, No. 2 (1986), pp. 4 – 5, 8.

Snow, V.E. and D.P. Birdsall. "Specific Parameters Used to Evaluate Hoof Balance and Support." *Proceedings of the American Association of Equine Practitioners* (1990), pp. 299 – 312.

Specht, T.E. and P.T. Colahan. "Surgical Treatment of Sand Colic in Equids: 48 Cases (1978 – 1985)." *Journal of the American Veterinary Medical Association*, Vol. 193, No. 12 (December 1988), pp. 1560 – 1563.

Spier, S.J. "Current Facts About Hyperkalemic Periodic Paralysis (HYPP) Disease." *The Quarter Racing Journal* (April 1993), pp. 44 – 47.

Spier, S.J. "Use of Hyperimmune Plasma Containing Antibody to Gram-negative Core Antigens." *Proceedings of the American Association of Equine Practitioners* (1989), pp. 91 – 94.

Spier, S.J. and G.P. Carlson. "Hyperkalemic Periodic Paralysis in Certain Registered Quarter Horses." *The Quarter Horse Journal* (September 1992), pp. 68 – 69, 120.

Spier, S.J., G.P. Carlson, et al. "Genetic Study of Hyperkalemic Periodic Paralysis in Horses." *Journal of the American Veterinary Medical Association*, Vol. 202, No. 6 (March 1993), pp. 933 – 937.

Spier, S.J., G.P. Carlson, et al. "Hyperkalemic Periodic Paralysis in Horses." *Journal of the American Veterinary Medical Association*, Vol. 197, No. 8 (October 1990), pp. 1009 – 1016.

Stabenfeldt, G.H. and J.P. Hughes. "Clinical Aspects of Reproductive Endocrinology in the Horse." *Compendium on Continuing Education*, Vol. 9, No. 6 (June 1987), pp. 678 – 684.

Stashak, Ted S. *Adams' Lameness in Horses*. Fourth Edition. Lea and Febiger, Philadelphia, 1987.

Stull, C. "Muscles for Motion." *Equine Practice*, Vol. 8, No. 4 (April 1986), pp. 17 – 20.

Subcommittee on Horse Nutrition, Committee on Animal Nutrition, Board of Agriculture, National Research Council, *Nutrient Requirements of Horses*. Fifth Revised Edition. National Academy Press, Washington DC, 1989.

Sullins, K.E., S.M. Roberts, J.D. Lavach, G.A. Severin, and D. Lueker. "Equine Sarcoid." *Equine Practice*, Vol. 8, No. 4 (April 1986), pp. 21 – 27.

Swaim, S.F. and A.H. Lee. "Topical Wound Medications: A Review." *Journal of the American Veterinary Medical Association*, Vol. 190, No. 12 (June 1987), pp. 1588 – 1592.

Swaim, S.F. and D. Wilhalf. "The Physics, Physiology, and Chemistry of Bandaging Open Wounds." *Compendium on Continuing Education*, Vol. 7, No. 2 (February 1985), pp. 146 – 155.

Swann, P. *Racehorse Training and Feeding*. Racehorse Sportsmedicine and Scientific Conditioning, Australia, 1985.

Swann, P. *Racehorse Training and Sports Medicine*. Racehorse Sportsmedicine and Scientific Conditioning, Australia, 1988.

Sweeney, C.R., C.E. Benson, et al. "Description of an Epizootic and Persistence of Streptococcus Equi Infections in Horses." *Journal of the American Veterinary Medical Association*, Vol. 194, No. 9 (1989), pp. 1281 – 1285.

Sweeney, C.R., C.E. Benson, et al. "Streptococcus Equi Infection in Horses — Part 1." *Compendium on Continuing Education*, Vol. 9, No. 6 (June 1987), pp. 689 – 693.

Sweeney, C.R., C.E. Benson, et al. "Streptococcus Equi Infection in Horses —

Part 2." *Compendium on Continuing Education,* Vol. 9, No. 8 (August 1987), pp. 845 – 851.

Sweeney, C.R., et al. "Equine Roundtable Discussion: Respiration." *Equine Practice* (May 1989), pp. 16 – 24. *Equine Practice* (June 1989), pp. 10 – 16. *Equine Practice* (July/August 1989), pp. 29 – 40.

Swenson, M.J., ed. *Dukes' Physiology of Domestic Animals.* Ninth Edition. Cornell University Press, 1977.

Tarwid, J.N., P.B. Fretz, and E.G. Clark. "Equine Sarcoids: A Study With Emphasis on Pathologic Diagnosis." *Compendium on Continuing Education,* Vol. 7, No. 5 (May 1985), pp. 293 – 300.

Templeton, J.W., R. Smith III, and L.G. Adams. "Natural Disease Resistance in Domestic Animals." *Journal of the American Veterinary Medical Association,* Vol. 192, No. 9 (May 1988), pp. 1306 – 1315.

Texas Veterinary Medical Association Annual Meeting. "Hyaluronic Acid Use in the Horse: A Roundtable Discussion." Schering Animal Health, February 1988.

The Veterinary Clinics of North America, Equine Practice, *Advanced Diagnostic Methods,* August 1991, Vol. 7, No. 2.

The Veterinary Clinics of North America, Equine Practice, *The Equine Foot,* April 1989, pp. 109 – 128.

The Veterinary Clinics of North America, Equine Practice, *Behavior,* December 1986, Vol. 2, No. 3.

The Veterinary Clinics of North America, Equine Practice, *Clinical Nutrition,* August 1990, Vol. 6, No. 2, pp. 281 – 293, 355 – 371, 393 – 418.

The Veterinary Clinics of North America, Equine Practice, *Clinical Pharmacology,* April 1987, Vol. 3, No. 1.

The Veterinary Clinics of North America, Equine Practice, *Exercise Physiology,* December 1985, Vol. 1, No. 3.

The Veterinary Clinics of North America, Equine Practice, *Management of Colic,* April 1988, Vol. 4, No. 1.

The Veterinary Clinics of North America, Equine Practice, *Parasitology,* August 1986, Vol. 2, No. 2.

The Veterinary Clinics of North America, Equine Practice, *Racetrack Practice,* April 1990, Vol. 6, No. 1.

The Veterinary Clinics of North America, Equine Practice, *Reproduction,* August 1988, Vol. 4, No. 2

The Veterinary Clinics of North America, Equine Practice, *Reproduction,* August 1988, Vol. 4, No. 2.

The Veterinary Clinics of North America, Equine Practice, *Respiratory Diseases,* April 1991, Vol. 7, No. 1.

The Veterinary Clinics of North America, Equine Practice, *Stallion Management,* April 1992, Vol. 8, No. 1.

The Veterinary Clinics of North America, Equine Practice, *Wound Management,* December 1989, Vol. 5, No. 3.

Thomas, H.S. "Using A Twitch." *American Farriers Journal* (July/August 1989), pp. 28 – 30.

Thompson, K.N., J.P. Baker, and S.G. Jackson. "The Influence of High Dietary Intakes of Energy and Protein on Third Metacarpal Characteristics of Weanling Ponies." *Equine Veterinary Science,* Vol. 8, No. 5 (1988), pp. 391 – 394.

Thomson, J.R. and E.A. McPherson. "Chronic Obstructive Pulmonary Disease in the Horse." *Equine Practice*, Vol. 10, No. 7 (July/August 1988), pp. 31 – 36.

Todhunter, R.J. and G. Lust. "Pathophysiology of Synovitis: Clinical Signs and Examination in Horses." *Compendium on Continuing Education*, Vol. 12, No. 7 (July 1990), pp. 980 – 991.

Traub-Dargatz, J.L., J.J. Bertone, et al. "Chronic Flunixin Meglumine Therapy in Foals." *American Journal of Veterinary Research*, Vol. 49, No. 1 (January 1988), pp. 7 – 12.

Traub-Dargatz, J.L. "Non-Steroidal Anti-Inflammatory Drug-induced Ulcers." *Proceedings of the American Association of Equine Practitioners* (1988), pp. 129 – 132.

Turner, A.S. "Local and Systemic Factors Affecting Wound Healing." *Proceedings of the American Association of Equine Practitioners* (1978), pp. 355 – 362.

Turner, A.S. and Tucker, C.M. "The Evaluation of Isoxsuprine Hydrochloride for the Treatment of Navicular Disease: A Double Blind Study." *Equine Veterinary Journal*, Vol. 21, No. 5 (1989), pp. 338 – 341.

Turner, T.A. "Hindlimb Muscle Strain as a Cause of Lameness in Horses." *Proceedings of the American Association of Equine Practitioners* (1989), pp. 281 – 290.

Turner, T.A. "Navicular Disease Management: Shoeing Principles." *Proceedings of the American Association of Equine Practitioners* (1986), pp. 625 – 633.

Turner, T.A. "Shoeing Principles for the Management of Navicular Disease in the Horse." *Journal of the American Veterinary Medical Association*, Vol. 189 (1986), pp. 298 – 301.

Turner, T.A., S.K. Kneller, R.R. Badertscher II, and J.L. Stowater. "Radiographic Changes in the Navicular Bones of Normal Horses." *Proceedings of the American Association of Equine Practitioners* (1986), pp. 309 – 314.

Turner, T.A., R.C. Purohit, and J.F. Fessler. "Thermography: A Review in Equine Medicine." *Compendium on Continuing Education*, Vol. 8, No. 11 (1986), pp. 855 – 861.

Turner, T.A., K. Wolfsdorf, and J. Jourdenais. "Effects of Heat, Cold, Biomagnets, and Ultrasound on Skin Circulation in the Horse." *Proceedings of the American Association of Equine Practitioners* (1991), pp. 249 – 257.

Turrel, J.M., S.M. Stover, and J. Gyorgyfalvy. "Iridium-192 Interstitial Brachytherapy of Equine Sarcoid." *Veterinary Radiology*, Vol. 26, No. 1 (1985), pp. 20 – 24.

Uhlinger, C.A., and M. Kristula. "Effects of Alternation of Drug Classes on the Development of Oxibendazole Resistance in a Herd of Horses." *Journal of the American Veterinary Medical Association*, Vol. 201, No. 1 (July 1992), pp. 51 – 55.

Uhlinger, C.A. "Equine Small Strongyles: Epidemiology, Pathology, and Control." *Compendium on Continuing Education*, Vol. 13, No. 5 (May 1991), pp. 863 – 868.

Valberg, S. "Metabolic Response to Racing and Fiber Properties of Skeletal Muscle in Standardbred and Thoroughbred Horses." *Equine Veterinary Science*, Vol. 7, No. 1 (1987), pp. 6 – 12.

Valberg, S. "Tying-Up Syndrome in Horses." *Hoof Print* (September/October 1991), pp. 35 – 36.

Van Den Hoven, R. "Mind Over Muscle." *Equine Veterinary Journal*, Vol. 23,

No. 2 (1991), pp. 73 – 74.

Vanselow, B.A., I. Abetz, and A.R.B. Jackson. "BCG Emulsion Immunotherapy of Equine Sarcoid." *Equine Veterinary Journal*, Vol. 20, No. 6 (1988), pp. 444 – 447.

Voges, F., E. Kienzle, and H. Meyer. "Investigations on the Composition of Horse Bones." *Equine Veterinary Science*, Vol. 10, No. 3 (1990), pp. 208 – 213.

Wagoner, D.M., ed. *Feeding To Win II*. Equine Research Publications, 1992.

Wagoner, D.M., ed. *The Illustrated Veterinary Encyclopedia for Horsemen*. Equine Research Publications, 1977.

Wagoner, D.M., ed. *Veterinary Treatments and Medications for Horsemen*. Equine Research Publications, 1977.

Wagoner, D.M., ed. *Breeding Management and Foal Development*. Equine Research Publications, 1982.

Waldsmith, Jim. The Equine Center. San Luis Obispo, California, personal communication.

Wanless, M. *The Natural Rider*. Summit Books, New York, New York, 1987.

Webb, S.P., G.D. Potter, et al. "Physiological Responses of Cutting Horses to Exercise Testing and to Training." *Equine Veterinary Science*, Vol. 8, No. 3 (1988), pp. 261 – 265.

Webbon, P.M. "Preliminary Study of Tendon Biopsy in the Horse." *Equine Veterinary Journal*, Vol. 18, No. 5, pp. 383 – 387.

White, G.W. "Adequan: A Review for the Practicing Veterinarian." *Equine Veterinary Science*, Vol. 8, No. 6 (1988), pp. 463 – 467.

White, N.A. "Thromboembolic Colic in Horses." *Compendium on Continuing Education*, Vol. 7, No. 3 (March 1985), pp. 156 – 162.

Wilson, G.L. and M. Mueller. *The Equine Athlete*. Veterinary Learning Systems Co., Inc., New Jersey, 1982.

Wilson, W.D. "Streptococcus Equi Infections (Strangles) in Horses." *Equine Practice*, Vol. 10, No. 7 (July/August 1988), pp. 12 – 25.

Wood, C.H., T.T. Ross, et al. "Variations in Muscle Fiber Composition Between Successfully and Unsuccessfully Raced Quarter Horses." *Equine Veterinary Science*, Vol. 8, No. 3 (1988), pp. 217 – 220.

Woolen, N., R.M. DeBowes, H.W. Leipold, and L.A. Schneider. "A Comparison of Four Types of Therapy for the Treatment of Full-Thickness Skin Wounds of the Horse." *Proceedings of the American Association of Equine Practitioners* (1988), pp. 569 – 576.

Yelle, M.T. "Clinical Aspects of Streptococcus Equi Infection." *Equine Veterinary Journal*, Vol. 19, No. 2 (1987), pp. 158 – 162.

Yovich, J.V., G.W. Trotter, C.W. McIlwraith, and R.W. Norrdin. "Effects of Polysulfated Glycosaminoglycan on Chemical and Physical Defects in Equine Articular Cartilage." *American Journal of Veterinary Research*, Vol. 48, No. 9 (September 1987), pp. 1407 – 1413.

Figure Credits

Figure 1–1. Don Shugart.
Figure 1–6. Don Shugart.
Figure 1–7. Cappy Jackson.
Figure 1–13. Courtesy of *The Quarter Horse Journal*.
Figure 1–17. Courtesy of *The Blood-Horse*.
Figure 1–20. Equine Sports Graphics, Inc.
Figure 1–27. Courtesy of the International Arabian Horse Association. Photo by Jerry Sparagowski.
Figure 1–29. Courtesy of the United States Trotting Association.
Figure 1–34. Courtesy of Don Stevenson.
Figure 2–1. J. Noye.
Figure 2–4. Courtesy of *The Blood-Horse*.
Figure 2–6. J. Noye.
Figure 3–4. Courtesy of the United States Trotting Association.
Figure 3–8. Courtesy of *The Blood-Horse*.
Figure 3–10. Cappy Jackson.
Figure 3–12. Cappy Jackson.
Figure 3–13. Cappy Jackson.
Figure 3–16. Courtesy of *The Blood-Horse*.
Figure 4–9. Courtesy of *The Blood-Horse*.
Figure 5–1. J. Noye.
Figure 5–6. Cappy Jackson.
Figure 5–9. Courtesy of *The Blood-Horse*.
Figure 6–1. Courtesy of the United States Trotting Association. Photo by George Smallsreed, Jr.
Figure 6–9. Courtesy of *The Blood-Horse*.
Figure 6–19. Courtesy of Dr. Jim Schumacher, Texas A&M University.
Figure 6–20. Cappy Jackson.
Figure 6–21. Courtesy of Nancy Zidonis, Equine Acupressure, Inc.
Figure 6–30. J. Noye.
Figure 7–1. Courtesy of *The Blood-Horse*.
Figure 7–8. Courtesy of The Horsemen's Journal. Photo by Bill Witkop.
Figure 7–13. Courtesy of the Girls' Barrel Racing Association of Indiana. Photo by Dick Wright.
Figure 8–1. Courtesy of *The Blood-Horse*.
Figure 8–5. Courtesy of Al Dunning Training Stables, Inc. Photo by Pat Hall.
Figure 8–9. Cappy Jackson.
Figure 10–1. J. Noye.
Figure 10–5. Dudley Barker.
Figure 10–14. Courtesy of Mimi Porter, Equine Therapy.
Figure 10–15. Courtesy of Dr. Dave Schmitz, Texas A&M University.
Figure 10–16. Courtesy of Dr. Dave Schmitz, Texas A&M University.
Figure 11–1. Courtesy of Dr. Ducharme, Cornell University.
Figure 11–4. Courtesy of Mimi Porter, Equine Therapy.
Figure 11–5. Courtesy of Mimi Porter, Equine Therapy.
Figure 11–6. Courtesy of Mimi Porter, Equine Therapy.
Figure 11–7. Courtesy of Mimi Porter, Equine Therapy.
Figure 11–8. Courtesy of Mimi Porter, Equine Therapy.
Figure 11–9. Courtesy of Mimi Porter, Equine Therapy.
Figure 11–10. Courtesy of Mimi Porter, Equine Therapy.
Figure 11–11. Courtesy of Mimi Porter, Equine Therapy.
Figure 11–13. Courtesy of Mimi Porter, Equine Therapy.

Glossary

abdomen, the cavity that lies between the diaphragm and the pelvis; contains the digestive organs, the liver, pancreas, kidneys, and spleen

abdominocentesis, withdrawal of fluid through a needle inserted into the abdominal cavity

abort, to expel a fetus before it is able to live outside the uterus

abrasion, a wound caused by the wearing away of the top layer of skin and hair by friction

abscess, a localized collection of pus in a cavity formed by the disintegration of tissues

acetylcholine, a chemical neuro-transmitter, which enables a neuron to fire

acrosome, the "cap" of the sperm cell which contains the enzymes necessary to penetrate the egg

actin filament, one of two types of filaments that make up a muscle fiber

acupressure, a form of acupuncture which seeks to stimulate specific nerve tracts and meridians without penetrating the skin

acupuncture, an ancient Oriental art which seeks to stimulate specific nerve tracts and meridians by needle penetration

acute, having short and relatively sudden course; not chronic

adenoma, a benign epithelial tumor in which the cells are derived from glandular epithelium or form glandular structures

adenosine diphosphate (ADP), product of the decomposition of the energy reserve of the muscles

adenosine triphosphate (ATP), represents the energy reserve of the muscles

adhesion, abnormal, firm, fibrous attachment between two structures, often formed as a result of inflammation

adjuvant, the liquid carrier that contains the organism in a vaccine

adrenaline, a powerful vasopressor that increases blood pressure and stimulates the heart muscle; also called epinephrine

aerobe, a microorganism that can live and grow in the presence of oxygen

aerobic, growing or taking place in the presence of oxygen

aerobic capacity, the ability to exercise without using anaerobic metabolism; increases with aerobic conditioning

agglutinate, clumping or massing together of cells or bacteria

agonist, a muscle opposed by another muscle, the antagonist

alcopecia, a loss of hair

alkalosis, increased alkalinity of blood and tissues; increased blood bicarbonate

allergen, a substance capable of causing allergy or hypersensitivity

allergy, a hypersensitive state acquired through exposure to a particular allergen; reexposure results in an altered capacity to react to the substance

alveolar macrophage, an immune cell which binds, internalizes, and inactivates microorganisms in the lungs

alveoli, a small cavity or pit, as in the air saccules of the lungs

amino acids, a class of organic compounds containing nitrogen; they form the building blocks of proteins

anabolic steroid, a chemical substance derived from testosterone; encourages protein-building

anaerobe, a microorganism that can live and grow in the complete, or almost complete lack of oxygen

anaerobic, growing or taking place in an environment lacking in oxygen

anaerobic threshold, the point at which lactic acid begins to accumulate in the muscles and bloodstream

analgesia, pain relief

anamnestic response, a state where the immune system "remembers" a foreign protein and responds quickly to further insult

anaphylactic shock, anaphylaxis, an unusually severe, life-threatening allergic reaction to a foreign protein or drug

anemia, a condition in which the number or volume of red blood cells, hemoglobin, and packed red blood cells is below normal

anesthetic, a drug or agent that is used to abolish the sensation of pain

anesthetize, to abolish the sensation of pain with or without a loss of consciousness

anestrus, a period of sexual quiescence during which there is an absence of observable estrus

angioedema, a profound hypersensitivity reaction characterized by sudden swelling of the respiratory tract

angle of the bar, the bottom of the foot where the hoof wall meets the sole; also called angle of the sole

angle of the wall, the bottom of the foot where the hoof wall meets the heel

angular limb deformity, abnormality in the growth plate of the limb; examples include toed-out, pigeon-toed, knock-knee, and bowlegged conformational faults

anhydrosis, an abnormal deficiency of sweat

antagonist, a muscle that counteracts another muscle, the agonist

anterior uveitis, inflammation of structures in the eye; characterized by pain, conjunctivitis, eye spasms, and tearing

antibacterial, able to kill or inhibit the growth of bacteria

antibiotic, a chemical produced by a microorganism that can destroy or inhibit the growth of other microorganisms

antibody, a complex protein molecule which combines with molecules of antigen; antibodies participate in the immune response which protects against disease

antigen, a substance which the immune system recognizes as foreign and causes formation of antibodies

antigenic drift, a minor change in the structure or makeup of a virus; this process is called mutation

anti-inflammatory, an agent which counteracts or suppresses fever and the inflammatory response

antimicrobial, able to inhibit the growth and development of microorganisms

antiseptic, an agent which prevents the decomposition of tissue by inhibiting the growth and development of microorganisms

antitoxin, an antibody to the toxin of a microorganism that combines with the toxin, neutralizing it

anus, the exterior opening of the rectum

arrhythmia, any variation from the normal heartbeat

arteritis, inflammation of an artery

artery, vessel through which oxygen-enriched blood passes away from the heart toward the various parts of the body

arthritis, inflammation of a joint

arthrodesis, surgical fusion of a joint

articular, pertaining to a joint

arytenoid cartilages, paired cartilages in the larynx, collapse of one or both is involved in roaring

arytenoid chondrosis, abnormal calcification and abscesses of the cartilage in the larynx; leads to exercise intolerance and respiratory noise

ascarid, intestinal roundworm, a parasite particularly of young horses

asphyxiation, suffocation

aspiration pneumonia, an infection caused by inhaling contaminated food or other substance into the lungs

astringent, a drying agent that causes contraction and shrinking of tissues, and stops the flow of discharge from a wound

asymptomatic, without symptoms

ataxia, the inability to coordinate voluntary muscle movements

atlanto-axial joint, see no joint

atlanto-occipital joint, see yes joint

atlas vertebra, the first cervical vertebra after the skull

atrophy, decrease in size or wasting away of a body part or tissue

axial compression, a force directly down the limb which squeezes the bones and joints together

axial tension, forces which pull apart

axis vertebra, the second vertebra after the skull

bactericide, an agent that destroys bacteria

bacterium, any microorganism in the class *Schizomycetes;* (plural: bacteria)

bar shoe, a therapeutic shoe in which the heels are joined by a bar, creating a larger base of support for the foot

bars, structures on the bottom of the foot formed by the hoof wall as it turns forward and inward at the heels; they run on each side of the frog and converge on each other

bascule, the rounding of the neck and back as a horse jumps an obstacle

base-narrow, a conformational fault where the distance between the center lines of the limbs at their origin is greater than the center lines of the feet on the ground

bastard strangles, the strangles bacteria spread to the lymph nodes of the intestinal tract, abdominal organs, or brain

bench knee, a conformational fault where the cannon bone is offset to the outside of the knee

bevelled shoe, see slippered shoe

bicarbonate, basic component of some salts; sharp increase may cause elevation of blood pH

biomechanical stress, all the forces applied to a bone during weight-bearing

biopsy, the process of removing tissue from living patients for diagnostic examination; a sample obtained by biopsy

blackflies, ear gnats which feed on blood in the ear pinnae; also called buffalo gnats; *Simulium*

bleeders, horses that bleed from the nose during a race due to exercise-induced pulmonary hemorrhage (EIPH)

bog spavin, excess joint fluid in the hock

bolus, a rounded mass of food or medicine which is given orally

bone marrow, the soft material filling the cavities of the bones; produces red and white blood cells

bone mineral content, the amount of minerals in a bone; a parameter of bone strength

bone spavin, a lameness originating in the hock which is characterized by either exostosis or cartilage destruction, particularly occurring on the inner surface of the hock

bots, the larvae of bot flies, which are parasitic in the stomach; *Gastrophilus sp.*

bowed tendon, damage to a tendon that results in inflammation and scarring

bowlegged, a conformational fault where the knees deviate away from each other; also called carpus varus

bradykinin, a strong vasodilator that increases the permeability of capillaries and constricts smooth muscle

breakover, the act of rolling the hoof forward, lifting the foot from the ground heel first, as the horse moves forward

broad spectrum, a wide range of activity, as in a wide range of bacteria affected by a broad spectrum antibiotic

bronchioles, the successively smaller airways in the lungs into which the bronchi divide

bronchitis, inflammation of one or more bronchi, often marked by fever, coughing, and difficulty breathing

bronchoconstriction, reduced diameter of a bronchiole

bronchopneumonia, inflammation of the lungs that begins in the bronchioles, which become clogged with mucopurulent exudate

bronchi, any of the larger airways, including the two main branches of the trachea, one going to each lung, also including the large airways inside the lungs

bucked knees, see over at the knee

bucked shins, microfractures on the front and inside surfaces of the cannon bone, usually occurring on the forelegs of young horses that are strenuously exercised

buffalo gnats, see blackflies

bursa, a sac or sac-like cavity filled with fluid and situated beneath tendons where friction would otherwise develop

bursitis, inflammation of the bursa

calf knee, a conformational fault where the knee is set too far back

camped out, a conformational fault where the hind legs are too far out behind

canker, chronic hypertrophy of the horn-producing tissues of the foot, beginning at the frog and extending to the sole and wall; characterized by foul-smelling, caseous, white discharge

capillaries, minute vessels that connect to the arterioles and venules, forming a network in nearly all parts of the body; their walls act as semipermeable membranes for the exchange of various substances between the blood and tissue fluid

capillary refill time, the time required for normal blood flow and color to return to an area of the gum pressed by a fingertip

capped hock, inflammation of the bursa over the point of the hock caused by trauma

carbohydrates, organic compounds containing carbon, hydrogen, and oxygen; the chief source of energy; including starches, sugars, and cellulose

carcinoma, a malignant new growth made of epithelium cells; a form of cancer

cardiac, pertaining to the heart

cardiac recovery index (CRI), a method of checking the heart rate recovery; the horse is trotted out 250 feet and the heart rate is counted after 1 minute from the start of the trot to determine if it has returned to the resting heart rate

cardiovascular system, the system formed by the heart, arteries, and veins; the circulatory system

carotid artery, the main artery of the neck, conducting blood to the brain

carpal, pertaining to the "knee" of the front leg

carpitis, inflammation of the synovial membranes of the bones of the knees, causing swelling, pain, and lameness

carpus, the "knee" of the front leg

carpus valgus, see knock-knee

carpus varus, see bowlegged

carrier, an animal that carries a recessive gene or the organisms of a disease without showing signs of the condition; the animal may transmit the gene to its offspring or the organism to another animal; see also adjuvant

cartilage, a specialized type of connective tissue found in the joints, ears, nose, throat, and ribs; may be a precursor to bone

caseous, resembling cheese or curd; cheesy

Caslick's surgery, a process of stitching a section of the labia together to prevent air and contaminants from entering the reproductive tract; also called episioplasty

catalytic enzymes, enzymes that trigger reactions within the body

cataract, a condition where the lens of the eye becomes opaque

catheter, a flexible tubular instrument for withdrawing fluids from or introducing fluids into the body, e.g., urinary catheter, indwelling intravenous catheter, etc.

caustic, burning, corrosive, and destructive to living tissue

cecum, the intestinal pouch between the large and small intestines; important for cellulose digestion

cell, the structural unit that is the living basis of all plant and animal life

cellular fluid, body fluid, composed mostly of water, which is both inside and outside of cells, and is constantly moving into and out of cells

cellulitis, inflammation and swelling of the subcutaneous tissue and muscle due to infection or trauma

cellulose, a carbohydrate that appears only in plants and is digested in the large intestine of horses by intestinal microorganisms; also called fiber

central core lesion, a common tendon injury which is associated with severe fiber disruption and hemorrhage, appearing as a black dot on an ultrasound image

central nervous system, the brain, spinal cord, cranial nerves, and spinal nerves; carries messages to and from the brain

cervical, pertaining to the neck, or to the neck of any organ or structure, such as the cervix of the uterus

cervical spine, the skeleton of the neck, made of seven vertebrae

cervicitis, inflammation of the cervix

cervix, the muscular, neck-like structure which separates the vagina from the uterus

chemotherapy, the treatment of disease by chemical agents

check apparatus, the network of muscles, tendons, and ligaments, which allows the horse to stand with little or no muscle effort, and to sleep standing up

chiggers, mites which cause trombiculiasis, characterized by small, crusty lesions; also called harvest mites

choke, a partial or complete esophageal obstruction created by swallowing too large a bolus of food or a foreign body

chorioptic mange, a skin disease caused by mite infection of the legs, frequently resulting in secondary infection and grease

chronic, a condition which persists for a long time with little change or progression; opposite of acute

chronic obstructive pulmonary disease (COPD), see heaves

cilia, minute finger-like projections whose whipping actions help maintain fluid transport over certain membranes

circulating antibodies, immune cells circulating in the blood and lymph

circumflex artery, the artery that runs around the bottom of the coffin bone

clinical diagnosis, diagnosis based on signs exhibited by the horse coupled with a physical exam

clot, a semi-solidified mass of blood

club foot, a foot configuration that may result in a high, upright heel and short toe; usually the result of a contracted tendon or nutritional deficiency in a foal

coagulate, to cause to clot, forming an insoluble fibrin clot

coffin bone, pedal bone surrounded by the hoof; also called P3, third phalanx

Coggins test, a test used to detect Equine Infectious Anemia antibodies in a blood sample

colic, acute abdominal pain due to a gastrointestinal disturbance

collagen, the predominant protein of the fibers of connective tissue, bone, and cartilage

collateral cartilages, the two cartilages on either side of the coffin bone

colon, the part of the large intestine extending from the cecum to the rectum; its length is about 10 – 12 feet

colony forming units (cfu), a bacterial colony created by rapid multiplication of a bacterium inoculated onto a nutrient medium

colostrum, the first milk after birth; important to the newborn foal's immune response

combined immunodeficiency disease (CID), a fatal disease; caused by a lack of an immune response in foals

common digital extensor tendon, a tendon located in front of the cannon bone

concentrate, high-energy feed, such as grains and pellets

concentration, the number of sperm cells in a semen sample

concentric contraction, a muscle contraction where the muscle thickens as it shortens

conception, the combination of the genetic material of the sperm and ovum

concussion, a violent jar or shock

congenital, existing at, and usually before, birth

conjunctivitis, inflammation of the delicate membrane that lines the eyelid

connective tissue, fibrous tissue that binds and supports various body structures

contagious, able to be spread from one animal to another

contagious equine metritis (CEM), a highly contagious disease which causes inflammation of uterine, cervical, and vaginal membranes; caused by *Taylorella equigenitalis*

contracted heels, a condition in which the foot is contracted and narrowed, caused by a lack of frog pressure and moisture

contracted tendon, a condition where movement of the affected limb is limited and the limb is not fully extended at rest; the horse stands on its toe or buckles at the fetlock

contraction, the reduction in size of a wound; also muscle movement

contrast radiography, injecting a radio-opaque dye into a part and taking an x-ray

contusion, an injury incurred without breaking the skin

convection, natural air circulation due to hot air rising and exiting out the top and cool air entering from the bottom

coon foot, a conformational fault in which the hoof and pastern angles are not identical, with the pastern sloping more than the front face of the hoof wall

COPD, chronic obstructive pulmonary disease, see heaves

coprophagy, manure ingestion

corium, modified vascular tissue inside the horn of the hoof which produces the horn: perioplic corium, coronary corium, laminar corium, sole corium, and frog corium

corneal ulcers, a defect in the epithelium of the cornea

coronary, encircling like a crown, as applied to blood vessels, ligaments, or nerves; the coronary band encircles the hoof

coronary band, where the hoof horn meets the skin of the leg

coronary corium, a dense bed of connective tissue with an elaborate blood and nerve supply underneath the coronary band; responsible for new hoof horn growth

corpus luteum, the mass of endocrine cells formed in the ovary at the site of a ruptured ovarian follicle

corrective shoeing, the practice of trimming and shoeing so as to correct a defect in the way of traveling or to reduce pain

cortex, cortical walls, the outer layers of bones

corticosteroids, hormones of the adrenal cortex or any other natural or synthetic compounds having a similar activity; they have a systemic and metabolic effect; inhibit the inflammatory process

cortisol, a natural steroid hormone secreted by the body in times of stress which suppresses the immune system

coupling, how the hindquarter muscles connect to the back at the lumbosacral joint

cowhocks, a conformational fault where the hocks are pointed inward when viewed from behind; the hocks are set closer in than the fetlocks

cracked heels, see scratches

cranial mesenteric artery, provides the main blood supply to the intestinal tract

crepitation, a sound like that of rubbing the hair between the fingers; caused by crackling from gas bubbles trapped under bruised or infected skin

cribbing, a vice of some horses in which it grasps the manger or other object with the incisor teeth, arches the neck, makes peculiar movements with the head, and sometimes swallows quantities of air

cross-protective antibodies, antibodies which will respond to variations of a virus strain, rather than only one strain

crude protein, percentage of protein contained in a feed

cryosurgery, the destruction of tissue by applying extreme cold; used to treat sarcoids

cryptorchidism, a condition in which one or both testicles are retained in the body cavity

Culicoides hypersensitivity, an allergic reaction to the bite of the *Culicoides* gnat; characterized by intense itching

culture, a growth of microorganisms or living tissue cells

curb, strain of the plantar ligament on the back of the hock, causes inflammation and lameness

cutaneous habronemiasis, see summer sores

cyst, any closed cavity or sac, lined by epithelium, particularly one that contains a liquid semi-solid substance or parasite

cytology, examination of cells

debride, to remove dead and dying tissue with scissors or a scalpel

deep digital flexor tendon, one of two tendons located at the back of the cannon bone

degenerative joint disease (DJD), arthritis

degenerative myocardial disease, progressive disease of the heart muscle

dehydration, condition resulting from excessive loss of body water

demineralize, to eliminate mineral or inorganic salts from tissues, especially bone

demodectic mange, a skin disease caused by demodectic mites living in hair follicles and sebaceous glands, causing tissue damage through the production of toxins

dens, part of the axis vertebra that hooks under the atlas vertebra

denude, to make bare by removing the epithelial covering

deoxyribonucleic acid (DNA), the genetic code present in every cell of the body

dermatitis, inflammation of the skin

desmitis, inflammation of a ligament

desmotomy, the cutting or division of ligaments

developmental orthopedic diseases (DOD), diseases of the bone in growing horses, including epiphysitis, osteochondrosis, osteochondritis dissecans

dew poisoning, see rain scald

dewormer, any of the many commercial products containing medications which destroy internal parasites; administered by stomach tube, oral syringe, or through feed

diagnosis, distinguishing one disease from another, or identifying a disease from its characteristics and/or causative agent

diagnostic ultrasound, see ultrasound

diaphragm, the muscle membrane separating the abdominal and chest cavities, lying behind and beneath the lungs

diarrhea, abnormal frequency and liquidity of fecal discharges

differentiation, process by which general cells develop into specialized structures during embryonic development

digestible energy, the portion of the gross energy in a feedstuff that the animal is able to digest and absorb

digestive tract, see gastrointestinal tract

digital cushion, a fibroelastic fatty pad forming the heel bulbs

dihydrostreptomycin, an antibiotic for infections in cattle

dilation, stretching or expanding

dimethyl sulfoxide (DMSO), an effective anti-inflammatory agent

disinfectant, chemical or physical agent used to kill bacteria on inanimate objects; too toxic for use on animals

dislocation, the displacement of any part, usually a bone

distal, farthest from the trunk

distal radius, the long bone above the carpus, or knee

distemper, see strangles

distension, being swollen or stretched from internal pressure

diuretic, agent that causes the secretion of urine

DL-methionine, a sulfur-containing amino acid

dorsal displacement of the soft palate, a condition where the soft palate rises upward above the epiglottis and partially obstructs normal breathing

dorsal laminar arteries, branches of the circumflex artery that feed the front of the hoof

dorsiflexion, an unnatural limb configuration where the fetlock sinks toward the ground due to fatigued musculotendinous attachments; results in overstretched flexor tendons

drench, dose of medicine given to a horse by pouring it into the horse's mouth

droplet nuclei, droplets of water in the air which contain bacteria or viruses

duct, passage with definite walls

dystocia, abnormal or difficult birth

ear plaques, small grey or white spots found on the inner surface of the pinna

early embryonic death (EED), death of the embryo before day 30 of gestation

Eastern equine encephalitis, see encephalitis

easy twitch, a plier-like clamp that puts pressure on the horse's nose; a form of restraint

eccentric contraction, a muscle contraction where the muscle gets thinner as it lengthens

echogenicity, the amount of gray in the projection on an ultra-sound screen; indication of tissue density

edema, accumulation of abnormally large amounts of fluid between the cells in the tissues

efficacy, the effectiveness of a medication or treatment

egg-bar shoe, an oval-shaped shoe which helps correct for navicular disease

egg count, the number of parasite eggs per gram of feces

ejaculation, emission of seminal fluid

elasticity, the ability of a bone to return to its original shape after being deformed by a stress

electrical muscle stimulation (EMS), high voltage electrical impulses which passively produce muscle contractions

electroanalgesia, electrically stimulating muscles to provide pain relief

electrolytes, salts in body fluids which are involved in various body functions, such as nerve impulses, oxygen and carbon dioxide transport, and muscle contractions

embolism, the sudden blocking of an artery by a clot or foreign material in the blood

embryo, in the horse, the unborn foal up to approximately 30 or 40 days of gestation

embryo transfer, a developing embryo is removed from its natural mother and implanted in the uterus of a host mother for the remainder of gestation

encephalitis, inflammation of the brain caused by an acute viral disease; three strains affect the horse: *Eastern equine e., Western equine e.,* and *Venezuelan equine e.;* also called sleeping sickness

encephalomyelitis, inflammation of the brain and spinal cord

endocrine, secreting internally; applied to various organs and structures which secrete hormones into the blood or lymph and have an affect on other parts of the body

endometrial cups, ulcer-like structures formed by the fetus in the endometrium of a pregnant mare; they secrete hormones necessary to maintain pregnancy

endometritis, inflammation of the endometrium

endometrium, the lining of the uterus

endorphin, a chemical released by the central nervous system to reduce and suppress the perception of pain

endoscope, an instrument for the visual examination of the interior of an organ such as the throat, trachea, or stomach

endotoxic shock, shock caused by large amounts of endotoxin in the bloodstream

endotoxin, a toxin that is present as a component of the cell walls of Gram-negative bacteria

energy molecules, ATP; the product of metabolism

engagement, the use of the hindquarters to allow the horse to achieve self-carriage, or to use them under the body for braking and thrust for sliding stops or quick turns

enkephalin, a chemical released by the central nervous system to reduce and suppress the perception of pain

enteric, pertaining to the intestines

enteritis, inflammation of the intestine, usually the small intestine

enterolith, a stone that develops in the intestine, formed by salt deposits around a hard object

enzyme, a protein that acts as a catalyst to produce or accelerate change in a substance, as in digestion of food

epidermis, the outermost layer of the skin

epiglottic entrapment, a condition where the epiglottis is trapped in the arytenoepiglottic fold, causing exercise intolerance, noisy breathing, and coughing

epiglottis, the thin plate of cartilage at the entrance to the larynx that prevents food from entering the larynx and trachea while swallowing

epinephrine, see adrenaline

epiphysis, a piece of bone that is separated by cartilage from the long bone in early life, but later becomes a part of the larger bone; it is at the cartilage growth plate that growth of the long bone occurs

epiphysitis, inflammation of the end of a long bone or of the cartilage that separates it from the long bone; more correctly called physitis

episioplasty, see Caslick's surgery

epistaxis, hemorrhage from the nose; nosebleed

epithelial, pertaining to epithelium

epithelialization, growth of new epithelium

epithelium, layer of cells of which skin and mucous membranes are formed

equine coital exanthema, a venereal disease caused by equine

Herpes virus-3

equine distemper, see strangles

equine Herpes virus (EHV), a respiratory virus with two subtypes, EHV-1 and EHV-4; causes rhinopneumonitis

equine tumor necrosis factor (TNF), a by-product of the inflammation caused by endotoxins

equine viral arteritis (EVA), an infectious viral disease characterized by fever, depression, limb edema, or abortion

erectile tissue, tissue containing vascular spaces that become filled with blood

erection, the state of erectile tissue when filled with blood; particularly of the penis

erythema, redness of the skin

erythema multiforme, "target" lesions caused by *Ehrlichia equi;* a form of hives

erythropoietin, a hormone which stimulates production of red blood cells in the bone marrow

eschar, a coagulated crust of skin debris which forms over the top of a rope burn

esophagus, canal extending from the pharynx to the stomach

estrogen, general term for any substance that exerts an estrogenic effect; formed naturally by the ovary, placenta, and testicles

estrous, pertaining to estrus

estrous cycle, the cyclic series of periods consisting of estrus, metestrus, diestrus, and proestrus

estrus, period of sexual receptivity in the female; heat

evaporation, transfer of water from a surface to the air

evaporative cooling, water vapor on the skin which is produced from the sweat glands pulls heat from the blood vessels, and the warmed water is then transferred to the air; a method of dissipating internal body heat

ewe-neck, a conformational fault where the topline of the neck appears to be put on upside down; instead of a crest, the neck has a dip in the neck along the topline

excretion, the act of eliminating the body's waste materials

exercise-induced pulmonary hemorrhage (EIPH), rupture of the capillaries in the lungs due to either previous lung infection or to obstruction of the upper airway; causes bleeding in the lungs, and sometimes from the nose

exostosis, an abnormal, benign growth projecting from a bone surface, usually capped by cartilage

exotoxin, a poison produced by a living organism

extender, formula used for semen dilution and preservation

extension, a movement that brings a limb forward and into a straight line

extensor, any muscle that extends a joint

extensor process, a bony protrusion at the top of the coffin bone to which the extensor tendon attaches

exudate, fluid or cells that have escaped from vessels into tissues or onto tissue surfaces, usually a result of inflammation

fartleks, continuous exercise over long distances but periodically changing speed

fascia, supportive sheets of fibrous tissue located between muscles or beneath the skin

fast twitch high oxidative (FTa), a muscle fiber type that burns glycogen in the absence of oxygen

fast twitch low oxidative (FTb), a muscle fiber type which cannot use oxygen to burn glycogen for energy production

fatigue state, the point at which a bone begins to lose its elasticity after being deformed by loading and unloading cycles

fatty acids, key components of fats; an important muscle fuel for aerobic metabolism

feathering, long hair on the back of the fetlocks of cold-blooded horses

fecal, relating to the bodily waste discharged from the intestines, consisting of bacteria, cells from the intestines, secretions (mainly of the liver), and food residue

fermentation, bacterial or enzymatic decomposition

fertile, able to produce offspring

fertilization, the union of the sperm cell and the ovum

fetlock, the area or joint of the lower leg above the pastern and below the cannon

fetlock valgus, see toed-out; also called splayfooted

fetlock varus, see pigeon-toed; also called toed-in

fetus, the unborn foal from approximately day 40 of gestation to birth

fibrin, elastic protein released during blood coagulation

fibroblast, cell which produces fibrin, or collagen

fibroblastic sarcoid, a sarcoid which often develops after a wound and resembles proud flesh

fibroma, benign tumor of fibrous tissue

fibrosis, an abnormal increase in the amount of fibrous connective tissue in an organ, part, or tissue; scarring

fibrotic myopathy, adhesions which form between muscle masses of the thigh, sometimes after an episode of myositis

fibrous connective tissue, tissue consisting of elongated cells, fibroblasts, and collagen

fibrovascular callus, a structure composed of fibrin; a scaffold for granulation tissue and more fibrin to repair an injury

field fitness test, a test to determine a horse's aerobic capacity by measuring $V_{200,}$ which is the horse's velocity at a heart rate of 200 beats per minute

fistula, an abnormal passage between two organs or from an internal organ to the surface of the body

fistulogram, the x-ray film taken of an area which was injected with a radio-opaque dye

flat feet, when the sole is not concave, which forces the horse to walk on the sole instead of the hoof wall, resulting in sole bruises

flexion, bending movement

flexion test, a diagnostic test for lameness where a specific joint is tightly flexed for 1 – 2 minutes, and the horse is trotted off

flexural deformities, a condition where the joint remains in flexion, for example, contracted tendons or club feet

float, to file down the teeth, removing the sharp edges

flora, various microorganisms inhabiting an individual

flushing, a weight-gain program instituted before breeding

focal ventral midline dermatitis, dermatitis on the abdominal midline caused by the horn fly, *Haematobia*

follicle, a small sac or cavity, such as in the skin from which a hair grows

follicle stimulating hormone (FSH), a hormone secreted by the anterior pituitary gland; stimulates follicular growth and controls estrogen secretion by the ovary; in the stallion, FSH stimulates sperm production

founder, see laminitis

founder ring, see laminitic rings

fracture, the breaking of a part, especially a bone

frog, wedge-shaped mass of tissue; lies between the bars of the horse's foot; absorbs shock upon the hoof's impact with the ground

full-thickness, a wound or burn which penetrates through the skin

fungus, plantlike organism that feeds on organic matter; responsible for the mycotic diseases, e.g., ringworm

gangrene, death of tissue, usually due to loss of blood supply

gaseous colic, colic caused by the build-up of gas in the intestines

gaskin, the area between the thigh and the hock

gastric, pertaining to the stomach

gastric ulcers, ulcers of the inner wall of the stomach

gastrointestinal tract, digestive tract through which food passes where nutrients are absorbed; consists of mouth, pharynx, esophagus, stomach, small intestine, cecum, large colon, small colon, rectum

gelding, a castrated male horse

gene, the functional unit of heredity carried by the chromosomes

genetic pool, all of the genes in a population

genital tract, reproductive tract; general term referring to the reproductive passageway and all of its associated organs

gestation, pregnancy

girth itch, see ringworm

gland, a secreting organ

glaucoma, eye disease marked by an increase in the intraocular pressure which causes changes in the optic disk

glucose, a simple sugar molecule derived from carbohydrates which is a principle source of energy

gluteal muscles, the muscle group over the croup and pelvis

glycine, an amino acid which functions as an inhibitory neuro-transmitter, preventing the next neuron from firing

glycogen, a chain of glucose sugar molecules which may be stored in the liver and skeletal muscles and/or used as muscle fuel

gonitis, inflammation of the stifle

Gram-negative bacteria, the type of bacteria that, during Gram's staining process, lose crystal violet stain when rinsed with alcohol; unlike the Gram-positive bacteria, which retain crystal violet stain because their cell walls are composed differently

granulation tissue, the formation in wounds of small rounded masses of tissue, composed of capillaries and connective tissue cells which grow outward to fill the wound defect; see second intention healing

granules, small particles or grains

grease heel, chronic inflammation of the skin on the fetlocks and pasterns

gut sounds, sounds heard with a stethoscope in the horse's abdomen; indicates intestinal activity and level of dehydration

harvest mites, see chiggars

heart rate, the number of times the heart beats in 1 minute

heart rate recovery, the time required for the heart rate to return to the resting rate after exercise; depends on fitness, weather, and level of exertion

heat increment, heat generated by digestion and metabolism of food

heat index, a combination of the environmental temperature and the humidity

heat stress, occurs when body temperature climbs above 105° F and the body cannot efficiently cool itself

heave line, a line between the flank and the thorax created by overdevelopment of abdominal muscles; caused by heaves

heaves, respiratory disturbance characterized by forced expiration of breath; caused by allergies and dust; also called chronic obstructive pulmonary disease (COPD)

heel fly, see warbles

hemagglutinin (HA) spikes, a specific sequence of amino acids on the surface of viral particles; the part of the virus that is recognized as foreign by the immune system

hematoma, a blood pocket due to a ruptured blood vessel

hemoglobin, oxygen-carrying red pigment of the red blood cells

hemoglobinuria, the presence of free hemoglobin in the urine

hemolysis, the destruction or breakdown of red blood cells

hemorrhage, the leaking of blood from a ruptured blood vessel

hemospermia, the presence of blood in the semen

hepatic, pertaining to the liver

hepatitis, inflammation of the liver

heritable, capable of being genetically inherited

hernia, a condition where an organ protrudes through the structure which normally contains it

high-frequency electroanalgesia (HFEA), a type of electroanalgesia which provides pain relief faster but for shorter periods than low-frequency electroanalgesia

hindgut, portion of the digestive tract, including the cecum and large intestine

hirsute, abnormal hairiness related to an endocrine disorder

histamine, a chemical compound which dilates capillaries, constricts the smooth muscle of the lungs, and increases secretion of the stomach

hives, small, flat-topped bumps which may coalesce into larger bumps, usually found on the neck and shoulders, caused by an allergic reaction; also called urticaria

hobbles, a restraining device which restricts leg movement

hoof tester, pincer-type instrument used to gently pinch the hoof to find any inflamed and sore area

hormone, a chemical substance produced in the body by a gland or body organ which travels in the blood or lymphatic system to a distant specific organ, to regulate the activity of that organ

horn fly, *Haematobia,* a gnat which causes dermatitis on the abdominal midline

horn tubules, hollow tubes of the hoof wall composed of keratin;

running parallel and vertical as they grow down from the coronary band

host, an organism that harbors or nourishes another organism

humerus, arm bone, extending from the shoulder to the elbow

hyaluronic acid (HA), thick lubricating fluid in the joints

hydrotherapy, the application of water in any form, internally or externally, in treating disease or illness

hygroma, a sac distended with fluid

hymen, a fold of mucous membrane which partially or completely covers the opening of the vagina

hyoid apparatus, the bones which attach the larynx to the base of the skull

hyperirritability, pathological responsiveness to slight stimuli

hyperkalemia, abnormally high potassium content of the blood

hyperkalemic periodic paralysis (HYPP), skeletal muscle weakness associated with hyperkalemia

hyperlipemia, high levels of circulating fatty acids

hyperplasia, an increase in the number of cells in a tissue or organs, excluding tumor formation

hypersensitivity, a state of altered activity in which the body reacts with an exaggerated response to a foreign agent

hyperthermia, a method of therapy which uses a radio-frequency current to heat and destroy sarcoid tissue

hypertrophy, overgrowth, general increase in bulk of a part or organ not due to tumor formation; use of the term may be restricted to denote greater bulk through increase in size, but not in number, of the individual tissue elements

hypothalamus, the part of the brain which regulates part of the nervous system, hormone activity, and many body functions

hypoxia, lack of oxygen

icterus, see jaundice

ileus, a condition where intestinal movement has stopped

immune system, the organs and cells in the body which protect it from foreign bodies such as bacteria and viruses

immunity, the power to resist infection

immunodeficiency, a deficiency in antibody response, leaving the animal susceptible to infection

immunoglobulins, group of proteins, including antibodies

immunotherapy, introducing a foreign protein into an area to draw the immune system's attention to another problem in the area

impaction, the condition of being firmly lodged or wedged

implantation, attachment of the placenta to the uterine endometrium between days 45 and 150 of gestation

impulsion, the energy and thrust exhibited by the horse in motion

in utero, in the uterus, before birth

inactivated vaccine, a vaccine where the virus particles are treated so they are unable to damage the tissues

incubation, period between acquiring an infectious disease and its clinical manifestation

indwelling catheter, see catheter

infection, abnormal multiplication of microorganisms in the body

inflammation, the response of tissue to injury or abnormal stimulation, usually involving a reaction which leads to healing

influenza, an acute viral infection involving the respiratory tract; characterized by inflammation of the nasal mucosa, pharynx, and conjuctiva

infrared thermography, non-invasive method of identifying areas of inflammation by "mapping" temperature differences in the tissues as related to increased or decreased blood flow and cellular activity

ingesta, consumed feed and fluids

inhalation, drawing air (or other substances) into the lungs

injection, forcing a liquid into a part, as into subcutaneous tissue, blood vessel, or muscle; a substance so forced

innervation, the distribution or supply of nerves or nerve stimulus to a part

insulin, a hormone produced by the pancreas; secreted into the blood to regulate sugar and fat metabolism

interactive system, a system in which all parts depend on the others for function

intercostal, between ribs

interference, striking of the inside of one leg with the inside of the hoof or shoe of the opposite leg; impact point may be from the coronary band up to the knee or hock

interval training, repeated sets of speed work and partial heart rate recovery periods; promotes lactic acid tolerance and increases speed

intestinal, pertaining to the intestines

intestinal flora, bacteria normally present within the intestine

intestinal threadworms, an internal parasite of foals caused by *Strongyloides westeri*; may cause foal diarrhea and scours

intestinal tract, the small and large intestines

intestinal torsion, twisting of the intestines

intra-articular, within a joint

intradermal (ID), within the skin

intramuscular (IM), within a muscle

intravenous (IV), within a vein

intussusception, the prolapse of one part of the intestine into the lumen of an immediately adjoining part causing blockage

inversion, the respiratory rate remains faster than the heart rate after exercise; an inverted horse appears to pant

irritant, an agent that produces irritation

isometric contraction, a muscle contraction where the muscle stays the same length

isoxsuprine hydrochloride, a peripheral vasodilatory drug which improves the blood flow to the foot of navicular horses

jaundice, yellowish discoloration of the mucous membranes of the body; also called icterus

joint, an articulation; the place of union or junction between two or more bones of the skeleton

joint ill, see navel ill

jugular furrow, the groove on each side of the neck in which the jugular vein is located; also called jugular groove

jugular pulse, the rhythmic expansion of the jugular vein in the neck that may be felt with the finger

keloid, a sharply elevated, irregularly-shaped, enlarging scar

keratin, an insoluble protein which is the principle constituent of epidermis, hair, horny tissues, and the enamel of teeth

killed vaccine, a vaccine where the viral particles are dead and are therefore incapable of damaging the tissues

knock-knee, a growth plate abnormality in the distal radius that results in the limb deviating outwards from the knee down; may result from dietary deficiency; also called carpus valgus

labia, the vulval lips arranged vertically on either side of the vaginal opening

laceration, a torn, ragged wound

lactation, secretion of milk from the mammary glands

lactic acid, a toxic by-product of anaerobic muscle metabolism; causes muscle fatigue and soreness

Lactobacillus, bacteria in the gut that produce very large amounts of lactic acid from fermentable carbohydrates

laminae, thin plates or layers; a latticework of tissue and blood vessels

laminitic rings, rings around the hoof that result from altered keratin production in an attack of laminitis; also called founder rings

laminitis, inflammation of the laminae within the foot; also called founder

larva, an early developmental stage, usually the feeding form of an animal such as an insect or worm

laryngeal hemiplegia, when one or both arytenoid cartilages of the larynx collapse into the airway due to nerve damage; causes exercise intolerance and perhaps a roaring noise; also called roaring

laryngo-palatal dislocation, separation of the larynx from the ostium of the soft palate; results in reduced airway efficiency

larynx, a structure composed of nine cartilages located at the top of the trachea; contains the vocal cords

laser, an acronym for Light Amplification by Stimulated Emission of Radiation; generated by electromagnetic waves of the same wavelength that are aligned in both time and space, and travel in nearly the same direction

lateral, on the side; the outside

lavage, washing out a cavity or wound with a stream of fluid

lesion, abnormal change in structure due to injury or disease

lice, host-specific skin parasites that inhabit the topline; this infestation is called pediculosis

ligament, band of fibrous tissue which connects bones and cartilage, and supports the joints

lime, calcium oxide, used as a disinfectant

liniment, an oily, soapy, or alcoholic liquid preparation used on the skin and applied with friction

lip chain, a chain which is passed under the upper lip and over the gum as a method of restraint

lipoma, a benign fatty tumor

live foal guarantee (LFG), breeding contract provision which guarantees the mare owner a live foal as a result of the purchased breeding; usually gives the mare owner the right to rebreed the next season to the same stallion if the pregnancy fails

lockjaw, see tetanus

long-toe – low-heel (LTLH), a long-toe – low-heel foot configuration where the hoof-pastern angle is broken; leads to many lameness problems

low-frequency electroanalgesia (LFEA), a type of electroanalgesia which provides pain relief for 1 – 3 days

lumbar, pertaining to the loins, the part of the back between the thorax and pelvis

lumbosacral (L-S) joint, at the top of the croup; pivots and rotates the hindquarters and pelvis forward under the body

lumen, cavity or channel within a tube or tubular organ

lymph, a transparent yellowish liquid containing mostly water and white blood cells, and derived from tissue fluids

lymphatic system, a system similar to the circulatory system which carries lymph from the tissues to the bloodstream

lysine, an essential amino acid for the growing horse

macrophage, an immune cell which binds, internalizes, and inactivates invading microorganisms in tissues

maiden mare, a mare that has not been bred

malabsorption, impaired intestinal absorption of nutrients

malignant, resistant to treatment; occurring in severe form, and frequently fatal; tending to become worse; in the case of a neoplasm, having the property of uncontrollable growth and/or recurrence after removal

malignant edema, a disease caused by *Clostridium septicum,* characterized by the formation of large amounts of gas in the muscles, creating a crackling feel beneath the skin

malnourished, suffering from imbalanced or insufficient nutrient intake

malnutrition, a nutrition disorder caused by either an imbalanced or insufficient diet, or due to poor absorption and utilization of nutrients

mammary gland, the udder; a collection of highly modified oil glands in the mare's inguinal region that collect nutrients and synthesize and secrete milk

mandibles, jaws

mange, a contagious skin disease caused by various types of mites

mast cells, cells which release chemicals such as histamine

mastitis, inflammation of the mammary gland

meconium, the first intestinal discharge of the newborn

meconium impaction, an impaction colic which occurs if the first fecal balls are not passed soon after birth

melanin, dark pigment of the body; protects the skin from sunburn from UV rays

melanoblasts, immature melanocytes; germinal cells

melanocytes, the cells responsible for producing melanin

melanoma, a neoplasm derived from melanoblasts; may occur in the skin of any part of the body, in the eye, or in the mucous membranes of the genitalia, anus, oral cavity, or other sites

membrane, a thin layer of tissue which covers a surface, lines a cavity, or divides a space or organ

meninge, the three membranes that envelop the brain and spinal cord

meningitis, inflammation of the meninges, usually a complication of a pre-existing disease; generally characterized by incoordination, compulsive movement, convulsions, and a high but fluctuating body temperature

mesentery, tissue that supports an organ, such as that which supports the small intestine

metabolic, pertaining to metabolism

metabolic alkalosis, a condition where the bloodstream is excessively alkalinized due to bicarbonate retention by the kidneys

metabolism, chemical changes in a cell which provide energy for vital bodily processes and activities

metastasis, the spread of neoplasms from the primary site to other parts of the body

metritis, inflammation of the uterus

microbes, see microorganisms

microfilaria, minute, prelarval stage of some parasites

microflora, see flora

micronutrient, any substance that plays a nutritional role in the body and is required only in minute quantities in the diet

microorganisms, microscopic organisms such as bacteria, viruses, molds, yeasts, and protozoa

milkshake, a sodium bicarbonate drench; may buffer the effects of lactic acid in the bloodstream

Millipore® filter, a filter used to reduce the amount of microorganisms in liquids

mineralization, deposition of minerals (such as calcium and phosphorus), into a bone or damaged soft tissue

mitochondria, "factories" within some muscle cells that use oxygen to break down fuel into energy

mixed sarcoid, a sarcoid that has both verrucous and fibroblastic sarcoid characteristics

modified live virus, a virus that has been raised in a laboratory under somewhat unnatural conditions and therefore does not have the disease-causing abilities of a virus in the natural state, but still stimulates production of antibodies

moonblindness, see periodic opthalmia

morphology, in semen evaluation, the examination of semen samples for normal sperm cell structure

motility, the ability to move; peristalsis when referring to the intestines; the ability of a sperm cell to move in a normal, forward manner; the percentage of sperm in a sample that are able to move normally

mucocilliary apparatus (MCA), a one-way flow of mucus on top of the epithelial cells which line the airways; an airway clearance mechanism

mucopurulent, containing both mucus and pus

mucosa, mucous membrane

mucous, relating to mucus or a mucous membrane

mucous membrane, membrane that lines the hollow organs, air passages, digestive tract, urinary passages, and genital passages

mucus, clear, viscous secretion of the mucous membranes, consisting of mucin, epithelial cells, immune cells, and various inorganic salts suspended in water

mud fever, see scratches

murmur, a periodic sound of short duration of cardiac or vascular origin

muscle, an organ which contracts to produce movement

muscle relaxant, an agent that aids in reducing muscle tension

muscle tremor, an involuntary trembling or quivering of a muscle

musculotendinous, a muscle and its complementary tendon

mutation, the process by which the genetic code is altered

myalgia, aching muscles

myofibroblasts, fibroblasts that act like muscle cells; they pull the full-thickness skin at the wound margins in, reducing wound size

myoglobin, a molecule contributing to the color of muscle and acting as a store of oxygen

myopathy, any disease of a muscle

myosin filament, one of two types of filaments that make up a muscle fiber

myositis, muscular inflammation; a common term to indicate disease of horses marked by a sudden attack of perspiration and cramping of the hindquarters, with the potential of passing light red to dark brown urine; occurs in horses that after engaging in continuous work, are rested, well-fed and then returned to work; also called tying-up

nasopharynx, the part of the pharynx above the soft palate

navel ill, in foals, an infection within the joints that entered through the umbilical cord and spread through the bloodstream; also called joint ill

navicular, a small bone in the foot of a horse; common term for disease of the navicular apparatus

navicular apparatus, collectively, the navicular bone, navicular bursa, and deep digital flexor tendon

navicular disease, chronic inflammation of one or more of the structures of the navicular apparatus

necrobiosis, cell death and scar tissue build-up

necropsy, post mortem examination

necrosis, the pathologic death of one or more cells, or of part of a tissue or organ; characterized by atrophy of the affected area

necrotic, pertaining to or affected by necrosis

neoplasm, tumor; an abnormal tissue that grows by cellular proliferation more rapidly than normal and continues to grow after the stimuli that initiated the new growth ceases

nerve, cord-like structure, visible to the naked eye, comprising a collection of nerve fibers which convey impulses between a part of the central nervous system and some other region of the body

nerve block, a diagnostic test; local anesthetic is injected into a nerve; if a lameness improves the source of pain is identified

neurectomy, cutting a nerve, especially the palmar digital nerves as a treatment for navicular disease

neuroma, a painful lump of nerve tissue that sometimes forms after a neurectomy

neuromuscular irritability, the ability of a muscle to respond to nerve impulses

neutralize, to make a substance neither acid nor base

neutrophil, a white blood cell readily stainable by neutral dyes

nits, the eggs of lice

no joint, the joint between the first and second cervical vertebrae; moves the head side-to-side; also called atlanto-axial joint

nociceptor, see pain receptor

nodule, small node or knot which is solid and can be detected by touch

non-steroidal anti-inflammatory drugs (NSAIDs), drugs which limit inflammation, edema, swelling, and pain

nuchal ligament, a fan-like structure forming the crest of the neck; extends from the base of the skull to the withers

nuclear scintigraphy, method of imaging an inflammatory condition by injecting a radioactive tracer material into the bloodstream; then a gamma camera "images" areas of injured bone or soft tissue which has a greater uptake of the tracer

nutrient medium, gel-like substance containing nutrients which grow and sustain microorganisms for laboratory identification

occipitus, the base of the skull

occult sarcoid, a flat sarcoid, having thick, rough skin

Onchocerciasis, a skin disorder which involves the larvae of *Onchocerca*, a parasitic worm; characterized by scaly, hairless lesions on the face, neck, or belly

ophthalmic, optic, pertaining to the eye

ophthalmoscope, instrument containing a perforated mirror and lenses used to examine the interior of the eye

opportunistic pathogen, an organism which does not usually cause illness until the immune system is depressed by another illness

organ, somewhat independent part of the body that performs a special function or functions

organization, replacement of blood clots by fibrous tissue

organophosphate, one of the phosphorus-containing chemicals which are used as drugs or pesticides

osmosis, diffusion through a semipermeable membrane that tends to equalize concentrations

ossify, to change or develop into bone

osteitis, inflammation of a bone

osteoblasts, cells that form new bone

osteochondrosis, a metabolic bone disease; incomplete maturation of growing cartilage in a joint, leading to cysts, fissures, or cartilage flaps

osteoclasts, cells that remove bone

ostium, a hole in the back of the soft palate through which a cartilage of the larynx fits during respiration

ovarian, pertaining to the ovaries or activity of the ovaries

ovary, one of the paired gonads in the female which contain ova (eggs)

over at the knee, a conformational fault where the knee is set too far forward; caused by excessive curvature of the radius; also called bucked knees

overtraining, exercising the horse too hard, too often without an adequate recovery period; characterized by weight loss or failure to gain weight, depression, exercise intolerance

ovulation, the release of an ovum from a mature follicle of the ovary

packed cell volume (PCV), the percentage of red blood cells in the blood

paddling, a gait defect in which the front foot is throw outwards during flight; common in horses that are pigeon-toed

pain receptor, sensory nerve terminal which responds to stimuli of various kinds; also called nociceptors

palmar digital nerves, nerves on either side of the pastern innervating the back third of the foot

palpation, feeling or perceiving by the sense of touch

papule, small, circumscribed, solid elevation on the skin

paralysis, loss or impairment of motor function in a part

parasite, plant or animal which lives upon or within another living organism at whose expense it obtains some advantage

parathyroid gland, small bodies in the neck or near the thyroid gland in the neck which secrete hormones

parotid, situated near the ear

parrot mouth, a congenital defect in which the lower jaw is too short or the upper jaw is too long

partial-thickness, a wound or burn which does not penetrate through the skin

particulate, composed of separate particles

passive immunity, disease resistance acquired though the transfer of antibodies from another individual

pastern, the area between the fetlock joint and the coronary band

pathogen, any microorganism or other substance that causes a disease

pathogenic, disease-causing

pathological, pertaining to pathology

pathology, the study of the nature of disease; the causes, development, and results of disease processes

pectoral, pertaining to the chest

pedal osteitis, coffin bone inflammation

pediculosis, infestation with lice

pelvic brim, the most anterior portion of the floor of the pelvis

pelvic flexure, narrowing segment of the large intestine situated on the left side of the abdomen

pelvis, the ring of bone, along with its ligaments, formed by the os coxae (the pubic bone, illiurn, ischium), sacrum, and coccyx

penis, the male organ of copulation; composed of veins and arteries, spongy erectile tissue, and a urethra

perineal, pertaining to the pelvic floor and the structures of the pelvic outlet

perineum, the area between the thighs, originating at the anus; in the male it ends at the scrotum; in the female at the mammary glands

periodic opthalmia, recurrent episodes of anterior uveitis, the most common cause of blindness in the horse; also called moonblindness

periople, a very thin layer of cells forming the protective, waxy covering of the hoof

peristalsis, worm-like movement by which the digestive tract propels ingesta

peristaltic action, pertaining to peristalsis

peritendinous, pertaining to the tissues surrounding a tendon

peritoneal lining, peritoneum, membrane lining the abdominal cavity

peritonitis, inflammation of the peritoneum

pH, symbol for measuring alkalinity and acidity; pH 7 is neutral, greater than 7 is alkaline, less than 7 is acid

pharyngeal lymphoid hyperplasia, inflammation and enlargement of lymphoid tissue of the nasopharynx and epiglottis; similar to tonsillitis in humans

pharynx, the cavity which joins the mouth and nasal passages to the esophagus and larynx

phonophoresis, using ultrasound over topical medication to encourage it to penetrate deep tissues

phosphocreatine, a compound of creatine and phosphoric acid; stored in and used by muscle cells as fuel for high-energy anaerobic muscle metabolism

photoaggravated vasculitis, inflammation of vessels made worse by sunlight

photophobia, abnormal aversion to light

photosensitization, excessive reaction of the skin to sunlight, resulting in swelling and inflammation

phrenic nerve, a nerve which passes directly across the heart muscle to the diaphragm; involved in thumps

phylloerythrin, a chemical which is a breakdown product of chlorophyll; accumulation in the skin causes photosensitization

physitis, inflammation of the end of a long bone or of the cartilage that separates it from the long bone; commonly called epiphysitis

pigeon-breasted, a conformational fault where the front legs are too far under the body; caused by a horizontal humerus

pigeon-toed, conformational fault where the feet point in because the forelegs are turned inwards; also called toed-in, fetlock varus

pigment, any coloring matter of the body

pineal gland, a gland in the brain behind the hypothalamus; may communicate with the photoreceptors in the eyes to determine the onset of estrus

pinnae, the parts of the ears which project from the head

pinworms, an internal parasite, *Oxyuris equi,* which causes itching and rubbing of the tailhead

Piroplasmosis, blood-borne protozoal disease transmitted by ticks; characterized by fever, depression, anemia, and limb and abdominal edema

pitting edema, a swelling which, when pressed with a fingertip, retains an impression of a pit

pituitary adenoma, a tumor on the pituitary gland

pituitary gland, an organ at the base of the brain which secretes and stores hormones that regulate most basic body functions

placenta, a vascular organ that surrounds the fetus during gestation; connected to the fetus by the umbilical cord and is the structure through which the fetus receives nourishment from, and eliminates waste matter into, the mare's circulatory system

plaiting, a gait defect where one foot crosses over the other, resulting in interference

plaque, any patch or flat area; a horny, dry growth

plasma, liquid portion of the blood in which blood cells and proteins are suspended

platelets, disk-shaped structures found in the blood of all mammals and chiefly known for their role in blood clotting

pleura, the membrane enclosing the lungs and lining the thoracic cavity

pleurisy, pleuritis, inflammation of the pleura with exudation into its cavity and upon its surface

pleuropneumonia, pneumonia accompanied by pleurisy

pneumovagina, the presence of air in the vagina; a common cause of infertility in mares; also called windsucking

pododermatitis, see thrush

polyp, protruding growth from mucous membrane

polypeptides, a compound of two or more amino acids

post-legged, a conformational fault where the hind legs are too straight

Potomac Horse Fever, a serious diarrheal disease caused by the bacteria *Ehrlichia risticii*

poultice, soft, moist, mass of the consistency of cooked cereal, spread between layers of muslin, linen, gauze, or towels, and applied to an area to create moist local heat or to counter irritation

precipitate, a solid separated from a solution or suspension

prepatent period, the period from ingestion of infective larvae to egg-producing adults

prepuce, the fold of skin that covers the glans penis

primary immunization, the initial vaccine which primes the cells that produce antibodies

process, a projection, as of bone

progesterone, hormone produced by the corpus luteum which quiets uterine muscle contractions

prognosis, the prospect of recovery from a disease or injury

progressive motility, the ability of a sperm cell to move in a normal, forward manner

prophylactic, prevention; an agent that tends to prevent disease

prostaglandin, stimulant to intestinal and uterine muscle, and mediator of the inflammatory cycle

protein, any of a group of complex compounds which contain nitrogen and are composed of amino acids

proteinaceous, pertaining to, or of the nature of protein

protozoa, primitive organisms which have only a single cell

proud flesh, exuberant granulation tissue

pruritus, itching

psoroptic mange, mange caused by a mite of the genus *Psoroptes;* occurs mainly on sheltered parts of the body, as on areas covered with long hair; also called scabies

psyllium hydrophilia mucilloid, a laxative which stimulates bowel movement and pulls fluids into the intestine; commonly known as Metamucil®

pulmonary, pertaining to the lungs

pulse, rhythmic throbbing of an vessel which may be felt with the finger; caused by blood forced through the vessel by contractions of the heart

pulsing electromagnetic fields (PEMF), two electromagnetic coils placed on opposite sides of the injured area to align the electro-magnetic field between them; allegedly promotes healing by improving oxygen supply

puncture, a wound that is deeper than it is wide

purpura hemorrhagica, a disease characterized by extensive collections of fluid and blood in tissues beneath the skin, occur-ring primarily on the head and legs; caused by an unusual allergic reaction to the bacteria responsible for strangles, *Streptococcus equi*

purulent, consisting of or containing pus; associated with the formation of, or caused by pus

pus, a liquid inflammatory product made up of immune cells and a thin fluid called liquor puris

pustules, visible collections of pus within or beneath the skin

pyloric sphincter, pylorus, tight band of muscle that regulates the juncture of the stomach with the small intestine

pyrogen, a fever-producing substance

quadriceps, the group of muscles covering the side of the thigh bone

quarantine, complete isolation from other horses

rabies, an acute infectious disease of the central nervous system, usually fatal in mammals

radiographs, x-ray films

radio-opaque, opaque to x-rays; shows white on a radiograph

radius, forearm bone

rain scald, dermatitis caused by *Dermatophilus bacteria;* also called dew poisoning

rectal examination, examination of organs or structures adjacent to the rectum by feeling for size, texture, and other characteristics through the rectal wall; also called rectal palpation

rectum, the terminal part of the digestive tract

recurrent, returning after intermissions

red blood cells, hemoglobin-carrying cells in the blood that transport oxygen

regeneration, natural renewal of a tissue or part

remodeling, addition of new bone in response to stress, or removal of bone in an area that is not undergoing stress

renal, pertaining to the kidney

renal papillary necrosis, death of kidney tissue due to the antiprostaglandin effects of NSAIDs combined with dehydration

replication, reproducing or duplicating, as of a virus

resorption, the removal of an exudate, blood clot, pus, bone cells, etc., by absorption

respiration, the act of inhaling and exhaling air to exchange oxygen and carbon dioxide between the atmosphere and the cells of the body

retained placenta, placenta which is not expelled within 6 hours after foaling

retention, holding onto a fluid or secretion which is normally excreted from the body

retropharyngeal lymph nodes, lymph nodes under the throatlatch

rhabditic dermatitis, itchy, painful dermatitis caused by *Pelodera strongyloides* larvae

rhinitis, inflammation of the mucous membrane of the nose

rhinopneumonitis, inflammation of the nasal and pulmonary mucous membranes; an infectious disease caused by an equine Herpes virus (EHV) subtype

rhinovirus (ERV), a respiratory virus for which there is no vaccine; symptoms include fever, swollen lymph nodes, and inflammation of the trachea and lower airways

rim pads, a pad between the hoof wall and the shoe

ringbone, bony enlargements and areas of new bone growth in the pastern or coffin joints due to degenerative joint disease

ringworm, a fungal disease causing circular patches of hair loss with scabby, flaking skin beneath; also called girth itch

roaring, see laryngeal hemiplegia

roughage, hay or pasture which provides fiber essential to intestinal function

ruminant, an animal which has a stomach with four complete cavities through which food passes during digestion; includes oxen, sheep, goats, deer, antelope

rupture, breaking or tearing of tissue

saccule, small bag or sac

saddle sore, an inflammation of hair follicles and skin caused by friction between the horse and the saddle

saline, relating to, of the nature of, or containing salt; physiological saline is a 0.9% sodium chloride solution

saliva, clear, alkaline, somewhat sticky secretion from various glands of the mouth; moistens and softens food for digestion

salve, a thick ointment

sarcoid, a benign tumor composed mainly of connective tissue which appears on the skin; the most common skin tumor of the horse

sarcoma, an often highly-malignant tumor made up of a substance similar to embryonic connective tissue

sarcoptic mange, the most serious type of mange usually affecting areas where the hair is thin (head, neck, and shoulders)

scabies, see psoroptic mange

scale, a thin layer of cornified epithelial cells on the skin

scalenus muscles, muscles connecting the last four vertebrae to the first rib; they raise the base of the neck

scapula, shoulder blade

scapulo-humeral angle, the angle between the shoulder blade and the arm bone, which should be at least 90°

scar tissue, tissue remaining after the healing of a wound or other healing process

scope, the degree of freedom (extension and flexion) of the limbs and body while the horse is in motion

scratches, dermatitis found (usually) on the back of the pastern which may have numerous causes; also called grease heel, mud fever, cracked heels

scrotum, the pouch which contains the testicles

scurfing, the process of forming thin, dry scales on the skin

seasonally polyestrous, having more than one estrous cycle per breeding season

second intention healing, healing by granulation, without sutures; scar tissue will form

secondary, a condition caused by or consequent to a primary condition

produce and give off cell products

bodies, immune cells found in body secretions, such ecretions in the nasal passages

sedative, a drug that reduces and controls excitement by its effect on the central nervous system

selenium, a trace mineral; toxicity causes tail and mane hair loss and, eventually, hoof sloughing

semen, fluid comprised of sperm cells and secretions of the testicles, seminal vesicles, prostate, and bulbourethral glands

semen evaluation, examination of semen for characteristics which indicate its fertility

semen extender, a formula used for semen dilution and preservation

semipermeable, permitting the passage of certain molecules and hindering the passage of others

septic shock, septicemia, a systemic disease caused by pathogenic microorganisms and their toxic products in the blood

sequestrum, a piece of dead bone that has been broken off or become separated from the sound bone

serotonin, a chemical released by the central nervous system which blocks pain impulses and reception by the brain

serous, pertaining to or resembling serum

serum, the clear liquid portion of the blood or any body fluid separated from its more solid elements; blood plasma with the fibrinogen removed

sesamoid, a small nodular bone embedded in a tendon or joint capsule

sesamoiditis, inflammation of the fetlock sesamoid bones usually involving both osteitis and periostitis

sheared heels, a syndrome where one heel bulb is higher than the other; results from improper trimming

sheath, a tubular structure surrounding an organ or part

shipping fever, disease related to stress of transport; symptoms include weakness, nasal discharge, discharge from the eyes, distressed breathing, and coughing

shock, a condition of acute circulatory failure due to loss of circulating blood volume; caused by septicemia, endotoxins, blood loss, colic, allergic reactions, or heart failure

shoe caulks, short protrusions from the underside of each heel of a horseshoe; used on racing shoes to provide better traction

sickle hocked, a conformational fault where the hind legs are angled beneath the horse

sign, evidence of a disease, as observed by someone other than the patient

silent heat, the mare does not display behavioral signs of estrus but she is ovulating

sleeping sickness, see encephalitis

slippered shoe, a shoe where the inside rim of the heel is thicker than the outside; also called beveled

slough, dead tissue in the process of separating from the body

slow twitch (ST), a muscle fiber type which uses oxygen to burn glycogen and fatty acids to produce energy

sodium bicarbonate, may reduce effects of acidic environment in the exercising muscle; baking soda

sodium chloride, table salt; an essential electrolyte

soft laser treatment (SLT), laser therapy which uses a broad laser beam to stimulate wound healing and provide pain relief

soft palate, a sheet of tissue arising from the bottom of the hard palate and extending back and up across the nasopharynx toward the epiglottis

solution, the homogeneous mixture of one or more substances dispersed in a sufficient quantity of dissolving medium

somatomedin, a hormone which regulates growth

spasm, a sudden, involuntary contraction of a muscle or constriction of a passage

spasticity, increase in the normal tone of a muscle

spavin, an exostosis, usually medial, of the tarsus of equids due to degenerative joint disease

spavin test, a test in which the affected leg is held acutely flexed for about 2 minutes, then released immediately before the horse is trotted; considered positive for bone spavin or stifle problems if lameness is markedly increased for more than the first few steps

speculum, an instrument for enlarging the opening of a canal or cavity to permit examination; for vaginal examination, a hollow tube, usually about 16 inches long and 1½ inches in diameter, used to examine the vagina and cervix

spermicidal, destructive to sperm

sphincter muscle, circular muscle fibers or specially arranged oblique fibers which partially or totally reduce the opening of a tube or the interior of an organ

spinous processes, upward projections of the vertebrae

splayfooted, see toed-out; also called fetlock valgus

splint, inflammation of one of the two small metacarpal bones that runs along the side of the cannon bone

spores, the reproductive elements of protozoa, fungi, algae, etc.

sprain, an injury in which some of the fibers of a ligament are stretched or ruptured

squamous, scaly or plate-like

squamous cell carcinoma, a malignant skin tumor derived from epithelial tissue; commonly called squames

sterile, infertile or barren; or, having no infectious microorganisms on its surface

sterility, the inability to produce progeny

sternothyrohyoideus, the strap muscle which runs from the hyoid apparatus, down the underside of the neck, and connects to the sternum; helps keep the larynx and trachea open during athletic demand

sternum, the bone connecting the cartilages of the ribs; the breastbone

steroid, any member of the class of compounds that includes sterols, bile acids, and sex hormones

stethoscope, an instrument for hearing sounds made by the heart, lungs, and other internal organs

stiffness, the ability of a bone to resist being deformed by a stress

stimulus, an agent or action which produces a reaction

"stock up," swelling of the lower legs; caused by poor circulation due to pregnancy or restricted exercise

stomach worm, the internal parasites, *Habronema sp.* and *Trichostrongylus axei*; abnormal migration of *Habronema* larvae causes summer sores, or cutaneous habronemiasis

strain, an overstretching or overexertion of some part of a muscle or tendon; the degree to which a bone deforms to a stress

strangles, an infectious disease of horses caused by *Streptococcus equi* bacteria which invade the upper respiratory tract; characterized by enlarged lymph nodes under the jaw and throatlatch, and mucopurulent inflammation of the respiratory mucous membrane; also called distemper

strangulate, overloaded with blood due to constriction

straw itch mite, a mite whose bite causes small wheals on the skin; commonly found in alfalfa hay or straw

Streptolysin O, a toxin which remains in the bloodstream after a *Streptococcus equi* infection (strangles); allergic response to this toxin causes purpura hemorrhagica

stress tetany, a visible form of hyperirritability; signs include muscle twitching or spasms, the limbs stiffen, and the horse is nervous or jumpy

strongyles, various parasitic roundworms (family *Strongylidae*) commonly called bloodworms

stud chain, a chain which is passed over the nose as a method of restraint

subchondral bone, bone which lies underneath joint cartilage and supports it

subclinical infection, an infection which has no clinical symptoms, but can be spread to others

subcutaneous (SubQ), beneath the skin

submandibular lymph nodes, lymph nodes under the jaw

subsolar corium, specialized skin tissue under the coffin bone which produces the sole and attaches it to the foot

sulci, the crevices of the frog

summer sores, sites of external inflammation caused by abnormal migration of *Habronema* larvae; also called cutaneous habronemiasis

superficial, near the surface; opposite of deep

superficial digital flexor muscle, the muscle attached to the superficial digital flexor tendon

superficial digital flexor tendon, one of two flexor tendons located along the back of the cannon bone

supportive treatment, that which is mainly directed at sustaining the strength of the patient

suppressor T-cells, cells of the immune system which suppress the action of other immune cells after the invader has been defeated

supraspinous, above a spine or spinous process

suspensory, a ligament, bone, muscle, sling, or bandage which holds up a part

suspensory desmitis, inflammation of the suspensory ligaments

swayback, a back deformity where the spine is concave when viewed from the side; common in older horses

sweat glands, glands near the skin surface which secrete sweat, which is composed of water, protein, and electrolytes

sweet feed, a concentrate grain mixture of corn, oats, barley, and molasses

symptom, evidence of a disease, as perceived and described by the patient; by definition, symptoms of a disease can truly only be found in humans

symptomatic, pertaining to or of the nature of a symptom

synchronous diaphragmatic flutter (SDF), see thumps

syndrome, a set of symptoms which occur together usually indicating a particular type of disease process

synovial capsule, the cavity containing synovia, or lubricating fluid, found in limb joints or bursae

synovial fluid, a viscous, transparent fluid, resembling the white of an egg, containing mucin and salts secreted by the synovial membrane and contained in joint cavities, bursae, and tendon sheaths for lubrication; reduces friction in the movement of joints, muscles, or tendons

synovial membrane, lining of a joint

systemic, relating to the entire organism as distinguished from any of its individual parts; pertaining to or affecting the whole body

teasing, showing a stallion to a mare to test her for sexual receptivity; especially useful when the mare exhibits no visible signs of estrus

tendinitis, inflammation of tendons and musculotendinous attachments

tendons, bands of strong fibrous tissue that connect muscles to bones

tenosynovitis, inflammation of the tendon sheath

tension, see axial tension

testicle, the male gonad inside the scrotum which produce sperm cells and testosterone

testosterone, the male hormone produced in the testicles and responsible for the development and maintenance of secondary sex characteristics

tetanus, an infectious disease in which tonic muscle spasm and hyperreflexia result in lockjaw and generalized muscle spasm; caused by toxin of anaerobic *Clostridium tetani* bacteria

tetany, localized spasmodic contractions of muscles; may cause twitching or convulsions; caused by subnormal levels of blood calcium

therapeutic, relating to the treatment of disease; curative

therapeutic index, in drug use, the margin between the safe dose of a drug that will effect a cure, and the toxic dose that will kill the patient

therapy, the treatment of disease

thermoregulation, temperature control

thermoregulatory center, that part of the brain which regulates internal body temperature within a very narrow range

third degree recto-vestibular laceration, occurs when a foal is delivered with a poorly aligned leg and the perineum is torn

thoracic, thorax, the chest; the part of the body between the neck and the diaphragm, encased by the ribs

thoroughpin, windpuff of the Achilles tendon behind the hock

thromboembolic colic, colic due to obstruction of an intestinal blood vessel

thrombophlebitis, inflammation of a vein

thrombus, a clot in a blood vessel or in one of the cavities of the heart; caused by coagulation of blood in the area of damage

thrush, a degenerative condition of the frog; results from moist and unhygienic conditions; also called pododermatitis

thumps, repeated contraction of the diaphragm in rhythm with the heartbeat; caused by low blood levels of calcium, potassium, and magnesium; also called synchronous diaphragmatic flutter (SDF)

thyroid gland, an organ that secretes the hormone thyroxine, which increases the rate of metabolism

thyroxine, a hormone which acts as a catalyst and has wide-reaching effects on metabolism, growth, and immunity

tied in, a conformational fault where the measurement at the top of the cannon bone is less than the measurement at the bottom

tilted vagina, a conformational fault where the labia sit high above the pelvic brim, the anus is pulled forward, and the vulva tilts horizontally; this often allows urine pooling on the vaginal floor

tipped vulva, a conformational fault where the vulva tilts forward horizontally, allowing feces to fall on the labia

tissue, an aggregation of similarly specialized cells united in the performance of a particular function

toed-in, see pigeon-toed; also called fetlock varus

toed-out, a conformational fault where the fetlock joint or carpus is rotated outwards; also called splayfooted, fetlock valgus, carpus valgus

topical, pertaining to a particular surface area, as in a topical ointment

torsion, twisting forces; twisting of the intestines in colic

toxemia, a general intoxication or poisoning sometimes due to the absorption of toxins formed at a local source of infection

toxicity, quality of being poisonous

toxin, a poison produced by a living organism (endotoxin) or that is an integral component of a microorganism (exotoxin)

toxoid, a toxin which has been treated to inactivate its toxic properties but can still stimulate an immune response

trace minerals, mineral micronutrients required by the body in small amounts, for example, copper, manganese, and zinc

trachea, the windpipe, descending from the larynx to the bronchi

tracheobronchitis, inflammation of the trachea and bronchi

tranquilizer, an agent that produces a quieting or calming effect, without changing the level of consciousness

transcutaneous electrical nerve stimulation (TENS), a method of electrically stimulating acupuncture points to provide pain relief

transfusion, the introduction of whole blood or blood component directly into the bloodstream

transition zone, the areas just above and below a healing tendon injury

transitional period, the period which occurs at the beginning and end of the breeding season, marked by erratic estrous cycles

transmission, a transfer of a disease, nerve impulse, or inheritable characteristic

trauma, a wound or injury

triglycerides, fat, composed of three fatty acids and one glycerol molecule

trombiculiasis, chiggar bites

tubule, a small tube

tumor, a mass of new tissue which persists and grows independently of surrounding structures and has no useful function

turbulence, departure in a fluid or gas from a smooth flow

twitch, a device used to restrain a horse by placing pressure on the upper lip; also the contraction and relaxation of a muscle fiber

tying-up, see myositis

udder, see mammary gland

ulcer, a hollowed-out space on the surface of an organ or tissue due to the sloughing of dead tissue

ulcerated, affected with or of the condition of an ulcer

ultrasound, use of reflecting sound waves as a diagnostic tool to "image" body parts or as a therapeutic tool to warm tissues

ultraviolet (UV) rays, light rays beyond the violet end of the light spectrum

upward fixation of the patella, when the ligament of the stifle is locked over the kneecap

urethra, the membranous canal for conveying urine from the bladder to the exterior of the body; also carries semen in the male

urethral extension surgery, surgery to "build" a urethral tunnel so urine is voided clear of the mare's reproductive tract

urinalysis, a physical, chemical, or microscopic analysis or examination of urine

urine, the fluid excreted by the kidneys, passed through the ureters, stored in the bladder, and discharged through the urethra; healthy horse urine is a pale and cloudy yellow color

urine pooling, collecting of urine on the vaginal floor; also called vesiculo-vaginal reflux (VVR)

urticaria, see hives

USP, United States Pharmacopeia

uterine biopsy, taking a tissue sample from the lining of the uterus to test for infection and abnormalities

uterus, the hollow, muscular organ, consisting of cervix, uterine body, and uterine horns

vaccine, a suspension of attenuated or killed microorganisms

administered for the prevention or treatment of infectious
diseases

vagina, the genital passageway that extends from the cervix to the
vulva

vaginal speculum examination, examining the vagina and cervix
using a hollow tube, usually about 16 inches long and 1½ inches
in diameter

vaginitis, inflammation of the vagina

vagus nerve, the two recurrent laryngeal nerve branches which
control the muscles which control the arytenoid cartilages of the
larynx; paralysis of the left branch is involved in roaring

vascular, pertaining to vessels

vasculitis, inflammation of vessels

vasoconstriction, diminution of blood vessels; leads to decreased
blood flow to a specific area

vasodilator, causing enlargement of blood vessels

vector, an animal or insect that transmits a disease-producing
organism

vein, a vessel through which the blood passes from various organs
or parts back to the heart

Venezuelan equine encephalitis, see encephalitis

verrucous sarcoid, dry, wart-like, horny sarcoids which may
resemble a cauliflower

vertebrae, the bone components of the spinal column

vesicular stomatitis, a localized inflammation of the soft tissues of
the mouth, containing blisters or other lesions

vesiculo-vaginal reflux (VVR), see urine pooling

vessel, any channel for carrying a fluid

vestibular seal, a barrier to uterine infection created by the back of
the vagina, the hymen, and the pelvic floor

vestibule, the vaginal area posterior to the hymen

villi, hair-like projections on certain mucous membranes

viral shift, the appearance of an entirely new strain of a virus due
to the combination of two different strains

virulent, exceedingly pathogenic or noxious

virus, a microscopic agent of infectious disease which lacks
metabolism and can reproduce only in living tissue or a culture
medium

volar annular ligament, a non-elastic band of connective tissue
running horizontally across the back of the fetlock

volatile fatty acids, an immediate aerobic energy source; produced
from roughage fermentation in the large intestine

vulva, the external genitalia of the female, comprised of the labia, the clitoris, the vestibule of the vagina and its glands, and the opening of the urethra and of the vagina

wall, a layer enclosing a space (such as the chest, abdomen, or hollow organ) or mass of material (such as the hoof wall)

warbles, a genus of insects called *Hypoderma* whose larvae migrate through the skin to the back and are seen as a nodule with a breathing pore; *Hypoderma* adults are also called heel flies

warts, skin tumors caused by a papilloma virus

water-soluble, able to be broken down by water

wave mouth, a condition of uneven teeth wear found mainly in older horses

weaving, a nervous condition or habit affecting horses suffering from boredom; the horse continually shifts its weight from one leg to another and sways the upper torso

wedge pad, a pad that is thicker at the heel than at the toe

weight-bearing, applying normal body weight to a limb

Western equine encephalitis, see encephalitis

wheals, smooth, slightly raised areas of the skin surface which are redder or paler than the surrounding areas

white blood cells, immune cells responsible for protecting the body from microorganisms

white line, margin of horn between the sole and the hoof wall; acts as soft cementing material between the wall and sole; line through which nails should be driven when shoeing

white pastern disease, dermatitis caused by a *Staphylococcal* bacteria

windpuffs, inflammation of a joint and/or tendon sheaths

windsucking, see pneumovagina

winging, a gait defect in which the front feet are thrown outwards from the knee; common in base-narrow, toed-out horses

winking, protrusion of the clitoris between the labia, frequently observed in mares in estrus

wobbler's syndrome, a disease that effects the cervical spinal cord and vertebrae of young horses; marked by incoordination

wolf teeth, small teeth that erupt in upper jaw, usually in front of the molars; vestigial premolar

x-rays, roentgen rays, electromagnetic vibrations of short wavelength that penetrate most substances to some degree, used to take radiographs of the body, thus locating fractures, etc.

yes joint, the joint between the atlas vertebra and the skull which moves the head up and down; also called atlanto-occipital joint

Index

W

X

Y